PRAISE FOR *THE WAHLS PROTOCOL*

"In *The Wahls Protocol*, Dr. Wahls provides elegant firsthand validation that diet truly represents the most powerful medicine. This book is totally supported by the most leading edge research and provides a beacon of hope when compared to the ever-changing landscape of pharmaceutical recommendations for multiple sclerosis."

—DAVID PERLMUTTER, M.D., #1 *New York Times*–BESTSELLING AUTHOR OF *Grain Brain*

"Groundbreaking! Once you understand why you need to eat for health, Dr. Wahls delivers a detailed road map, guiding you step by step. This will be life changing for many."

—ROBB WOLF, *New York Times*–BESTSELLING AUTHOR OF *The Paleo Solution*

"Whether or not you struggle with autoimmune diseases, I can't recommend *The Wahls Protocol* highly enough. Dr. Wahls provides a clear, in-depth, copiously researched dietary and lifestyle protocol to help you take charge of your health and your life. An absolute must-read book."

—JJ VIRGIN, CNS, CHFS, *New York Times*–BESTSELLING AUTHOR OF *The Virgin Diet*

"Terry Wahls is a hero to many for her discovery that a nourishing ancestral diet can heal multiple sclerosis. In *The Wahls Protocol*, Terry sets forth a straightforward plan for achieving good health through good food. Not just for MS patients, *The Wahls Protocol* is a fascinating tale that proves the wisdom of Hippocrates: 'Let food be thy medicine.' Try it, it works!"

—PAUL JAMINET, PH.D., AUTHOR OF *Perfect Health Diet* AND
EDITOR-IN-CHIEF OF THE *Journal of Evolution and Health*

"I've long recommended that anyone diagnosed with MS who is also interested in health and healing research the work of Dr. Wahls online, but the game has now changed. *The Wahls Protocol* will be the go-to resource for anyone suffering from MS or another autoimmune condition who is ready to fight back. Dr. Wahls outlines a clear-cut, stepped approach to dietary and lifestyle changes—supported by her extensive research and testing of the plans—that will put anyone on a path to better health. Whether you have MS or not, *The Wahls Protocol* is a gold mine of easy-to-follow, real-food nutritional guidelines that will leave you feeling so amazing it'll make you wonder how you ever ate any other way." —DIANE SANFILIPPO, B.S., N.C., *New York Times*–BESTSELLING AUTHOR of *Practical Paleo*

"*The Wahls Protocol* is one 'ah-ha' after another of how Terry Wahls' realizations may help you in your health journey. Not only will you be captivated by what you read, you'll also learn how to be healthier. Highly recommended."

—DR. TOM O'BRYAN, CREATOR OF "A GRAIN OF TRUTH: THE GLUTEN SUMMIT"

"Terry Wahls' new book is one of the most important books on health ever written. That's not a hyperbolic statement, just plain fact. If doctors would take this incredible information to heart (and into their practices), the health crisis in this world would be over—the cancer industry crushed and the rise in autoimmune conditions would fall. True health reform is contained within these pages. I cannot recommend a book any more highly. Bravo, Dr. Wahls!"   —LEANNE ELY, C.N.C., *New York Times*–BESTSELLING AUTHOR OF *Saving Dinner*

"Terry Wahls does an amazing job at highlighting the importance of micronutrients (vitamins, minerals and essential fats) as an integral part in preventing and reversing disease. Her story is incredible and brings hope to millions needlessly suffering. *The Wahls Protocol* is a must read for anyone looking to reverse autoimmune conditions naturally."

—MIRA CALTON, C.N., AND JAYSON CALTON, PH.D., AUTHORS OF *Rich Food, Poor Food*

"The best treatment for multiple sclerosis, autoimmunity, and chronic disease is teaching people how and why to eat and live for optimal health. By combining the latest science with the all-important factors of nutrition, exercise, and healthy lifestyle, *The Wahls Protocol* goes beyond conventional treatments and empowers you with real solutions."

—ANN BOROCH, C.N.C., AUTHOR OF *Healing Multiple Sclerosis: Diet, Detox & Nutritional Makeover for Total Recovery*

"Dr. Wahls engages us with her personal story of triumph over multiple sclerosis while educating us on the importance of a nutrient-dense diet for our cellular health. You will find yourself drawn in and inspired to take control of your own health as Dr. Wahls shares her experiences, knowledge, and compassion. The three levels of *The Wahls Protocol* provide a concrete plan—including both feasible diet and lifestyle changes—to help you on your road to recovery."   —SARAH BALLANTYNE, PH.D., AUTHOR OF *The Paleo Approach*

"*The Wahls Protocol* is essential reading for anyone suffering from a chronic disease and wanting to regain their health. All the therapies which restored Dr. Wahls to well-being are described in detail and are succinctly summarized in the appendices. The huge amount of scientific information, clear explanations, and practical advice make this book an invaluable resource and indispensable reference."

—ASHTON EMBRY, PH.D., PRESIDENT OF DIRECT-MS

"Only Terry Wahls, M.D., could have written a book as important as *The Wahls Protocol*. Her discovery of a path to recovery from disabling multiple sclerosis after failing to respond to the traditional medical approach is not only a story of great personal triumph, but a manifesto of hope for many others with various chronic illnesses for which drug therapy has not worked. This is a book that provides a program that can be applied by anyone who is searching for solutions to health challenges."

—JEFFREY BLAND, PH.D., PRESIDENT AND FOUNDER OF THE PERSONALIZED LIFESTYLE MEDICINE INSTITUTE

The
WAHLS
PROTOCOL

*A Radical New Way to Treat All Chronic
Autoimmune Conditions Using Paleo Principles*

TERRY WAHLS, M.D.
with Eve Adamson

AVERY
a member of Penguin Group (USA)
New York

Published by the Penguin Group
Penguin Group (USA) LLC
375 Hudson Street
New York, New York 10014

USA · Canada · UK · Ireland · Australia
New Zealand · India · South Africa · China

penguin.com
A Penguin Random House Company
First trade paperback edition 2014

Most Avery books are available at special quantity discounts for bulk purchase for sales
promotions, premiums, fund-raising, and educational needs. Special books or book excerpts also
can be created to fit specific needs. For details, write: Special.Markets@us.penguingroup.com.

The Library of Congress has catalogued the hardcover edition as follows:

Wahls, Terry L.
The Wahls protocol : how I beat progressive ms using Paleo principles and functional
medicine / by Terry Wahls, M.D., with Eve Adamson.
p.   cm.
ISBN 978-1-58333-521-5
1. Wahls, Terry L.—Health.   2. Multiple sclerosis—Patients—Rehabilitation.
3. Physicians—Diseases—Biography.   4. Multiple sclerosis—Exercise therapy.
5. Multiple sclerosis—Diet therapy.   I. Adamson, Eve.   II. Title.
RC377.W34   2014   2013043692
616.8.'34—dc23
ISBN 978-1-58333-554-3 (paperback)

Printed in the United States of America
9   10   8

BOOK DESIGN BY TANYA MAIBORODA

To Jackie,
who has sustained me
through the challenges and joys of this life

A NOTE TO THE READER

MANY OF THE Wahls Warriors who generously contributed their stories and are quoted in this book have included their actual names and locations, but a few prefer to remain anonymous, so some names and locations have been changed to protect the privacy of those who desire it.

Nutrient composition of recipes and menus were calculated with Nutrition Data System for Research (NDSR) Database Version 2012 © Regents of the University of Minnesota, at www.ncc.umn.edu/products/ndsr.html. Nutrient totals include all ingredients except those listed as optional. When a choice of ingredients is presented, the nutrient composition for the first item was used in the calculations. Reasonable effort has been made to check the accuracy of this data; however, variations in natural and manufactured foods as well as deviations from the stated recipe or menu ingredients, amounts, and preparation methods will impact the nutrient composition. All nutritional values should be considered approximate. Conclusions regarding the nutritional adequacy of the diets are based on the sample menus shown and the current nutritional recommendations for women in my age group (51 to 70 years), who have higher calcium intake requirements than premenopausal women, or men under the age of 71. Note that nutritional recommendations are otherwise relatively similar between age groups. Always consult your health care provider to discuss your personal diet and nutritional needs and have these concepts adapted and personalized to your circumstances.

Disclaimer

Medicine and nutrition are ever-changing sciences. As new research and clinical experience broadens our knowledge, changes in nutrition recommendations, treatment, and drug therapy are required. The authors have checked with sources believed to be reliable in their efforts to provide information that is complete and generally in accord with the standards accepted at the time of publication. However, in view of the possibility of human error or changes in medical sciences, neither the authors nor the publisher nor any other party who has been involved in the preparation or publication of this work warrants that the information contained herein is in every respect accurate or complete, and they are not responsible for any errors or omissions or for the results obtained from the use of such information. Readers are encouraged to confirm the information contained herein with other sources.

The Food and Drug Administration has not evaluated any of the statements made on my websites, in my lectures, or in my books. This is education and not intended to diagnose, treat, cure, or prevent any disease. This book is based upon my review of hundreds of basic science studies, animal model studies, hundreds of human clinical trials, my experience in my primary care clinics and traumatic brain injury clinics, my own self-experimentation over the last ten years, and our clinical trial.

Trademark Notice

The terms Wahls Protocol™ program, Wahls™ diet, Wahls Paleo™ diet, and Wahls Paleo Plus™ diet are the trademarks of Dr. Terry Wahls LLC. Whenever the terms Wahls Protocol, Wahls Diet, Wahls Paleo, or Wahls Paleo Plus are used in this book, they are referring to the Wahls Protocol™ program, the Wahls™ diet, the Wahls Paleo™ diet, and the Wahls Paleo Plus™ diet.

CONTENTS

Introduction   1

Part One | BEFORE YOU GET STARTED

Chapter 1: The Science of Life, Disease, and You   19

Chapter 2: Autoimmunity: Conventional Versus Functional Medicine   46

Chapter 3: Getting Focused   67

Part Two | EATING FOR YOUR CELLULAR HEALTH

Chapter 4: The Wahls Diet 101   85

Chapter 5: Mastering the Wahls Diet   106

Chapter 6: Wahls Paleo   149

Chapter 7: Wahls Paleo Plus   188

Part Three | GOING BEYOND FOOD

Chapter 8: Reduce Toxic Load   219

Chapter 9: Exercise and Electricity   232

Chapter 10: What About Drugs, Supplements, and Alternative Medicine?   261

Chapter 11: Stress Management   295

Chapter 12: Recovery   310

Epilogue: The End of My Story, the Beginning of Yours   331

Wahls Recipes   335

Appendices:

Appendix A: The Wahls Protocol Complete Food Lists   366

Appendix B: Nutrient Comparison Tables   381

Appendix C: Resources   384

Acknowledgments   391

Notes   394

Index   413

INTRODUCTION

I USED TO RUN marathons and climb mountains in Nepal. I've competed multiple times in the American Birkebeiner 54-kilometer cross-country ski marathon (once while pregnant), earned a black belt in tae kwon do, and won a bronze medal in women's full contact free sparring at the trials for the 1978 Pan American Games in Washington, DC. I used to feel invincible.

Then I developed multiple sclerosis. After decades of troubling symptoms I tried to ignore, I was finally diagnosed in 2000. By that time, the disease had a good footing in my central nervous system. My decline progressed rapidly. Within two years of my diagnosis, I could no longer play soccer with my kids in the backyard. By fall 2003, walking from room to room for my hospital rounds exhausted me, and by summer 2004, my back and stomach muscles had weakened so much that I needed a tilt/recline wheelchair. Within three years of initial diagnosis, my disease had transitioned from relapsing-remitting multiple sclerosis into secondary progressive multiple sclerosis. In that phase, disability slowly progresses despite increasingly aggressive therapy. By 2007, I spent most of my time lying in a zero-gravity chair. I was 52 years old.

Everyone with multiple sclerosis has a story—the years of clues and strange symptoms that finally, in retrospect, make sense. It is in the nature of most neurological and autoimmune diseases that symptoms accumulate slowly, bit by bit, over the course of decades. This is what happened to me. As a doctor, I was compelled to find answers: a diagnosis and a cure. As a patient, I was compelled to save my own life.

Like most physicians, I was always focused on quickly diagnosing my patients, and then using drugs and surgical procedures to treat them—that is, until I became a patient myself. Conventional medicine was failing me. I saw that. I was heading toward a bedridden life. Since the beginning of our profession, physicians have used self-experimentation, either to prove a scientific point or to treat themselves when the conventional treatments were of limited value. In that tradition, and in the face of this chronic, progressive disease for which there was no cure, I began to experiment on myself. What I didn't expect were the stunning results I got from my self-experimentation: I not only arrested my disease, I achieved a dramatic restoration of my health and my function. What I learned changed forever how I saw the battling worlds of health and disease.

More than a hundred years ago, Thomas Edison said, "The doctor of the future will give no medicine, but will interest his [or her] patients in the care of the human frame, in a proper diet, and in the cause and prevention of disease." This became my new course, my passion, and my mission. I understood health and disease in an entirely new way. I became a new person, both physically and emotionally, both personally and professionally. I also became passionately committed to helping other people become new people, too.

My Diagnosis

The stress and pressure of medical school may have been what triggered my first symptoms in 1980, years before I had any idea what they were. I would eventually call them "zingers"—intense stabs of facial pain. They lasted just a moment and would come randomly, sometimes in waves, the episodes building over a week or two and then gradually fading over the next several. They were most likely to happen during my busiest and most brutal hospital rotations, with shifts lasting thirty-six hours and allowing for little sleep. Over the years they became steadily worse, like electrical pain that felt like a 10,000-volt cattle prod sticking me in the face.

At the time, I thought the episodes of face pains were an aggravation, nothing more. I thought it was an isolated, unexplained problem—one of those medical mysteries that don't really require solving. Even as a doctor, I didn't think much about it. I was too busy with my own patients to dedicate too much diagnostic thought to myself. I certainly never suspected an autoimmune problem.

This was my first symptom, but it was not likely the moment when multiple sclerosis began its relentless march through my central nervous system. For at least a decade before then, probably two, my brain and spinal cord had been under siege from friendly fire—my own immune system attacking the myelin that insulated my nerves. I couldn't feel it at first. I couldn't feel it for years. Nevertheless, it was happening.

As the years passed, I became a mother, first to my son, Zach, then my daughter, Zebby. The rigors of parenting and full-time work distracted me, but my multiple sclerosis clock was ticking. This was a clock I did not hear, even though alarms of visual dimming and the zingers were going off. I fully expected to be an active, adventurous, vibrant woman for at least forty more years. I imagined mountain climbing with my children, even as a white-haired old grandma. I never thought my unexplained symptoms would have anything to do with something as basic as my mobility or as crucial as my thinking.

One evening at a dinner party, I was talking to a neurologist and I happened to mention that I perceived the color blue somewhat differently in my right and left eyes. Blues were a bit brighter when I used my right eye than if I used the left. She seemed interested.

"You'll have multiple sclerosis someday," she said. It was the first time anyone had said those words. My father died the next morning, and so her words were forgotten in the chaos of grief. Years later, I recalled those prescient comments.

The day my wife, Jackie, noticed I seemed to be walking strangely, I didn't believe her. I didn't even notice until she insisted we go for a three-mile walk to the local dairy for ice cream. By the time we got back, I was dragging my left foot like a sandbag. I couldn't pick up my toes. I was exhausted, nauseated, and scared. I scheduled an appointment with my physician.

Many people who are ultimately diagnosed with multiple sclerosis go through a similar experience. Symptoms develop slowly over years, and diagnosis may take additional years once physical problems manifest and become obvious.

I spent the next few weeks going through test after test, dreading each result. Some tests involved flashing lights and buzzers. Others involved more electricity and more pain. There were more blood tests. I said little and feared much. Everything came back negative, but there was clearly something wrong with me.

Finally, we were down to the last test: a spinal tap. If there were oligoclonal-band proteins (an indicator of excessive amounts of antibodies) present in the spinal fluid, then the diagnosis would be multiple sclerosis. But if this test was also negative, then I likely had what they call "idiopathic degeneration of the spinal cord" (meaning they don't know the cause). In the long list of potential diseases I had faced, this seemed like the best option. I was hopeful.

When I got up the next morning, I knew that the results should be in my chart. I could get into the clinic medical records from my home computer through remote access. I brought up my medical record on the screen and went to the laboratory section. Positive. I stood up. I paced. Two hours later, I logged onto the system and checked again. Five times I looked up my results, hoping they would somehow change. They never did.

It was official: I had multiple sclerosis.

My Decline

In summer 2000, I moved with Jackie and my children from Marshfield, Wisconsin, to Iowa to accept a joint appointment as assistant professor at the University of Iowa and chief of primary care at the VA hospital. I was newly diagnosed with multiple sclerosis. I was taking Copaxone, which my physician had prescribed for the MS, and I relied entirely on my physicians for treatment decisions. I had been trained as a doctor and conditioned to believe that doctors know best. Besides, what did I know about multiple sclerosis? It wasn't my area. I was seeing the very best people and getting the very best treatments available, so I assumed I was doing all that I could do.

I was determined not to let my diagnosis influence my new job. I was in a leadership position with plenty of challenges, and I loved it. I enjoyed teaching, and the kids were thriving in their new home. I thought I was doing pretty well, and so did my doctors. I even began to imagine I might never get much worse. I dreamed I might not even have to confess to my children that I had multiple sclerosis.

Then my right arm and hand became weak. My doctors gave me steroids to suppress my immune cells, and my strength slowly returned, but it was the beginning of a slow, steady decline. I could see it, Jackie could see it, and so could the kids. They've since admitted that sometimes it was embarrassing to have me around because I was less and less mobile. Sometimes they wished I wouldn't attend their activities, and that made me feel guilty for wanting to be there. It was a strain on the whole family, and I felt responsible. It was all my fault. I was supposed to be the provider, and I was slowly losing my ability to manage my own body. It had been only two years since my initial diagnosis.

Then something happened that changed my life. In 2002, my neurology doctor at the Cleveland Clinic noted that I was slowly getting worse and suggested I check out Ashton Embry's MS charity website, Direct-MS, at www.direct-ms.org. Dr. Embry is a geologist with a Ph.D. whose son has MS. Dr. Embry's son improved dramatically by changing his diet, so Dr. Embry became an active and vocal proponent of the link between diet and multiple sclerosis. This was the first I'd heard of such an idea—or, at least, the first time I paid attention. Although it sounded a little like "alternative care" to me—and, being a conventional doctor, I didn't put much stock into what I saw as fringe medical practices—this was a suggestion from my *neurologist*, so I took her seriously. I decided to check it out.

Dr. Embry's website was full of scientific references, which I began to read one by one. The articles were from peer-reviewed journals, written by scientists from highly respected medical schools. This wasn't "soft science." This wasn't "fringe." This was legitimate research. It was difficult science, too. A lot of it was in fields outside my expertise, or it relied on basic science concepts that hadn't been part of my medical training. I had trouble absorbing everything, and the MS-related brain fog didn't help. There was so much new information—how did I not know about any of this? After a lot of intensive reading, I determined that Dr. Embry was not a charlatan and that maybe he was on to something. What if diet could have a major impact on MS? After years of leaving my health in the hands of doctors while continuing to decline, this idea fascinated me. I could control what I ate. It seemed too easy and too good to be true. I had to know more.

Dr. Embry's website was the first place I heard about Dr. Loren Cordain. Dr. Cordain linked changes in the human diet to the development of chronic disease in Western society. He had published a number of articles and had also recently published a book for the public called *The Paleo Diet: Lose Weight and Get Healthy by Eating the Foods You Were Designed to Eat*, which was much easier reading than the technical scientific papers.[1] I began to absorb information more quickly: molecular mimicry, leaky gut, lectins, immune modulation (I'll talk about all these things later in this book). I began to see where Dr. Embry and Dr. Cordain were going with their theories. I began to consider that what we eat has a major, rather than a minor, influence on how our bodies work.

I was particularly interested in the idea that excessive carbohydrates and sugars in our modern diet lead to excess insulin and inflammation. The evidence that the original human diet could possibly improve my MS was compelling, but switching to this kind of diet would be a major change for me. I had been a vegetarian since my college days and I loved my beans and rice. I loved making bread. Could I really cut out grain, dairy, and legumes, the current staples of my diet?

But I wanted to arrest my disease more than anything else. I wanted to keep walking, working, and playing with my kids. I decided to try it. Meat was back on the menu, and I gave up the now-forbidden foods I loved so much. At first the smell of meat was nauseating to me. I started slowly, adding meat to soup in small amounts. With time, it got easier.

I was hopeful about this change, but despite this switch to a Paleo Diet, my decline continued. I couldn't play soccer in the backyard with my kids without falling. I couldn't take long hikes with the Cub Scouts and Girl Scouts. Then it became harder to take even short walks with Jackie. Fatigue became more and more of a problem. I was disappointed, at times despondent, and tears came at inconvenient times. But I was determined. Some of the entries on Embry's website said that recovery took five years. I realized I could not expect an overnight miracle, so I stuck with the changes. Even if progress would be slow, it was still something I could do for myself, and that came with its own sense of empowerment.

Meanwhile, I rearranged my schedule to avoid walking. My doctor told me that it was time to get a scooter, and then changed his mind and suggested a tilt/recline wheelchair because of the worsening fatigue. He also suggested I try taking mitoxantrone, a form of chemotherapy. When that didn't help, I switched to a new, potent immune-suppressing medication called Tysabri; but before I went in for my third injection, Tysabri was pulled from the market because people were dying from the activation of a latent virus in their brains. After this, my doctor suggested that I take CellCept, a transplant medicine, which would suppress my immune cells. I often had mouth ulcers after that. My skin was grayish. I started every day tired, and despair gnawed at me each night as I lay in bed. Jackie, Zach, and Zebby were my lifeline. Jackie would hold me and tell me we'd get through everything together. We often discussed our kids and how they were absorbing the ways that we dealt with what was happening. For their sakes, I didn't want to let my discouragement and fatigue show.

Though I had resisted getting the tilt/recline wheelchair, it actually felt liberating once I had it. I was able to go outside and stroll (or rather, roll) with my family as we hiked around the county park or the neighborhood. It did make my life easier. It weakened my back muscles, however, and the more those muscles atrophied, the more time I spent in bed. I didn't talk about it much, but I thought it likely that eventually I would become bedridden. Sitting at my desk at work was exhausting. Then I found a zero-gravity chair, designed like the NASA chairs used during space flights. When I was fully reclined, my knees were higher than my nose and gravity held me in the chair. I had one for my office and another for my home. That helped with the fatigue a great deal, but this wasn't how I wanted to live my life. I just couldn't accept that this was my future.

Taking My Life Back

Getting into that wheelchair triggered something. I realized that conventional medicine was not likely to stop what was happening to me. I still hoped that the Paleo Diet would make a difference, but I hadn't seen much of a change thus far. I decided to go back to reading the medical literature. I wanted to know if there was something more, some other avenue, something the doctors had overlooked. I had come to accept that recovery was not possible, but maybe I could slow things down. I was through ceding my power to doctors and not seeing results. I needed to be more forward thinking. I vowed to research and study and exhaust every avenue, just in case there was some other answer for me out there, something that would delay a little longer the inevitable life in bed.

At first, I began to read all about the latest clinical drug trials going on, but then I realized that those all involved medications that I'd be unable to get. This kind of knowledge would only be theoretical. So I started to think outside the box. I knew how science worked—I knew that studies on mice and rats are always the source of tomorrow's treatments, but that it's typically years, often decades, before anything becomes a matter for a clinical trial, let alone a standard of care. This was the cutting edge of the cutting edge, so I began to look there. I wanted to know what the brightest minds were thinking and how they envisioned the future of diseases like mine.

Each night I would spend a few minutes searching www.pubmed.gov for articles about the mouse model for MS. I knew that brains afflicted with MS shrink over time, so I also began reading about the animal models of other conditions with shrinking brains. I researched Parkinson's disease, Alzheimer's dementia, Lou Gehrig's disease (amyotrophic lateral sclerosis, or ALS), and Huntington's disease. I discovered that, in all four of those conditions, the mitochondria—small subunits within cells that manage the energy supply for that cell—stop working well and lead to early death of brain cells, causing shrinking of the brain. More searching led me to articles in which mouse brains and their mitochondria had been protected using vitamins[2] and supplements like coenzyme Q, carnitine, and creatine.[3]

I didn't have anything to lose, so I decided to take action. I translated those mouse-size doses into human-size ones, then made an appointment with my primary-care doctor. She looked over my list and decided the supplements were likely safe. She entered each one into my medication list, one by one, to check for potential adverse interactions with my medication list. There were none. I was excited about starting my new, experimental vitamin-and-supplement routine. I began to take them and was disappointed when nothing happened. After a couple of months I stopped taking them, and a few days later I couldn't get out of bed. When I resumed the supplements, I could get up again. They were helping after all!

This was a ray of hope. Obviously, I thought, my body was getting something from those supplements that it wasn't getting without them—something it needed.

Discovering E-Stim

Next, I discovered electrical therapy. I got the idea by reviewing a research protocol that used electrical stimulation of muscles to treat people who'd become paralyzed due to an acute spinal injury. The purpose of this therapy, known as e-stim, in the research was to maintain bone health and quality of life for these patients. Reviewing that research protocol made me wonder if the electrical stimulation might slow down my disability. I talked to a physical therapist who used this technology, and he warned me that it was painful and exhausting for the athletes who did it. He wasn't sure if it would help me, but he was willing to give it a test session.

During my first session, the therapist had me lie on my belly and applied the electrodes to my left paraspinous back muscles. I lifted my left leg off the table and held it there as he dialed up the electrical current. If felt like bugs racing across my skin. He kept dialing up the current. The bugs raced faster. It became more and more electrical, and then painful. After a minute my therapist asked if he could turn up the current again. This is the typical procedure because the brain releases endorphins and nerve growth factors that make the e-stim more comfortable, so after a few minutes patients can typically tolerate a higher dose of electricity. When that was done, we did my quadriceps muscles on my left leg, where I suffered particular weakness. After it was over, I had completed thirty minutes of "exercise" that was more rigorous than what I had been able to do in years. I began a regular regimen of e-stim therapy.

Discovering Functional Medicine

Every night, after everyone else was sleeping, I searched the Internet, looking for more information that might help me. One night I stumbled onto the web page for the Institute for Functional Medicine and was immediately intrigued. Its goal was to provide clinicians like myself with a better way to care for people with complex chronic disease by looking at how the interaction between genetics, diet, hormone balance, toxin exposures, infections, and psychological factors contribute to the development of disease or the improvement of one's health and vitality.

This was exactly what I had been searching for since I'd hit the wheelchair. The institute had textbooks, conferences, and continuing education courses for physicians and other health care professionals. One course captured my attention immediately: *Neuroprotection: A Functional Medicine Approach for Common and Uncommon Neurologic Syndromes*. I ordered it and began studying, night after night. Although it was difficult at first, that functional medicine course taught me that I could improve the condition of my mitochondria and my brain cells. It gave me an entirely new way of thinking about brain health and how it relates to whole-body health. Although it wasn't the way I was trained, it made sense to me. It was all logical and scientifically supported, so it resonated with me as a doctor, but it also fit into the context of my experience as an MS patient.

I also understood that it was likely that I had a genetic vulnerability, or several, that had increased the likelihood that I'd develop multiple sclerosis. I finally had a much deeper understanding of the significance to the brain of leaky gut, food allergies, toxins, mitochondria that were not providing enough energy for the cell, neurotransmitter problems, and the impact of having inefficient enzymes for the metabolism of B vitamins and sulfur. Based on what I now knew, I had a much longer list of vitamins, minerals, amino acids, antioxidants, and essential fatty acids that I understood were helpful for mitochondria and brain cells. I finally understood why my brain was on fire, under attack by my immune cells, and I also had some ideas about what I could do to cool the fires of inflammation that were raging there. My worldview was changing. I immediately began to plan and implement lifestyle changes that went far beyond anything I'd been doing before. The seeds for the Wahls Protocol, although not yet named, were sown.

But how would I do it? I had a long list of nutrients, but was I really going to take huge fistfuls of pills every day? And would that even work? The Paleo Diet suggested that food was the best source, but many functional medicine concepts relied on supplements. Our Paleolithic ancestors didn't take supplements, obviously. The Paleo Diet had taught me to eliminate certain foods but didn't necessarily tell me how to get the precise nutrients I now knew I needed. Functional medicine helped me to determine what nutrients I needed with their list of advised vitamins and supplements to take but didn't necessarily tell me how to get them.

If I could get those same nutrients I was taking in pill form from the food I was eating, I reasoned, those nutrients might be more effective than the synthetic versions of the nutrients I was taking. In addition, I might also pick up many additional compounds—maybe thousands of compounds—that had yet to be named, that contributed synergistically to the effectiveness of a particular vitamin or supplement because they existed along with the nutrients in the original package. (Most vitamins in nature are actually a family of related compounds that are all biologically active in our cells.) I realized that I needed an eating plan specifically designed to maximize my mitochondrial and brain function—an eating plan that went beyond anything I'd already encountered. It would incorporate Paleo principles, functional medicine concepts, and my own research. Maybe that would jump-start the changes in my body I desperately wanted to see and feel.

I stared at my new list of the nutrients functional medicine suggested I needed for better brain health and wondered: Which foods contain these nutrients? I had no idea. I showed my list of nutrients to my registered dietitian friends, but they didn't know where to find those things in the food supply, either. Next I went to the health science library. I couldn't find any answers there, and so I went back to the Internet and began searching once again. With more work, I finally developed a long list of new foodstuffs to add to my diet that seemed to match up nutritionally. I began to add these to every meal.

That's when things really began to change in my brain and body.

Generating the Proof

I was just about to start a new position as the primary care doctor for the polytrauma unit, treating veterans with head injuries. It was a job I wasn't sure I could do, and Jackie and I both wondered whether the hospital had assigned me the position in order to force me to face the fact that I could no longer work. Instead, I surprised everyone, including myself. After just three months practicing the new diet, gradually increasing my e-stim exercises, and practicing daily meditation and a simple self-massage, I could walk between exam rooms using just one cane. After six months I could walk throughout the entire hospital without a cane. But it wasn't just my body that had changed. I experienced and saw the world very differently. The old me—the conventional internal medicine physician—had been struck down like Paul on the way to Damascus. The old me, who had relied on drugs and procedures to make my patients well, who had been made progressively more feeble by my illness, had been replaced with someone who understood intellectually and physically that disease begins at the cellular level, when cells are starved of the building blocks they need to conduct the chemistry of life properly, and that the root of optimal health begins with taking away the things that harm and confuse our cells while providing the body with the right environment in which to thrive. I finally understood what I had to do to provide my cells with all the building blocks of life they needed to heal. I was doing it, and it was working.

This completely altered how I practiced medicine. I began teaching residents and patients in our primary care clinics how to care for themselves in a way I had only just discovered as optimal, using diet and health behaviors for diabetes, high blood pressure, high cholesterol, mood disorders, post-traumatic stress disorder, and traumatic brain injury instead of relying only on drugs. The residents learned that diet and lifestyle are powerful treatments, often as effective, if not more so, than drugs. The patients in the traumatic brain injury clinic were also eager to learn what things they could do to speed the healing of their brains. In patient after patient, I watched symptoms and the need for drugs decrease as diet and lifestyles improved.

The many people I helped notwithstanding, however, anecdotal evidence wasn't good enough for me. There was no question that the medical establishment wouldn't believe, let alone endorse, my protocol without a clinical trial. I felt compelled to apply the same rigor to my own work that I had required when researching what to do for myself. I needed definitive tests to determine whether this would help others. I decided to begin the long, complex, and expensive process of doing a clinical trial to prove that my new protocol didn't just work for me—that it would work for anyone with a similar affliction. That meant designing a clinical trial, writing the grant, securing funding (in a world that funds less than 2 percent of grants), and getting my study approved by the Institutional Review Board (the committee that oversees research at the VA and university). In less than eighteen months, I achieved the seemingly impossible. On October 6, 2010, we enrolled our first patient.

In fall 2011, a group organizing a local TEDx talk asked me to submit a proposal to speak. For those not familiar with TEDx, it is an offshoot of TED, which stands for Technology, Entertainment, Design. This is a set of nonprofit conferences on a variety of topics that are filmed and available for public viewing on the Internet. TEDx is similar. Conferences are organized locally but are also available to view for free online, and speakers are not paid. Millions of people view the TED and TEDx talks, however, and many have gone viral. I would have eighteen minutes to tell my story and explain how I designed a diet specifically for my mitochondria and my brain. I agreed.

In my TEDx talk, I explained the specifics of my intensive nutrition plan, and I challenged people to become ambassadors for their mitochondria and to eat for health. At the end of November, that TEDx talk, "Minding Your Mitochondria," was placed on YouTube. It spread into the Paleo community, the MS community, and the functional medicine community. Within a year, that lecture had more than 1 million views. I'd touched more lives than most physicians or scientists will touch in their lifetimes. I felt like I was helping to change the world for the better, and that was exhilarating, but I wanted to do even more.

My mission was never clearer. I needed to continue to do the research so I could reach my physician colleagues and eventually change the standard of care. I needed to continue to teach the public because I believe the public will soon be far ahead of the medical community when it comes to understanding the power of food to reclaim and maintain health.

The next step was to write this book.

Meanwhile, I've expanded the lab, we have additional studies under way, and our preliminary results continue to be very exciting. We have published our first paper, "A Multimodal Intervention for Patients with Secondary Progressive Multiple Sclerosis: Feasibility and Effect on Fatigue,"[4] showing that the protocol can be implemented by others safely and lead to a clinically and statistically significant reduction in fatigue. More papers are on the way, describing the effect on mood, thinking, walking ability, nutritional status, and MRI findings. We have several other trials in the works so we can continue to refine and improve and disseminate information about the limitless potential of this lifestyle.

I still have multiple sclerosis, but now I also have my life back.

Your Story

It will take many years and millions of dollars for us to do clinical trials that can prove that the Wahls Protocol is effective for multiple sclerosis and other chronic diseases. I am busy writing and submitting grants to conduct those studies. In the meantime, I invite you to read my book, take my story to heart, and talk to your family and your physician about the protocol. Because here's the most important thing I want you to realize: Your doctor cannot cure your autoimmune disease. Your medication can only ease your symptoms, sometimes with side effects that make you feel even worse. But this is not the end of the story. The power of healing is within you. All you need to do is give your body what it needs and remove what is poisoning it. You can restore your own health by what you do—not by the pills you take, but by *how you choose to live*. When you eat and live in accordance with the needs of your cells, your body can finally concentrate on healing, and that is when the dramatic changes will happen for you.

The purpose of my years of self-experimentation was to determine exactly what the body needs to fight back against autoimmune disease. The result is the Wahls Protocol: a systematic and aggressive intervention into your body's downward spiral. It is a mending of your broken biochemistry that comes not from your doctor or your pharmacist but from you, making changes that are entirely under your control. It is a restoration of your body's healing power generated by altering what you eat and do each day. You don't have to wait until all the proof comes in and is vetted by the medical community. You don't have to wait until a "food prescription" becomes part of the standard of care in your conventional doctor's office (which I believe someday will happen—it is the only rational course). You can have this information *right now.* Food is the bedrock of health. Our food choices can either lead to disease or create health and vitality.

As you implement the Wahls Protocol, you will likely begin noticing that your thinking is clearer, your moods are better, and your energy is coming back. Those over their ideal weight will find that their weight normalizes without hunger. In my clinics, when people come back in three months, everyone who has fully implemented the diet has begun noticing all these things. For the next three years, I typically see my patients "youthen"—they look younger and younger each time I see them as their cells revitalize and their bodies become healthy once more.

If I can rise up from a tilt/recline wheelchair by changing the way I live my life, consider what the people you love, your community, your country, and the world would look like if everybody began eating and living to optimally fuel their cells. We could restore health and vitality to the world and dramatically lower the cost of health care, saving billions of dollars. What choice will you make? How will you choose to live the rest of *your* life? With disability? Or with vitality? It's all up to you.

Part One

BEFORE YOU GET STARTED

Chapter 1

THE SCIENCE OF LIFE, DISEASE, AND YOU

Y OU HEAR THE DOCTOR say those words—*multiple sclerosis*—and you wonder if your life will ever be the same. Maybe you aren't entirely sure what it means, but you've seen it—you've seen the people in wheelchairs who can't seem to remember things, who have a hard time even using their hands. Or maybe you are already there, your mobility declining or seemingly lost. Maybe you think that you are on the downhill slope and there is no climbing back up. Not in your condition.

Or perhaps you have a different kind of autoimmune disease, like rheumatoid arthritis or lupus. Maybe you are also saddled with obesity or severe allergies, food intolerances or celiac disease, diabetes or a heart condition. Perhaps you also must endure depression or anxiety or attention deficit disorder. All you really know is that the days of feeling good, feeling like yourself, seem far behind you. Your body doesn't work the way it should, and neither does your brain.

You have probably seen a doctor, and maybe you have a diagnosis. Physicians treat your symptoms, but they cannot cure chronic diseases like multiple sclerosis, depression, high blood pressure, diabetes, or even obesity, for that matter. You may be prescribed a list of pharmaceutical interventions to ease your symptoms, but this may only exacerbate your problem long term because of medication side effects and the worsening nutrient depletion that may accompany long-term medication use. Medications for autoimmune disease *do not cure the disease*. Their only purpose is to make you feel a little better, which might work, and possibly slow the progression, which also might work. Or not.

Perhaps you are losing hope. I want to restore your hope.

This book is about hope. My overarching message couldn't be more straightforward: *You don't have to be a victim.* The disease or condition you have is already happening, but there are many significant things you can do to slow, halt, or even reverse your symptoms. Medication can't take away your autoimmune disease, *but your body can heal itself*—if you give it the tools.

Disease is not a simple cause-and-effect condition. It is a complex melding of forces, both genetic and environmental. Fortunately for all of us, the environmental aspect is of much greater significance than the genetic, and you can start doing something about your environment today. The lifestyle you choose can actually repair your broken biochemistry and restore your vitality. That's big, big news for anyone with an autoimmune or any other chronic disease. *You* can turn your life around. Not your doctor. Not your pharmacist. Not that bottle of pills. *You*. The power is in your hands.

When chronic disease is the result of a *deficiency*, drugs aren't going to solve the problem. As I'm sure you realize, multiple sclerosis is not a deficiency of the latest multiple-sclerosis-disease-modifying drug like Copaxone, just as fatigue is not a deficiency of wakefulness-promoting drugs like Provigil or even caffeine, and depression is not a deficiency of antidepressants like Prozac. No, these problems are not deficiencies of drugs, but they are triggered by deficiencies *in your cells* that lead to broken biochemistry and impaired signaling between your cells. When you look at chronic disease in this way, it's obvious that you should treat the cellular deficiencies that cause diseases to develop in the first place instead of just treating the symptoms, which is what most conventional pharmaceutical treatments do.

Unless you understand what your body actually needs to function and heal, however, then you can't possibly make wise decisions about what you should do to keep your body going. You might decide to take someone else's advice about diet—advice that might be motivated by wanting to help you to lose weight or gain strength. It might even be based on political, environmental, spiritual, or ethical concerns. Unless you understand what your body actually needs, you won't know what advice to take and what advice to leave. You won't know what foods to choose. You won't know which diet is the right one for your condition. You won't know how to fuel your own cells for optimal health.

I challenge you to stop believing everything you read and everything everyone tells you, and to learn something about biology and biochemistry so you can make your own decisions. When considering nutrition at the cellular level, we have plenty of scientific studies to guide us. We don't know everything there is to know about nutrition yet—not by a long shot—but we do know a lot about how to facilitate many of the biochemical repairs we need. Science has already demonstrated that when you give your cells more of what they need, your cells will thrive, even heal. If you deprive them of essential nutrients, they will deteriorate. They might not die—at least, not right away—but they'll soon begin to falter in their functionality, and that is exactly where problems start.

As a doctor and a scientist as well as a patient, I base the decisions I make for my own health and for the health of others on science. I would never ask anyone to just "believe me." I want you to understand *why* I designed the Wahls Protocol the way I did. If you don't understand why you must make the dietary and lifestyle changes I suggest, you might not be willing to stick to them. The results you'll experience by following the Wahls Protocol speak for themselves, of course, but an informed and proactive patient is an empowered patient. I want to empower you, so before we begin—before I give you even one bit of advice about what you should or shouldn't be eating, drinking, or doing—let's take a look at what's really going on in your body.

What Creates Health?

You are made of cells. A cell is the unit that makes up a living organism. Some organisms consist of only one cell, like an amoeba. Some, like human bodies, consist of trillions of cells. Cells come in different sizes and shapes, and they all do different things, but they are, essentially, the building blocks that make up our bodies.

WAHLS WARRIORS SPEAK

My first multiple sclerosis–related episode at age 33 involved facial numbness and vertigo, and for the next seven years, I experienced increasing fatigue and heat intolerance. I used Copaxone for five years but went off it when I ran out of tolerable injectable space. Over the next eight years, I experienced a decline in energy, a massive decline in heat tolerance, and an increase in brain fog and fatigue, so much so that working two days a week was all I could muster.

I found the Wahls Diet completely by accident, when I ran across the TEDx talk online. I started the diet in July 2012 and called my son after two weeks to say I felt as if I had new eyeglasses—everything was sharper and clearer than it had been for years. I have had such an improvement in my mental clarity and fatigue that I feel like I should pinch myself! I really am still in shock that I have energy again and do not need a nap every day. The quality of my sleep has improved and when I do nap, it is for 10 minutes. When I awaken, I am as energetic as I was in the morning. You can see why I think it is miraculous!

—Jan W., Steamboat Springs, Colorado

Cells, however, don't work under just any conditions. They need certain nutrients in order to do the work of keeping you alive and healthy. Without those nutrients, the cells begin to malfunction, even die. Where do those nutrients come from? They come from the food you eat—nowhere else. If you aren't providing the right nutrients and environment for your cells, then they won't work as well as they could, and a malfunction at the cellular level could eventually impact any aspect of your health. Your genetics may determine *what* goes wrong, but when the cells aren't getting what they need, the body doesn't work right, and *something* (usually many somethings) will go wrong somewhere.

People often wonder whether health is mostly a matter of genetics. Do your cells work well or poorly depending on your DNA? If it were all up to your genes, then what you eat and how you live wouldn't matter very much. However, we know this is not the case.

Living in Iowa, we hear a lot about corn and see a lot of corn, and so I use this as an example reflecting my Midwestern roots—an example of how important fuel is for your mitochondria and, by extension, your cells, your organs, and your entire body, including your brain. A packet of seeds can all contain the same DNA, but if you plant a handful of corn seeds in rich black Iowa soil and you toss another handful onto a toxic trash heap topped with a thin layer of dirt, the seeds will grow into much different plants. The seeds planted in the rich Iowa soil will be tall, sturdy, and lush, with healthy ears of corn. The seeds planted in the trash heap, if they sprout at all, will be spindly, pale, and probably unable to produce much, if any, corn because there were not enough nutrients to nourish the plant. Same DNA, completely different result.

Your cells—and you—are like that corn. If your cells don't get the nutrients they require to function properly and aren't protected from harmful toxins, you will wilt. Your mitochondria won't produce enough energy (more about mitochondria in a moment), or won't produce energy efficiently, and that can trigger a cascade of dysfunctional biochemical reactions that can eventually launch a chronic disease process. (I will talk more about how the toxins trip up your chemistry in chapter 8, "Reduce Toxic Load.")

Don't get me wrong: Genetics do play a role. Our cells rely on enzymes to facilitate the chemistry of life, and how we make those enzymes is determined by our genes—that is, our DNA. We know that there are hundreds of different genes, maybe more, that could each slightly increase the chance that someone will develop multiple sclerosis. These could affect a number of relevant factors: whether some enzyme doesn't work very well, whether some process interferes with inflammation control, whether toxins are managed sufficiently or nutrients are fully absorbed, the effectiveness of your hormones, and even the effectiveness of your neurotransmitter production.

Very few conditions, however, are caused solely by a single mutation in our DNA. The vast majority are caused by the interaction of multiple genes—sometimes as many as fifty or even a hundred—that shift the efficiency of our enzymes in response to our environments, including nutritional deprivation or toxic exposure. Environment largely determines which genes are silent, or "turned off," and which are active, or "turned on." For example, you may have

> ## WAHLS WORDS
>
> Epigenetics is the science of understanding how the environment deter-
> mines which genes are active, or "turned on," and which genes are inac-
> tive, or "turned off." Currently, hundreds of millions of dollars are being
> poured into epigenetics research because epigenetics is thought to hold
> the answers to why we develop chronic diseases like cancer and diseases
> of aging. Much more information will be forthcoming in this field, but why
> wait for scientists to develop new, expensive drugs based upon epigenetics
> when you can learn how to optimize the environment for your genes right
> now, using the Wahls Protocol?

a propensity to develop cancer, but if your body is fully nourished and not exposed to excessive toxins, you are far less likely to develop cancer, even with that propensity. Or if you do develop cancer, your white blood cells may be strong enough to kill the cancer cells as soon as they develop and you won't ever experience symptoms or be diagnosed. Or if you do get cancer, you will have a much better chance of beating it. Through optimal lifestyle choices, you can keep the most harmful genes in the "off" position and the most health-promoting genes in the "on" position.

The bottom line is that your DNA will play a remarkably small role in whether or not you develop a particular disease like multiple sclerosis, even if it runs in your family. It's the epigenetics that determine which genes turn on, and that determines your risk. Scientists believe that environment determines 70 to 95 percent of the risk of developing autoimmune problems, obesity, heart disease, and mental health problems.[1] "Environment" means what you eat, what you drink, what you breathe in, what you bathe in, how you move, and even how you think and interact with people. What really matters is how your genes interact with the accumulation of your choices. This is what will determine whether you have good health or develop a chronic disease. The key is to know how to shift the odds toward achieving the most optimal health, given the genes that you were born with, by making your internal environment—your cellular environment—as favorable as possible.

WAHLS WORDS

The scientific term for a mutation in a DNA sequence is *single nucleotide polymorphism*, or *SNP*. We know that people with specific SNPs ("snips") that affect the production of enzymes for handling the B vitamins or sulfur are more likely to have heart disease, brain disease, mood problems, and/ or autoimmune problems. It is often possible, however, to overcome problem enzymes by using a specific nutritional regimen once we know which enzymes are affected and which vitamins and which forms of the vitamins or foodstuffs can help the person bypass that particular SNP. If a disease or condition runs in your family, that's a sign that you and your relatives might have a particular SNP. A functional medicine doctor can make some predictions about the SNPs based on family history and genetic testing, and can recommend a personalized plan of action. (See chapter 12, "Recovery," for more information.)

We are still learning how lifestyle factors like prior infections, diet, environmental pollutants, amount and type of exercise, stress, vitamin D levels, hormone balance—even attitude and approach to life—can turn on harmful genes, interfere with our biochemical factories, and lead to harmful changes in nutrient absorption, hormone production, neurotransmitter function, and more, but we do know that a genetic propensity may never come to anything if the body stays healthy and fully nourished. Cellular dysfunction caused by a lack of proper nutrients and/or the presence of toxins, however—including those the body generates during times of excessive stress—can be all it takes to flip the genetic switch.

In other words, genes are not your destiny. You get to decide how you live, and that means you have a lot of control over which genes will become active. Even if you already have a chronic disease like MS, it's not too late to intervene. Correcting your lifestyle now can do more than just arrest disease progression; in many instances, it may even reverse it. Healthier choices can turn off those harmful genes and turn on the most health-promoting ones.

Fueling Your Cells

This brings us back to the cell. Cellular fuel comes from the food you eat. This is one of the most important things I want you to take away from this book: *What your cells use to fuel the chemistry of life comes directly from what you feed yourself.* The food you eat has everything to do with how well your body functions, how likely it will be that your genetic susceptibilities will be activated, and whether or not you develop a chronic disease—as well as how well you are able to come back from the disabilities that a chronic disease has inflicted on you.

If you put sugar into the gas tank of a car, the car isn't going to run right. If you are missing half of the parts in an "assembly required" toy, it's not going to work. This is not a new concept, but for some reason people tend not to apply it to our cells. They have some general concept that "you are what you eat" or that certain foods are "healthy" or "unhealthy," but really, it's more concrete than that. Your diet directly correlates to your cells' ability to function.

I'll say it again: Cellular nutrition is everything. It is the very basis of health. It all comes down to the cell, because when cells malfunction, eventually organs malfunction. When organs malfunction, eventually *you* malfunction. The disease you have today began in your cells, and while the susceptibility to that disease might have a genetic component, whether those genes get turned on or turned off has everything to do with what you are giving your cells and what you aren't giving them. It's never too late to turn your cellular dysfunction around, but unless you know how to do this, based on what cells actually require, you're just guessing about what you should or shouldn't do.

You're probably used to hearing about giving your body what you need, but I believe a better question is: Are you giving your *mitochondria* what they need? This is where it all begins—with cellular health. If you want to be healthy, strong, and sharp, then your cells have to be healthy, and your cells won't be healthy unless their (that is, your) mitochondria are healthy. That is how you start at the very root, the very beginning of the dysfunction in your body. That is how you turn your health around.

Mitochondria aren't something you would typically read about in a diet

WAHLS WARRIORS SPEAK

My diagnosis with multiple sclerosis was a true wake-up call, but Dr. Wahls has created a wonderful road map for teaching the importance of nutrition. My improvements have been dramatic! Not only has my physical stamina improved greatly, to an extent I cannot overemphasize, but I have experienced drastic improvements with my balance, fatigue, mental clarity, and decreased neuropathy pain, and the list goes on and on. It is truly amazing. I have not used my cane since April 2011. I do still have MS issues. I still lose my balance and fall sometimes. I still have optic neuritis sometimes. I still get fatigued, but it is all 10,000 percent better than it was! Dr. Wahls has proven how profoundly food affects our physical bodies, our disease, and our mental outlook and clarity. The Wahls Diet really does prove the old adage "you are what you eat."

—Pam J., Pecatonica, Illinois

book. They are more a subject for a medical text. The word isn't catchy; it doesn't roll off the tongue. Mitochondria aren't sexy. They are the cellular workhorses. Yet, they are *incredibly important* for your life and health. Without mitochondria, a cell would be like the chassis of a car. It might look like a cell, but without an engine, it's not going to do much. It won't keep you running, and it won't shuttle the trash out the exhaust pipe. And, like any engine, mitochondria need fuel. Not just any fuel—high-quality fuel.

To fully understand how this works, I want you to understand what a cell is, exactly, and in particular how a cell is fueled by the organelles inside it called mitochondria.

Maybe you remember having to draw a cell on a high school biology test, but you may not remember what you drew. Generally, a cell contains a nucleus, which contains DNA, or the genetic instructions for the organism. The nucleus is the heart of the cell, where all the information lives. However, there are other things floating around in that cellular space, including the engines that power the cell. Those engines are called mitochondria. The singular term is *mitochondrion*.

THE EVOLUTION OF MITOCHONDRIA

About 1.5 billion years ago, when the only life-forms on Earth were bacteria, small bacteria invaded larger bacteria; but instead of harming their hosts, these smaller bacteria benefited them by generating energy more efficiently for the host.

The effect of these small "invader" bacteria was to open the door to specialization, so that the larger bacteria were able to evolve into even larger, multicellular organisms that eventually became animals. The smaller bacteria evolved into mitochondria. Interestingly, a similar process seems to have happened with plants: cyanobacteria engulfed smaller bacteria that were capable of photosynthesis, which evolved into plants having chloroplasts—organelles in which photosynthesis occurs. These potent, nutrient-packed, energy-generating chloroplasts are one of the reasons why fresh leafy green vegetables are so good for us to eat.

Most cells in your body contain mitochondria. Some contain many more mitochondria than others. The more energy that a particular cell needs, the more mitochondria it requires to churn out that energy. For example, your brain, retina, heart, and liver cells contain a lot more mitochondria than most other cells in other parts of your body because thinking, seeing, pumping blood, and processing toxins are all high-energy activities.

Cells need fuel for multiple functions: building, maintaining, repairing, and eliminating toxic waste. Toxins can come from medications, pesticides, herbicides, and pollution, as well as from the by-products of basic cell functioning (every engine has its waste products). Too much toxicity can overwhelm cells and organs, but fortunately, your versatile and hardworking mitochondria are busy powering the cells that do the processing of fat-soluble toxins, converting them into a water-soluble form that can be eliminated by your equally hardworking liver and kidneys.

Mitochondria also orchestrate cell death. All cells die eventually, and timely cell death is crucial for health. When the mitochondrion gives the signal, the cell opens up to a flood of calcium, which kills it in a sort of cell

MITOCHONDRIA IN CELL LIFE AND DEATH

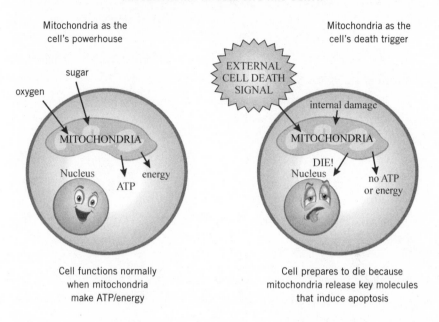

Mitochondria as the
cell's powerhouse

Mitochondria as the
cell's death trigger

Cell functions normally
when mitochondria
make ATP/energy

Cell prepares to die because
mitochondria release key molecules
that induce apoptosis

"suicide" or pre-programmed cell death. (The technical name for this is *apoptosis*.) The cells that do not die when their time is up will continually grow at the expense of all other cells, becoming cancerous tumors.

You should also know a little bit about ATP. Mitochondria produce a compound called ATP (adenosine triphosphate), which stores energy in the bonds between its molecules. ATP helps your body create proteins and antibodies. It is the fuel used to power the chemistry that is used by our cells for all that they do. Without it, your cells couldn't function as they should and could perish prematurely. Just like some cars need unleaded fuel and some cars need diesel fuel and other kinds of vehicles like jet airplanes need their own kind of fuel, cells need a particular kind of fuel to operate, and ATP provides it.

To produce ATP efficiently, the mitochondria need particular things: glucose or ketone bodies from fat (more about this in chapter 7) and oxygen are primary. Your mitochondria can limp along, producing a few ATP on only those three things, but to really do the job right and produce the most ATP molecules, your mitochondria also need thiamine (vitamin B_1), riboflavin (vitamin B_2), niacinamide (vitamin B_3), pantothenic acid (vitamin B_5), minerals (especially sulfur, zinc, magnesium, iron, and manganese), and antioxidants. Mitochondria also need plenty of L-carnitine, alpha-lipoic acid, creatine, and ubiquinone (also called coenzyme Q, coenzyme Q10, CoQ, or CoQ10) for peak efficiency.[2] They also need to be protected from toxins like lead, mercury, and arsenic.

If you don't get all these nutrients, or if you are exposed to too many toxins, your ATP production will become less efficient, which leads to two problems:

1. Your cells will produce less energy, so they may not be able to do everything they need to do.
2. Your cells will generate more waste than necessary, in the form of free radicals.

Without the right nutrient sources to fuel the ATP production in the mitochondria—which in turn produces energy for the cellular processes required to sustain life—your mitochondria can become starved. The cell then can't do its job very effectively. Furthermore, if the mitochondria are too strained, they will begin to disintegrate. With fewer mitochondria in a cell, there are greater demands from the existing mitochondria for the necessary energy. This strain on mitochondria can send a signal to the nucleus that it is time to die, and then the cell will "commit suicide" prematurely. That leads to more rapid aging in the organs and in the body as a whole, especially in the brain, where mitochondrial action is so important. This can eventually lead to "brain fog" (confusion, memory loss, feeling "out of it") and even shrinking of the brain.

LET'S SUMMARIZE WHAT we've learned so far: When your mitochondria are working at peak performance, your cells have the energy they need to function so your body can work the way it's supposed to, without having to compensate for deficiencies in energy and nutrients. Your cells will produce fewer free radicals, minimizing cellular damage. The proper diet will facilitate this entire process. An improper diet derails this process, leading to mitochondrial strain, rapid aging, and more and worsening chronic disease(s).

WAHLS WORDS

All chemical processes involve some waste, and free radicals are some of the trash your body produces in order to make the energy you need. Free radicals are molecules with an open place for an electron that creates a "dangling" bond, making them highly chemically reactive. Free radicals can cause problems in your cells because they scavenge for something to oxidize (in other words, destroy) to get rid of the dangling bond. The free radicals cause problems by changing the shape of a protein, cell membrane, or your DNA, thereby changing its function. If a cell gets too damaged by free radicals, it can stop working correctly and even die prematurely. Too much premature cell death eventually results in rapid aging of your internal organs and of you.

Antioxidants to the rescue! Antioxidant compounds from plants act by stimulating the production of enzymes in our cells that will neutralize those free electrons before they can damage our cells. They make the biochemical machinery much more efficient and effective at protecting the cell from the free radicals.

Imagine what your house would look like if you never cleaned it or threw away any trash. Eventually, trash and dirt would clog up your vents and plumbing, interfere with your electrical system, and cause rot and decay to the structure until your home is no longer livable. Antioxidants are your cleanup crew, your cellular housekeepers, and they keep the free radicals at bay. They sweep up the trash created by ATP production. (I'll talk later about the best dietary sources for antioxidants.)

Signs of Mitochondrial Starvation

Now, you may be realizing how important your mitochondria are to your health, and you are right! You may also be thinking that you need more nutrients so your mitochondria will have what they need to produce ATP—

nutrients like B vitamins and minerals and coenzyme Q and antioxidants. You are probably correct about that, too: Most people don't get enough of the nutrients their cells need.

But how do you know whether your mitochondria are properly nourished? You can't look in the mirror and see your mitochondria or assess their health. There are, however, a few clues that I've discovered in my practice—signs and beacons to indicate that your mitochondria probably aren't getting what they need to keep your system up and running at peak capacity:

- **You experience fatigue.** If you always feel exhausted and low on energy, even when you've gotten enough sleep, your mitochondria may be starved for the vitamins, minerals, and antioxidants they need to produce energy at the cellular level. Low energy at the cellular level can translate to low energy you can actually feel.

- **You eat a high-sugar, high-starch diet.** Too much white flour, sugar, and high-fructose corn syrup can "gum up" your mitochondria, diminishing efficiency. Sugars and refined starches affect your body detrimentally in two ways: (1) They are high in calories but low in nutritional quality, so you can fill up without getting the nutrients you need, starving your cells; and (2) they encourage the growth of unfavorable bacteria and yeasts in your gut, which can lead to a lot of other problems. (I'll talk more about this throughout the book.)

- **You are over 50 years old.** Your ability to manufacture coenzyme Q, an important nutrient for healthy and efficient mitochondria, slowly declines with age. As you pass 50 years, your mitochondrial efficiency also slowly declines, particularly if your nutrition is suboptimal.

- **You are on statin drugs.** Statin drugs help lower cholesterol, so many doctors recommend them for people at risk for heart disease or who have uncontrolled cholesterol. Some doctors even recommend them as preventive medicine. The statin class of drugs that are commonly prescribed to lower cholesterol, however, make it more difficult for cells to manufacture coenzyme Q. Because cholesterol tends to be higher in older people, they are the ones most likely to be on statin drugs, and older people (over the age of 50) already often have problems manufacturing coenzyme Q, further compounding the issue. Several studies have shown that improving the level of coenzyme Q reduces symptoms in patients with neurodegenerative brain disease.[3] If you have been prescribed statins, don't go off them without talking to your doctor, but you might want to consider this information and increase your coenzyme Q intake to compensate.

- **You take prescription or over-the-counter medication regularly.** Many common prescription and over-the-counter medications can deplete your B vitamin, mineral, and coenzyme Q supplies. The longer you are on the medications, the more depleted these levels may become. Some of the medications that interfere with coenzyme Q include:
  - tricyclic antidepressants
  - benzodiazepines
  - sulfonylureas
  - thiazide diuretics
  - beta blockers
  - acetaminophen (Tylenol)

Medications that can interfere with B vitamin absorption and your metabolism include:

  - diuretics
  - metformin and other common diabetic medications
  - birth control pills
  - medications that lower stomach acid
  - certain antibiotics
  - benzodiazepines
  - tricyclic antidepressants
  - NSAIDs (nonsteroidal anti-inflammatory drugs, such as ibuprofen)
  - aspirin
  - proton pump inhibitors like Prilosec

- **Diuretics and medications that lower stomach acid may also interfere with the absorption of minerals.** The nutrient depletion associated with long-term medication use may be a factor in why so many diseases continue to progress when treated with medications.[4]
- **You have chronic migraine or tension headaches.** There is a correlation between chronic tension headaches and mitochondrial dysfunction.[5]
- **You have a chronic disease.** The list of health problems linked to mitochondria not working well is growing every day and now includes diabe-

tes, heart failure, hepatitis C, fibromyalgia, schizophrenia, mood disorders, epilepsy, strokes, neuropathy, memory problems, and autoimmune disease.[6]

Chronic disease is the most obvious manifestation of long-term mitochondrial dysfunction. When your mitochondria aren't powering your body correctly, everything begins to malfunction in a negative spiraling chain reaction that eventually relates to cell aging, organ dysfunction, and chronic disease. Science increasingly shows that mitochondrial strain is at the root of most of the chronic diseases afflicting modern society. Want to grow healthier? Then restore your mitochondria to the healthiest function possible for you.

If any or all of these symptoms or categories apply to you, your mitochondria will benefit greatly from a tune-up. Every aspect of the Wahls Protocol program will benefit your mitochondrial function, either directly or indirectly, but none more so than the improvements you will make to your diet. You are

WAHLS WARRIORS SPEAK

I was diagnosed with relapsing remitting MS in January 2003, when I was 46, although I had the disease many years earlier. I stuck with traditional medicine for years. I have been on Avonex, Tysabri, and Copaxone, but continued to decline. My neurologist suggested Gilenya, but I was reluctant to go on it because of recent deaths and dangerous side effects, so I started looking for another way. This led me to Dr. Terry Wahls.

I've been practicing the Wahls Diet for six months now, and also use the e-stim device. I am clearer mentally, my decline has stopped, and I have some strength returning. The color in my legs is better and I exercise 20 to 30 minutes a day, meditate, breathe deeply, and spend time outside. Dr. Wahls is my role model and heroine on several fronts. (I am also a gay mom with two young adult children of my own.) I had asked doctors for years about diet, exercise, and stress, and they blew my questions off. I so appreciate the depth of her research and her willingness to relate her personal experience. She is a lifesaver!

—Ann P., Houston, Texas

going to start flooding your body with the B vitamins, minerals, antioxidants, and amino acids that your body needs to keep your mitochondria well fed so that every aspect of your health, from the cellular level on up, can begin to repair itself.

Your New Prescription: Food

Your cells have approximately 4,000 different enzyme systems with more than 1,000 different chemical signals, performing trillions of chemical reactions every second.[7] More than 250 different nutrients have been identified and likely there are thousands more that scientists have not yet identified that are important to enjoying optimal health.[8] Are you getting them all? Probably not.

And is your gut capable of properly digesting the food you eat and absorbing the nutrients you need into your bloodstream, providing your cells with a sufficient supply of the vitamins, minerals, essential fatty acids, and antioxidants they need to thrive? This may also be a problem for you.

Biochemistry is complex, and the workings of the human body are unimaginably intricate and involved. Although we have some idea of the nutritional requirements of mitochondria, we don't yet fully understand every single mitochondrial requirement, nor do we fully understand all the nutritional needs of every cell type in our body. When I talk about "global nutrition," or what our bodies need overall, understand that while we know we have these nutritional needs for thousands of different functions, we still don't understand it all.

But nature does. This is why we can't have optimal health by relying only on vitamins and nutritional supplements on top of our usual diets. Real foods contain all the secrets we don't yet understand, and that is why the Wahls Protocol is specifically designed to use real foods in very particular ways in order to fulfill the vast nutritional requirements of your cells—even the thousands of requirements we don't yet understand.

What we do know is that when vitamin, mineral, and antioxidant levels in the body fall below optimum levels, we see a clear decline in health. This isn't just theory. Case in point: Dr. Bruce Ames, a biochemist who studies nutrition at the cellular level, provides evidence that illustrates how an individual is much more likely to have more rapid aging and the development of cancer with inadequate vitamin and mineral levels, even if she or he is okay short term.[9] For example, when the supply of vitamin K is limited, your body will prioritize how to use the limited supply. It will make proteins that will clot your blood if you are cut, but it will not make the proteins you need to maintain flexible blood vessels and heart valves. So although you won't bleed to death if you get an injury today, if your deficiency continues over the long term, you will develop stiffness in your heart valves and/or high blood pressure.[10] The result could be that in the future you may need heart surgery to replace your heart valves, or you may need to take blood pressure medication.

There was an interesting study that measured the blood levels in seniors of over thirty-one different vitamins, minerals, essential fats, and antioxidants that were thought to impact the health of the brain, in order to examine the impact of these nutrients on both brain size and thinking capacity. The Oregon Brain Aging Study looked at 104 adults (mean age 87). The researchers analyzed blood levels of various nutrients, brain size as measured by MRI, and thinking ability as measured by various neuropsychological tests, and then did regression analysis to measure the relationship between nutrient levels, brain size, and cognitive performance.[11] The results were illuminating. High levels of vitamins B_1, B_2, B_6, B_9, B_{12}, C, D, E, and fatty acids were the most powerful predictors of brain health. Additionally, high levels of vitamins A and K and antioxidants corresponded with increased brain volume and better thinking capacity.

The study also looked at detrimental substances, or "antinutrients." Notably, the more trans fat (hydrogenated vegetable oil) in the blood, the smaller the brain and the lower the thinking capacity, as determined by how well the subjects performed thinking tasks.[12] In other words, spending all of your calories on foods packed with the nutrition your brain needs is likely the most powerful thing you can do to protect your brain. If you want a smaller brain that thinks poorly, eat more antinutrients like the trans fat–laden processed foods. Eat fast food daily or even just three times a week and you are well on the way to early dementia!

Food can't do everything. I want you to understand that up front. I still have multiple sclerosis and I still have lesions in my cervical spinal cord. Some scarring and degeneration is permanent. Quite a lot more degeneration may not be permanent after all, however. My lesions no longer keep me from walking. You can see them on an MRI, but they do not affect me the way they once did. Food can directly influence the firestorm of destruction inside your body. Will you continue to fuel the fire, or will you douse it by infusing your body with the particular and extensive nutrients it needs to best fight its way from the debilitating effects of an autoimmune condition back toward steadily greater health and vitality?

Micronutrients Your Brain Needs Now

Cellular nutrition is crucial for overall health, but of particular interest to those with MS and other diseases that impact the brain is nutrition that specifically targets brain health. Your brain is an amazing and complex organ, and it needs a lot of resources in order to function properly. One of the most important structures to repair and maintain in your brain is myelin, and myelin is the very thing that the immune system attacks in people with MS.

Myelin is the fatty insulation around the nerve cells. There are ten billion brain cells with ten trillion connections. All that connective wiring must be insulated with myelin. However, your doctor probably didn't tell you which nutrients your brain cells need to function optimally, not to mention repair damage. Your doctor probably doesn't even know about this, as physicians receive very little nutrition training. However, I know. To make healthy myelin, you need to consume thiamine (vitamin B_1), folate (vitamin B_9), cobalamin (vitamin B_{12}), omega-3 fatty acids (in particular, docosahexaenoic acid, or DHA), and iodine. (Later in the book I'll tell you what foods you need to eat to be sure you have all these essential building blocks on hand.)

Your brain also depends on neurotransmitters. These are the molecules our brain cells use to talk to one another. When neurotransmitters malfunction, the result can be depression, anxiety, irritability, and increased pain. Many physicians give patients with mood problems drugs like Prozac to boost the production of particular neurotransmitters, but oftentimes patients don't get much relief, in part because they aren't eating the building blocks the brain cells need to make the neurotransmitters in the first place. The Prozac can't work as well if your brain doesn't have the building blocks it needs to run the chemistry of the brain. For proper neurotransmitter function, your brain cells need, in particular, certain amino acids, sulfur, and pyridoxine (vitamin B_6).[13]

BRAIN CELLS: WHERE THE BUILDING BLOCKS DO THE WORK

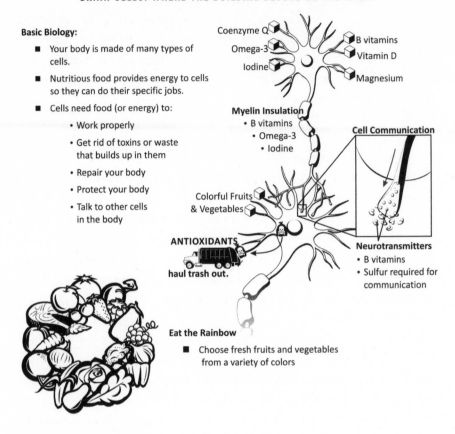

Basic Biology:

- Your body is made of many types of cells.
- Nutritious food provides energy to cells so they can do their specific jobs.
- Cells need food (or energy) to:
  - Work properly
  - Get rid of toxins or waste that builds up in them
  - Repair your body
  - Protect your body
  - Talk to other cells in the body

Coenzyme Q
Omega-3
Iodine

B vitamins
Vitamin D
Magnesium

Myelin Insulation
- B vitamins
- Omega-3
- Iodine

Cell Communication

Colorful Fruits & Vegetables

ANTIOXIDANTS
haul trash out.

Neurotransmitters
- B vitamins
- Sulfur required for communication

Eat the Rainbow
- Choose fresh fruits and vegetables from a variety of colors

When I first began researching the nutrients that fuel the proper biochemistry of cells, especially brain cells, I identified the micronutrients that scientists had said were important to either mitochondrial efficiency[14] or to optimal function of brain cells.[15] I have listed the micronutrients and their main functions for you here. I have also listed food groups that are excellent sources for the calories consumed based upon the food itself (as opposed to those foods with vitamins added back after processing).[16] Keep in mind that synthetic vitamins do not have the same shape as naturally occurring vitamins, and they don't occur within the context of all the other elements in whole food. In addition, I have listed a key antinutrient that has been associated with worsening brain health.

Beyond Food: The Wahls Protocol

Food is the core component of the Wahls Protocol, and cellular as well as brain-targeted nutrition can determine what happens to your health for the rest of your life. It is not the entirety of the Wahls Protocol, however, and it is not the only thing I changed in my life in order to drastically reverse my symptoms. Many other factors led to my continuing recovery. These include targeted toxin reduction, electrical stimulation of muscles, a regular and appropriate exercise program, a few key supplements, and a commitment to a targeted program of stress reduction.

These round out the Wahls Protocol and are all things you can do for yourself. Combined with an improved diet, you can give your body the best possible shot at healing. Throughout this book, I will take you step by step through the various components of the Wahls Protocol that I developed to help myself and that I systemized to help others, but here's a preview of the basic elements:

The Wahls Diet

This is the crux of biochemical restoration. I'll walk you through the steps that will take you from your current diet, which may be lacking in some of the potent nutrition your cells require for health, to eating the Wahls way. There are three levels, and you can start wherever you are most comfortable. The most basic level, the Wahls Diet, involves adding some things and taking some things away. The next level, Wahls Paleo, gets a little bit stricter. Finally, Wahls Paleo Plus is for those who want serious and rapid intervention. The dietary steps may sound difficult at first, but you'll be eating great natural whole foods, including lots of vegetables, fruit, meat, poultry, seafood, nuts, seeds, and even some surprising foods you might never have considered trying before. You won't be hungry; in fact, you'll be required to eat a *lot* of food, and if you are overweight, you'll find those extra pounds melting away (a bonus of the Wahls Protocol!). Don't be nervous. You don't have to make the changes all at once. I'll talk you through them so you understand exactly what you are doing and why before you try anything radical.

Table 1 · List of Nutrients Critical to Brain Cell Health

Nutrient	Main Function	Top Food Sources for Nutrients[17]
Vitamin A, retinol (animal form of vitamin A)	Involved in synthesis of visual pigments in the retina	Cod-liver oil, liver
Vitamin B_1 (thiamine)	Facilitates use of glucose, generation of myelin	Organ meat, seeds, nuts
Vitamin B_2 (riboflavin)	Helps produce mitochondrial energy	Liver, greens
Vitamin B_3 (niacin)	Helps produce mitochondrial energy	Liver, chicken
Vitamin B_6 (pyridoxine)	Aids in neurotransmitter production	Fish, greens
Vitamin B_9 (folic acid)	Facilitates myelin generation	Liver, greens, asparagus
Vitamin B_{12} (cobalamin)	Facilitates myelin generation	Liver, shellfish
Vitamin C	Fights infection, supplies intracellular antioxidants	Greens, citrus
Vitamin D	Aids in proper reading of the DNA, protects cells in the brain	Cod-liver oil, sunlight
Vitamin E	Promotes cell signaling; protects cholesterol-carrying molecules from oxidation; reduces brain cell death, which protects against aging	Nuts, seeds, avocado
Iron	Helps supply oxygen to the brain	Organ meat, greens, molasses
Copper	Promotes iron/copper balance involved in higher brain functions	Organ meat, shellfish, nuts, seeds
Zinc	Aids in perception	Liver, shellfish, nuts, seeds
Iodine	Involved with intelligence and myelin production	Seaweed, seafood, iodized sea salt
Magnesium	Stabilizes cells against excess glutamate (too much stimulation)	Greens, raw soaked nuts, seaweed
Selenium	Protects against oxidative stress	Brazil nuts, sunflower seeds, seafood, seaweed
Lycopene, lutein, zeaxanthin, alpha- and beta-carotene, beta-cryptoxanthin	Antioxidants, which protect cell membranes and mitochondria	Brightly colored vegetables and berries
Carnitine	Assists with energy production in mitochondria	Heart, kidney, liver, beef, and all other meats, including poultry

Nutrient	Main Function	Top Food Sources for Nutrients[17]
Lipoic acid	Assists with energy production in mitochondria	Heart, kidney, liver
Coenzyme Q	Assists with energy production in mitochondria	Heart, kidney, liver
Creatine	Assists with energy production in mitochondria	Organ meat, wild game
Pantothenic acid (vitamin B$_5$)	Assists with energy production in mitochondria	Liver, mushrooms, avocado
Vitamin K	Helps strengthen myelin and blood vessels	Greens
Cholesterol	Strengthens cell membranes, promotes hormone production	Animal fats
Alpha-linolenic fatty acid (ALA) (vegetarian form of omega-3 fatty acids)	Helps to generate cell membranes and myelin	Walnut, flax, and hemp oils
Omega-3 fatty acids, eicosapentaenoic acid (EPA), docosahexaenoic acid (DHA) (animal forms of omega-3 fatty acids)	Helps to generate cell membranes and myelin, lowers excessive inflammation	Wild herring, salmon, grass-fed meats
Omega-6 fatty acids, linoleic acid (LA), arachidonic acid (AA)	Helps to generate cell membranes and myelin, signals molecules to communicate between cells (Too much can lead to excessive inflammation; must be in balance with omega-3 fatty acids.)	Seeds and nuts (LA); organ meat, meat (AA)
Gamma-linolenic fatty acid (GLA)	Lowers inflammation	Borage, primrose, hemp oil
Harmful Antinutrients		
Trans fats	Increase the damage to cell membranes and mitochondria	Partially hydrogenated fats, food fried in vegetable oil (especially fast food)

Toxic Exposure

The modern world is chemically burdened and many of those chemicals interact with our cells, often thwarting the natural chemical processes. I'll explain how many of these chemicals are associated with the leading causes of disability and disease in America. I'll help you identify where your exposures to these chemicals lie and the specific steps you can take to reduce your exposure. I'll also explain how your body processes the toxic chemicals and eliminates them. Most important, I'll give you the specific steps to take to safely strengthen and optimize your body's toxin elimination systems so that you can slowly and safely reduce the body burden of toxins that are stored in your fat.

Exercise and E-Stim

Your brain and your body need you to use your muscles and *move*, even if you have a degenerative disease. Exercise is important to maintaining the proper balance of hormones in the brain and in the body. It also keeps muscles from atrophying. When you have a chronic disease, it's also important to do enough, and not too much, and to do the right kinds of exercise for your needs. After I talk about exercise, I'll also tell you all about electrical stimulation, or e-stim, a process that had a dramatic effect on my mobility as well as my mood.

Supplements, Medications, and Alternative Medicine Treatments

I strongly believe that most nutrition should come from food, but, depending on your particular needs, you could benefit from certain supplements; I'll tell you which ones I recommend and which ones I believe are contraindicated. I'll also talk about your medications and whether you should or shouldn't go off them as you begin the Wahls Protocol. Finally, I will give you my conventional-doctor-turned-functional-medicine-advocate perspective on alternative medicine treatments you might want to try and those I believe you should avoid. Learn what's proven and what's merely speculation, as well as what's safe and what might not be.

Stress-Reduction Techniques

Stress reduction is absolutely critical for optimizing your body's ability to heal. The stress response causes a cascade of changes in the body that can be highly beneficial in the short term and drastically destructive over the long term. I'll explain exactly why and how you can get yourself back out of fight-or-flight mode.

Looking Back over Your Life

I hope you can still remember a time when you felt well. You could work or play all day and you felt happy, or at least normal, in your body. At some point, however, you probably noticed some subtle changes. Perhaps you noticed that you couldn't move as freely or think as clearly, or you began to experience pain. These very outward symptoms were a signal that your biochemistry was changing. The signaling between your cells was gradually becoming confused.

You could recognize that you didn't feel well, though you may not have been able to explain precisely what was amiss. You eventually saw your doctor, who performed an examination and conducted blood tests but found nothing wrong. Perhaps you were told to come back in a year. When you did, you felt a little worse than you did the year before, but all your tests still looked okay and the doctor continued to say you were "fine." Perhaps this dance went on for years, perhaps decades, before your body finally suffered enough damage that a test or two began to come up abnormal. Finally, your doctor began to investigate more seriously. And perhaps, at long last, you were given a diagnosis. Your doctor had not been trained in functional medicine, and so opportunities to recover your vitality were missed, but the inexorable process of biochemical decline was happening all along, through all those years of negative test results and doctors reassuring you. Your body began to produce and accumulate incorrectly made molecules in your cells and your organs. To you, it probably felt like the music of your life slowly began to deteriorate, note by note, losing the melody and harmony, moving from a beautiful symphonic concert to chaotic noise. That's how it felt to me.

The most exciting thing about the Wahls Protocol is that it puts your care back under your control. It's so easy to feel helpless, lost, and dependent on doctors and family members when your health declines. The Wahls Protocol offers you a chance to wean yourself off excessive dependence on others. You will still need to take your medications, at least for now. You will still need to do as your doctor asks. You will likely still need help from your family—but who doesn't? However, there is much you can do on your own, and that will only increase if you follow the Wahls Protocol. You have a future, and it doesn't have to be a dark one.

In Viktor Frankl's powerful and moving book *Man's Search for Meaning*,[18] he states that we all have a choice about how we will respond to the events in our lives. He says that between every event and our response is a space. In that space, we show the strength of our character. After I was diagnosed with MS, I resolved to get up every day, go to work, and do my job, however fatigued I was. I determined which things I could still do, rather than focusing on what I couldn't do. I decided I would do everything in my power to slow my descent. Remember, at that time, my doctors all told me that functions, once gone, were lost forever—that once you hit secondary progressive MS, it is a long, slow, steady, inevitable decline. When I started this journey, I was only hoping to slow the decline.

I couldn't have done what I did—get back out of my wheelchair, not to mention develop the Wahls Protocol and begin teaching it to others—if I hadn't made that initial decision not to give up but to keep pushing and living and being who I was, apart from my disease. This is what I want for you: to choose life rather than disability, and to choose your own well-being and health over sickness, even if it sounds difficult, even if you don't want to get out of bed.

The beauty of the Wahls Protocol is that no matter what deficiencies you might have or what faulty enzymes might be at work in your body—and no matter what you have been eating and drinking and doing and thinking up until now, even as recently as yesterday—you can still shore up your body and begin to replenish your cells. This is a new paradigm, and ironically it's exactly the way your body was originally intended to function. Your cells determine if you will continue to decline or begin to heal. With healthier cells, you become stronger, smarter, and younger. I see it in my primary care, therapeutic lifestyle, and traumatic-brain-injury clinics every week.

I call my patients and the many others who have written to me to tell me about their success "Wahls Warriors," because they are fighters and they are winning at taking back their lives. You can be one of them. It's not too late for any of the good things you still want for your life. You can start over. This can be your new beginning. Will you join us?

Chapter 2

AUTOIMMUNITY: CONVENTIONAL VERSUS FUNCTIONAL MEDICINE

WHAT IS IN a name? What *is* a disease, exactly? Diseases seem real and specific to those who have them or fear they have them because, as patients, we understand diseases according to what they do to us and how they make us feel. This is logical, after all: What we feel is all we know. In my body, multiple sclerosis was causing degeneration in my spinal cord, and I could feel the results: a slow loss of mobility, brain fog, and episodes of horrific pain.

Although MS looks like a particular condition on the outside, at the cellular level MS is not so different from other autoimmune diseases like rheumatoid arthritis and systemic lupus; chronic diseases like diabetes and heart disease; and even from mood disorders like depression, autism, and schizophrenia. My biochemistry was malfunctioning, and in my case these dysfunctional processes began in the cells in my brain and spinal cord. But that root cause—cellular dysfunction—has everything in common with other diseases that have other names.

At the most basic level, scientists are discovering that nearly all of the chronic diseases that cause so much suffering and are steadily driving up the cost of health care all share mitochondrial dysfunction, excessive inflammation, high cortisol levels, and other markers of broken biochemistry. In a very real sense, we all have the same disease because all disease begins with broken, incorrect biochemistry and disordered communication within and between our cells. For health to return, the chemistry must revert to normal, and communication within and between our cells must be restored. This is true for every disease.

Whether you are diagnosed with multiple sclerosis or rheumatoid arthritis or systemic lupus or inflammatory bowel disease—or whether you are told your symptoms are "idiopathic" (meaning we don't know what is causing them)—depends largely on how your disease looks on the outside. Inside, the distinction between these autoimmune diseases is, frankly, fairly arbitrary, although there are different ways to view, think about, and understand what is happening when cellular dysfunction gains a foothold. As a conventionally trained doctor, I learned one way; in my studies of functional medicine, I learned a different way. However, the fact remained that inside the body, health problems begin in the cells.

But I know my patients. They want a diagnosis. They want to know *what they have.* This is a very typical response, to which I am quite sympathetic. I wanted to know what I had, too. I wanted a name, something to blame, something to cure. It's part of how the human mind works. We want to separate out and define and categorize things, to better understand them.

Let's take a step back from all of that for a moment and try to think outside the box. To help you do this, I'm going to explain something that most doctors know but many patients don't totally understand: The truth is that diagnoses are simply names we put on conditions, based on the parts we can actually quantify, like symptoms, test results, and which medications improve or worsen symptoms, as well as through a process of elimination. If it's not *this* or *this* or *this,* then it must be *that.* This stems from the impulse to categorize and name, but it doesn't actually mean that one disease is something completely different from another disease.

What many people also don't know is that the names we put on chronic diseases are frequently specifically the result of studies that look at what treatments, most often pharmaceutical, will make a difference in the symptoms. In other words, when specific symptoms are relieved by a specific drug, then scientists often name the disease based on this information alone. Everyone who gets relief of symptom X by taking drug Y has disease Z.

Sometimes it isn't a drug that causes a defined population to improve (or worsen) in a predictable way. Sometimes it is a surgical technique or another treatment or therapy. Whatever it is, if it has an effect on symptoms, then that defined population gets a name for their particular type of illness, along with a specific treatment that eventually becomes the "standard of care," which means it is the generally accepted treatment for that condition. That is how, for hundreds of generations, physicians created diagnoses, naming conditions like multiple sclerosis, diabetes, congestive heart failure, asthma, depression, and inflammatory bowel disease. They were not yet able to look into the biochemical workings of the cells to understand the root cause of these diseases or how similar, at the cellular level, all these diseases really are.

It's important to understand this so you don't give your diagnosis more power than it deserves: Diagnoses are often based on the external effects of treatments and historical observations rather than on the biochemical processes that cause the disease themselves. As our understanding deepens about disease processes and treatments, diseases are reclassified, treatments adjusted, and often new diseases named. Sometimes one disease is divided into several, or several diseases are merged into one.

Because they are not based on all the information, however, and because they are based on our human need to name things, one could argue that these classifications are mostly a matter of semantics. Physicians have been classifying diseases on the basis of physical examination and laboratory testing results for hundreds of years now, and we do this to guide both the clinical research we do to understand how diseases progress over time and to develop better treatments. This is all good science, but it's not the whole picture.

To do our scientific studies of disease, scientists follow a precise research protocol. We always have a tightly defined group of patients and a tightly controlled intervention (preferably a drug or a very specific procedure so it can be easily reproduced), so there are fewer variables to study. This makes the results seem more concrete and objective, but that's not really necessarily true. The research is easier to do and to analyze this way, making it easier to show if the study intervention works or not; but the effectiveness of any given drug to relieve symptoms doesn't necessarily have anything to do with what's really wrong with your broken biochemical pathways that are at the root of many of your symptoms.

Let me say this again in yet another way: *The names we first put on most chronic diseases are the result of observations made prior to the scientific understanding of the biochemical workings of individual cells.* Billions of dollars are spent by the National Institutes of Health and by the drug industry studying disease symptoms and drugs to control those symptoms. By contrast, very little is spent to study how to create optimal health and vitality through lifestyle choices that can lead to healthier biochemistry and, consequently, healthier people.

This may seem counterproductive to you. It certainly does to me.

Fortunately, we are beginning to understand the disordered biochemical pathways that lead to the broken chemistry at the root of many chronic symptoms across many diagnoses. I believe that eventually this will change the way all diseases are diagnosed. Unfortunately, although science is finally uncovering how those broken pathways disrupt the biochemistry of cells and disease, most conventional physicians are still using the traditional models of disease based on symptoms instead of addressing the disordered pathways that are at the root of the problem. The old ways govern the standard of care. As a result, most conventional physicians are focused on symptoms that can be improved by drugs or surgery instead of trying to create more health and vitality in their patients by improving the biochemistry of the cells through optimal lifestyle choices.

This is the realm of functional medicine: to discover and treat the root causes of broken biochemistry by looking at the physiological systems for everything from the cells to the organs to the entire organism, and addressing the causes of the problems at their root. This is why I have embraced this form of medicine. I believe it is the only sensible way to correct biochemical dysfunction so you can return to health, rather than simply easing symptoms with drug therapy.

Conventional medicine still has its place. I still do conventional diagnosing in my clinic and still write medication prescriptions for my patients. It is useful to a point. However, I now add a second layer: I diagnose the person's health behaviors, exposure to toxins, stress level, nutrition quality, and exercise level. I try actively to create more health and vitality in my patients by increasing their knowledge about what they can do on their own. This is where the Wahls Protocol differs from conventional treatment, more closely resembling the functional medicine model. I help my patients reset their broken biochemistry by teaching them to fix how they move and what they eat. Then I help them minimize toxins and improve their hormone balance, and we work from there, untying the biochemical knots so the cells can work the way they were intended to work. In turn, this allows the body to work the way it is meant to work.

WAHLS WARRIORS SPEAK

I am a registered dietitian who understood cognitively the role of diet for health, but it wasn't until after my diagnosis with relapsing remitting multiple sclerosis that I began experimenting with whole foods and specifically anti-inflammatory foods that I noticed a change in my body. My first symptom was optic neuritis (inflamed optic nerve). Subsequently, I experienced paresthesias (painful sensations due to diseased nerve transmission) in my legs and severe fatigue. Then I got numbness in my feet and I had difficulty remembering recent information. After seeing Dr. Terry Wahls speak via her TEDx video clip, I felt pushed to another level. I increased my intake of the foods she suggested, including fish (I was previously a vegetarian), and I eliminated gluten and dairy. I began to feel more energy and focus and noticed a distinct reduction in my symptoms. Then I went further, eating even more kale and other nervous system and mitochondrial substrates, as the Wahls Diet suggests.

I now feel even better than I did before. I am so grateful that a Western-trained physician is promoting what I have been trying to convey to doctors for years: that diet is more powerful than drugs in the long term. I am so grateful to see clinical research beginning to back this up so that others in the medical profession will begin to see credibility in what we already know in our bodies and minds.

—Marla B., RD, LD, CNSD, Chicago, Illinois

This is what I want to do for you, but first I want you to understand what is going wrong in your body. Let's look first at autoimmune disease in general, and then at multiple sclerosis in particular, through the lenses of both conventional and functional medicine.

What Is an Autoimmune Disease?

First, let's consider autoimmunity. In biology, *auto* means "self" and autoimmunity is a condition in which the immune cells become confused and begin attacking cellular structures of the person's own body. All of our cells have receptors on the cell membrane that allow the immune cells to recognize our cells as part of our own bodies. When the body doesn't see or sense these "self" receptors, it interprets a structure or substance as foreign and a possible threat. Is it a virus? Bacteria? An object that shouldn't be there? Your body doesn't know. It only knows "self" and "not self," and if it is "not self," it must then determine whether something is "not self but safe to ignore" or "not self and dangerous." Your immune cells will ignore "self" molecules and the "not-self-but-safe" molecules, but the immune cells are terribly threatened by anything seen as "not self and dangerous," and they will vigorously attack these molecules in an attempt to damage or destroy the dangerous foreigner so it can't harm the body and endanger survival.

It's a good system—when it works. It helps to keep you healthy by attacking the legitimately dangerous viruses and bacteria that can invade your system. With autoimmunity, however, the wires get crossed and, for some unknown reason, the immune cells mistake proteins that are genuinely "self" as foreign, and more specifically as "not self and dangerous." The results can be devastating. Which structures the body attacks determines what kind of autoimmune condition the person has. When the body attacks the myelin—the fatty sheath around nerve cells—resulting in nervous system damage, then we say that person has multiple sclerosis. If the immune cells attack the skin, resulting in rashes, blisters, and other visible skin conditions, we may name the condition psoriasis, eczema, or a blistering condition such as bullous pemphigoid. If the body attacks lung tissue, resulting in wheezing and constricted airways, then we call it asthma. If it attacks the thyroid, resulting in a wide range of symptoms related to thyroid function, then we may call it autoimmune thyroid disease. If it attacks the joints, resulting in pain and stiffness, then the person may be diagnosed with rheumatoid arthritis or systemic lupus. Although all these diseases present differently, the root cause for the more than 140 different types of autoimmune conditions is the loss of tolerance of "self" in the body, and the attack by the immune cells on "self," causing the symptoms of the disease.

Actually, autoimmune disease may be a factor in more diseases than previously thought. Research is revealing that there may be an autoimmune component to a host of other chronic conditions, like heart disease and high blood pressure, migraines, and mood disorders. Research is ongoing in this area, and I believe we've only scratched the surface in understanding the effects of autoimmunity on our bodies.

Why would the complex and intelligent human body mistakenly attack its own tissues? There is a conventional view of autoimmune disease, and then there is a functional medicine view. Let's consider both.

The Conventional
View of Autoimmune Disease

The conventional medicine view of autoimmune disease says that the body has lost the ability to recognize its own internal protein components as native components of itself, but that we don't know why. Scientists are aware that all chronic disease states begin as the result of broken chemistry and confused signaling between cells. Autoimmune disease is like scrambling a few notes in the middle of a grand symphony. As more and more notes are scrambled, the harmonies and melody are increasingly lost until there is no semblance of the original score and what was once beautiful music just sounds like noise.

That's frustrating for scientists, but because medicine is a practice of action, conventional medicine focuses on slowing the progression of disability, usually through drug therapy. This is the only proven way, according to published research, to make any consistent favorable impact on the progression of an autoimmune disease, so that is what doctors do: They try to help. They assess the patient and they pull out their prescription pads (or laptop computers, as is increasingly the case today) and they send their patients off to the pharmacy.

The drugs conventional doctors prescribe for an autoimmune disease make the immune cells weaker so that they cannot attack the body as vigorously. All of the disease-modifying drugs for MS and the other autoimmune conditions focus on blocking some part of the body's immune response, using various mechanisms. Some disease-modifying drugs for autoimmune disorders act as a poison to rapidly dividing cells (the immune cells are some of the most rapidly dividing cells in the body) so that they cannot work as effectively at attacking (or protecting) the body. Some disease-modifying drugs are designed to block a specific pathway in the immune process.

Because our immunity has evolved to play a protective role through multiple channels, however, all drugs that target our immune cells will have an extensive list of side effects, many of them having major negative impacts on quality of life. We are blocking a major natural function in the body, and even though this function isn't working properly, the body doesn't like this. Some of the side effects of these drugs include fatigue, joint pain, achiness, depression, and mouth sores. There is a slightly higher risk of infection (because the immune system is being suppressed) as well as a feeling of general malaise, because making the immune cells less effective generally results in making *all* cells somewhat less effective.

Essentially, autoimmune drugs blunt the body's activity, in both a negative and a positive way. Symptoms of the autoimmune disease may improve, but people on immune-suppression drugs may feel acutely worse in other ways while taking drug treatment. Many stay on the treatment no matter how bad they feel because of the looming probability of becoming progressively more disabled by the disease progression if the disease is unchecked.

This is the treatment conventional medicine offers the autoimmune patient: a slowing of the progression of disability at the cost of feeling somewhat or even a lot worse right now.

The Functional Medicine
Perspective on Autoimmunity

There is another view of autoimmune disease, and this is the view on which I've based the Wahls Protocol. The problem with the conventional focus on drugs is that study after study has shown that diet, toxin exposure, and activity level account for 70 to 95 percent of the risk for autoimmune disease, mental health issues, cancer, and, in fact, most chronic diseases. Drugs do not improve the quality of your diet. They do not reduce your toxin exposure—and often increase it. And they certainly don't increase your activity level. Rarely will they help lower the chronic stress you feel in your life.

Functional medicine looks more deeply at the reasons why the body has lost its tolerance to its own proteins in the first place. We know that if proteins change their shape and no longer fit into the recognition receptors, the body may not recognize them and they'll look threatening and ominous. They will more likely look like "not self and dangerous." Functional medicine seeks to know why and how this happens. What biochemical reactions have gone wrong that led to the development of these misshapen proteins? What is the exact nature of the broken chemistry, and what are the environmental factors that triggered or worsened the condition?

There are theories about why autoimmune disease happens. One theory is that the proteins that the body no longer recognizes actually change because of oxidation when a sugar molecule, a heavy metal ion (like from lead or mercury), or even a virus or bacteria particle gets attached to the protein. The most common oxidizer is glucose (eating a diet high in sugar and carbohydrates can increase the frequency of this). When the protein is oxidized, it changes its shape, and in genetically susceptible individuals the protein now looks like a dangerous foreign invader. The immune cells attack.

Immune system hyperreactivity is another issue of interest in a functional medicine approach. A cell need only change a small amount for a highly reactive immune cell to get suspicious. We know that there are many factors that increase the reactivity of immune cells. These include the amount and proportion of omega-3 and omega-6 fatty acids and antioxidants in the diet, carbohydrate content of the diet, food intolerances, toxic load in the body, hormone levels, and the presence of chronic infections. All these things can make the immune cells hyperreactive. Therefore, we want them less irritated so they are less likely to go berserk and begin attacking oxidized proteins in the body. A nearly infinite number of possible injuries (from toxins, hormones, and infections) to the proteins in our blood and our cells can occur—but our immune cells have only a limited number of responses they can make to this damage.

Another way the immune cells can get activated to attack the self is through molecular mimicry. That is when viruses and bacteria have evolved

WAHLS WARRIORS SPEAK

After the birth of my first son in 2006, I ended up in the hospital with a bad staph infection. After it was finally "gone," I started having weird symptoms: tingling in my back, breathing difficulties, and cold feet. I was told initially that I had anxiety, or that I drank too much coffee. Finally, after my entire right side went numb in 2009, they did an MRI and immediately sent me to a neurologist, who just threw my chart on the table and said, "The good news is you don't have a tumor and the bad news is you have multiple sclerosis. Would you like Copaxone daily injections or Avonex?" He told me I would be fine for about ten years, then slowly progress. Nice bedside manner. I was 27 years old.

I started the Wahls Diet in May 2012 and my progression has definitively slowed. My mood is 100 percent better, which is awesome, and I am able to exercise again, which I had not been able to do because of the fatigue. I now treat my food as my medicine, and if it is not going to heal me, I don't eat it. My family is so grateful for Dr. Wahls's work because they have their mom and wife back!

—Karen K., Elk Grove, California

to share some of the same amino acid sequences that are in our cellular proteins in order to hide from our immune cells. They mimic our definition of "self" to hide from our immune cells so as to set up a chronic low-grade infection.[1] When our immune cells finally recognize that an infection is happening and the immune system begins to attack those infections, however, it also begins to attack "self." This is one mechanism by which chronic infections may lead to an autoimmune disease in the genetically susceptible person.

Treatment of an autoimmune disease with functional medicine involves optimizing the body's environment to minimize immune hyperreactivity rather than restricting normal immune activity through pharmaceutical intervention, as a conventional approach recommends. The way we do this is to infuse the body with things it needs and remove things that cause harm. We focus on that 70 to 95 percent: A nutrient-dense diet of whole food relatively free of allergens and sugar, toxin elimination, appropriate physical activity, rebalancing of stress hormones, and the resolution of chronic infections are the first lines of defense against autoimmune disease. These environmental alterations help to restore tolerance in the body by slowly coaxing the body into a healthier and healthier state. The lack of a precise environmental cause for MS may be the reason why few conventional physicians use therapeutic lifestyle changes— that is, diet, exercise, and meditative practices—to treat their MS patients, but that doesn't stop the functional medicine physician from employing these treatments. A functional medicine doctor may still recommend pharmaceutical intervention but does not limit the approach to this. We believe we can do more, and the results, like those from my clinical trials, prove it's true.

Many of the patients I see in my clinical practice have been able to steadily reduce their prescription medications the longer they are on the Wahls Protocol. I see the same thing in our clinical trials. As you feed your cells what they need, your cells will rebuild you, molecule by molecule. Blood pressure improves, fatigue lessens, and the need for disease-modifying drugs often declines over the next three years. This is true whether the disease is a classical autoimmune problem like multiple sclerosis or a chronic disease like obesity or diabetes or post-traumatic stress disorder.

Note, however, that *we do not stop medications before cellular healing has eliminated the need for the medication.* Once blood pressure drops, blood sugars improve, mood brightens, energy is good, and fatigue is gone, then I begin a conversation about what drugs need to be continued and what could be gradually, carefully tapered and perhaps, if all goes well, eventually stopped.

It's important to understand, however, why, for some patients, medication remains important. If the patient is still not well while adapting to lifestyle changes, medication limits how much additional collateral damage will occur during these positive changes, and should therefore be continued. Combined with the intensive nutrition and lifestyle changes, continued use of medication will create a more favorable environment for the cells. Even if the medication results in a low level of side effects or toxic exposure in the body, as medications often do, the good that your current medication regimen does for the autoimmune process is more significant than the harm it may cause. Eventually, as the body is rebuilt, replacing incorrectly shaped molecules with

WAHLS WARRIORS SPEAK

In December 2011, at the age of 56, I received my third diagnosis of relapsing-remitting multiple sclerosis [RRMS] since experiencing my first "diagnosable" episode in August 2011. After months of testing and obtaining second and third opinions, I accepted my diagnosis from a neurologist at Mt. Sinai. I was shown on my MRIs that my lesions were significant, and some looked "old." I may have been living with RRMS for the past 30 years. In early January 2012, I began a treatment of Copaxone and started the Wahls Diet. Over time, I was able to decrease the daily injections to weekly, and stopped them altogether in June 2012. My neurologist told me that whatever I was doing to heal, it wasn't the Copaxone. Everyone who has seen me this past year concurs that I am doing something right and am on the road to recovery and beyond!

—*Debra K., Accord, New York*

correctly made and shaped molecules, the rate of worsening slows, then stops, and often better and better health and vitality ensue; but stopping medication too early will very likely disrupt this process. Each person is unique, and how quickly his or her health is stabilized and improves will be unique. It will depend on the burden of less effective enzymes (DNA), the burden of poor lifestyle factors (diet, exercise, toxins, hormone balance, etc.), the burden of prior and current infection(s), and how much work he or she does to optimize all lifestyle factors. Your personal physician or a functional medicine doctor is the one who can help you determine when and if medication should be reduced or tapered.

About Multiple Sclerosis

Now that you understand a little bit more about the differing perspectives on autoimmune disease in general, let's consider multiple sclerosis in particular.

MS was first described by French physician Jean-Martin Charcot back in 1868, and although we've known about this condition for more than a hundred years, there is still a lot we don't understand about how the disease gets started, how it progresses, and why. Although the majority of people with multiple sclerosis are diagnosed initially with relapsing-remitting multiple sclerosis, in which periods of disability come and go, within fifteen years of diagnosis, 80 percent will transition to the more severe form of the disease, secondary progressive multiple sclerosis, in which disability becomes permanent and inevitable in spite of therapy.

There are several theories about why someone develops multiple sclerosis, but MS is generally thought to be related to some genetic vulnerability that interacts with many unknown environmental factors. Numerous studies have shown that it is the interaction of multiple genes and the environment that determine whether someone will develop MS. There have been nearly a hundred genes identified that slightly increase the odds for getting MS. Yet no study has definitively identified precisely which problem is the cause of MS,[2] or why the problem develops in the first place.

When the disease is triggered, immune cells begin attacking and damaging myelin and other parts of the brain, leading to shrinking brain and problems with balance, vision, and/or muscle strength. Over the years, as symptoms accrue, doctors are finally able to diagnosis these symptoms as multiple sclerosis.

The highest rates of MS are found in Europe, Canada, the United States, and southern Australia. Epidemiologic evidence suggests that people who develop this disease probably acquired an infection before the age of 15 that, because of a genetic vulnerability, was not completely cleared from the body. If the person who suffered from the infection is also exposed to particular environmental factors (whatever they might be) and is genetically vulnerable (in some way not clearly understood), the immune system will commence destruction to the brain and spinal cord. In other words:

Genetic vulnerabilities + Environmental triggers = Onset of MS

That appears to be the formula, and the more genes you have that put you at risk, the smaller the dose of environmental triggers you will require to develop the symptoms that will be ultimately diagnosed as multiple sclerosis. The disease may not rear its ugly head or show on the surface for decades, but inside the body the process of silent damage has already begun its inexorable march.

As the immune cells attack the myelin, which wraps around the wiring connecting cells in the brain and in the spinal cord, the transmission of information down the long arms of the nerve cells slows. As the damage to the myelin progresses, the nerve cells can become so damaged that they can no longer transmit information at all. When that happens, the loss becomes permanent.

Types of MS

According to current diagnostic criteria, there are now four subtypes of MS, categorized by the way in which the disease presents and progresses.

Most people—80 percent—will be initially diagnosed with relapsing-remitting multiple sclerosis, or RRMS. This form of the disease involves acute episodes of worsening symptoms, called relapses, which are followed by gradual improvements as the brain and spinal cord add sodium channels to the nerve cells, allowing them to transmit information again, albeit more slowly than before. In addition to the relapses, which have obvious symptoms, the person with RRMS will often develop silent lesions (lesions that have no apparent symptoms), which can be seen on MRI scans of the brain.

The majority of people diagnosed with RRMS will convert to a different form, called secondary progressive MS (SPMS), within twenty years of initial diagnosis. When that happens, the person often stops having acute relapses and remissions. Instead, there is a gradual worsening of the MS-related symptoms and increasing disability. There is only decline. (This is what happened to me.) Approximately 10 to 15 percent of MS patients are initially diagnosed with another form called primary-progressive MS (PPMS). They never have acute worsening and remissions. They experience only a gradual decline from the beginning. Another 5 to 10 percent will have progressive-relapsing MS

(PRMS) and experience steady decline, with occasional superimposed attacks of worsening MS symptoms but without experiencing periods of improvement.

Conventional Treatment for MS

Because multiple sclerosis is an autoimmune disease, the mainstay of treatment is suppression of the immune cells with progressively more potent drugs—usually the "ABC-R" drugs, which are Avonex, Betaseron, and Copaxone, or the drug Rebif. These are meant to slow progression, but rarely does the MS sufferer return to a state of good health or vitality. This is the nature of most autoimmune diseases.

Even if we take as truth the notion that genetic vulnerability plus environmental triggers equals MS, scientists are still seeking to understand the exact nature of the genetic vulnerabilities and why they are not all the same in every person with MS. There are some theories that currently influence treatment.

One theory is that multiple sclerosis is actually a vascular disease. Dr. Paolo Zamboni has described chronic cerebrospinal venous insufficiency (CCSVI) in the setting of multiple sclerosis and as the cause of MS.[3] CCSVI is the narrowing of the veins that drain the brain. The consequence is that the backing up of pressure in the veins leads to an excess deposit of iron in the tissues, increasing inflammation and oxidative stress, thereby contributing to the development of MS symptoms.

Although the typical conventional treatment for MS often involves immune-suppressing drugs, Zamboni reports that doing angioplasty to open the blockages has been associated with an acute reduction of MS-related symptoms. He further reports success treating fatigue with angioplasty—that is, using a balloon or stent to open up the narrowed blood vessel in an outpatient procedure.[4] This is certainly interesting and, on the surface, sounds promising. A simple surgical procedure to correct MS? It almost sounds like a miracle. For some, dramatic improvement is immediately noticeable following angioplasty. Some subjects find that the reduction in symptoms is relatively short-lived, however, necessitating multiple angioplasties to reopen the blood vessels.[5] Furthermore, there has been controversy about whether CCSVI is present at an increased rate in those with MS over those without MS. Some scientists have found no significant increase in CCSVI[6] in MS patients.

This is just one of several conventional approaches that prescribe surgery or pharmaceuticals to relieve MS symptoms. They do not address the initial cause of the dysfunction, so they cannot ever actually cure it. If MS is related to CCSVI, what caused the veins to narrow in the first place? Once again, conventional medicine stops short at symptom relief—and when it comes to MS, symptom relief is notoriously ineffective.

Functional medicine, on the other hand, sees MS and its treatment in a different way.

The Functional Medicine Approach to Treating MS

Conventional medicine has divided MS into four types, but even within the four types, the way MS presents is widely variable because the damage can occur anywhere in the brain and spinal cord. If the damage occurs to the nerves that carry information from the sensory organs, then abnormal sensations will result. The person may have poor vision, poor balance, or problems with pain, like the face pain I experienced. If the damage occurs to the nerves that are going between the brain and the muscles, then problems with weakness and/or poor coordination will result, which often impedes mobility. Because the damage is often spotty, people can develop a uniquely abnormal pattern of walking, standing, or using their hands.

These are all characteristics of what we call multiple sclerosis, but here is the interesting part: When we look at the level of our cells, autoimmune conditions share six common characteristics, regardless of the specific diagnosis:

1. Mitochondria are strained, producing energy inefficiently and producing too much waste, as I explained in the last chapter. This leads to too many free radicals in the body, which damage the cells.
2. The immune cells are too reactive, leading to excessive inflammation throughout the body.

3. The immune cells specifically attack "self," or cell structures that belong to us.
4. Toxins such as lead, mercury, and pesticides stored in the body and chronic low-grade infections, such as Lyme disease or even periodontal (gum) infection, worsen autoimmune-related symptoms.
5. Low vitamin D and excessive stress hormone levels are present, both of which worsen inflammation.
6. Deficiencies or excesses of particular vitamins, minerals, essential fatty acids, and antioxidant phytonutrient molecules are common.

Functional medicine looks at MS less as a specific disease and more as a system-wide malfunction that shares a commonality with a broad range of chronic diseases. This turns treatment on its head, because defining the problem and therefore the "solution" is no longer about which drugs relieve specific symptoms and much more about correcting mitochondrial strain, immune cell irritability, toxin load in the body, stress hormone balance, and infections. Accomplish that, and you've helped a host of diseases and

WAHLS WARRIORS SPEAK

I felt immensely better within three weeks of beginning the Wahls Diet! My cognitive functioning and energy levels felt like they had returned to what they had been pre–MS diagnosis. I realized that I had not been aware of how foggy my brain had become until I was out of the fog. I no longer needed naps in the middle of the afternoon after moderate outings, exercise, or company. My balance is improving. Urinary frequency, urgency, and incontinence are fading. My double vision when overheated has changed to reduced color saturation in one eye. The nighttime muscle tension in my legs has significantly reduced. I have fewer issues with insomnia.

When I tell people how well I feel, they sometimes ask if I am in remission. I say no, I believe that I am actually healing. The most recent MRI showed no new lesions and my doctor allowed me to go off Betaseron.

—Sally B., Lansing, Michigan

unexplained chronic symptoms and yet-to-be-diagnosed problems, no matter what you call them. You will reduce the severity of symptoms for many kinds of autoimmune diseases, not just MS. You'll also reduce symptoms of many other chronic diseases, like mood disorders, obesity, high blood pressure, and heart disease. You do that by fixing the cells, which can then fix the body.

For example, let's look at Zamboni's theory, which I explained earlier. Even if cerebrospinal venous insufficiency is related to MS, the fact is that blood vessels develop clogging of the veins or arteries for a reason: It is part of their attempt to heal and repair the damage caused by environmental insults, narrowing the vein. Scientists have identified thirty-eight discrete steps that occur as blood vessels transition from healthy to being significantly clogged.[7] Some of the insults that can contribute to the development of clogging of the veins or arteries include:

1. Toxins such has heavy metals, pesticides, and solvents[8]
2. Chronic low-grade infections such as a chlamydia bacteria and Epstein-Barr virus[9]
3. Insufficient vitamins, minerals, antioxidants, and essential fats (micronutrients)[10]
4. Food allergies and sensitivities[11]
5. Hormonal imbalance[12]
6. Sleep disruption[13]

Knowing this, are we really saying that the only answer to a clogged or narrowed blood vessel is angioplasty or surgery of some type? These are all the same factors that lead to mitochondrial dysfunction, and that can be altered through environmental changes: diet, toxin removal, exercise, elimination of allergens—all the factors the Wahls Protocol addresses without drugs and without surgery.

Why treat clogged arteries with balloon angioplasty or bypass if lifestyle changes can have the same effect without the risks of surgery—especially if the procedures will often need to be repeated multiple times? Why treat fatigue with surgery when, in my clinical practice, I see a reduction in fatigue as *the very first thing people notice* after starting the Wahls Protocol? Patients often report significant reduction in fatigue within three months, and sometimes within days or weeks.

Every time the blood vessel is manipulated with the stent or balloon, microscopic damage occurs. Our immune cells will create inflammation as they repair the microscopic damage caused by the stent, and this inflammation has the potential to reclose the blood vessel. There is also the potential for acute unintentional damage to the blood vessel, such as a rupture, which can be fatal, not to mention the potential for a surgical error.

Functional medicine's prescription—and my preference as both a physician and a patient—is to use intensive lifestyle management to allow blood vessels to begin healing and reopen any blockages there may be throughout their vessels—whether or not this is a particular "cause" of multiple sclerosis. (I believe it is more likely just another symptom of immune cells attacking the body inappropriately—in this case, the blood vessels.)

Life is a series of self-correcting chemical reactions. Therefore, once you have optimized your cell chemistry, the body will often begin to heal itself in remarkable ways, even when scientists don't understand the exact nature of what was wrong in the first place. Yes, functional medicine seeks to find an underlying cause, but it is less focused on naming and categorizing because this can result in a narrowed view of what is really going on.

What This Means for You

As science advances and scientists consider chronic diseases at the cellular and biochemical levels, they are increasingly noting the commonality between chronic diseases, in particular the common threads across the entire autoimmune spectrum. No matter what disease you look at, at the cellular level you can see that mitochondrial strain leads to excess free radicals and damage to our cells, organs, and bodies, worsening the disease in question, and that our immune cells create too much inflammation that also damages our cells, organs, and bodies.[14]

When I was in medical school, I was taught to diagnose based upon the patient's story, physical examination, and laboratory findings. I learned to distinguish many diseases that scientists who study the cellular biology and biochemistry of our diseases now recognize as different manifestations of the same illness. For example, excessive inflammation is a factor in many if not all psychiatric disorders.[15] Excessive inflammation is also a factor in heart disease, high blood pressure, stroke, and cancer.[16] Inadequate vitamin, mineral, and antioxidant content in the blood increases the likelihood that an individual will have one of the top ten causes of death and disability.[17] Relatively low vitamin levels increase the probability of cancer, accelerated aging, and multiple chronic disease states by interfering with hundreds of steps in our biology.[18] High blood pressure, the clogging of arteries, and heart disease all exhibit strained mitochondria, too much inflammation, and immune cells that are attacking the blood vessels—and many are now theorizing that these conditions have an autoimmune component.[19]

Furthermore, the same problems of strained mitochondria, excessive inflammation, immune cells that are attacking other cellular structures, and toxin overload have been observed in obesity, metabolic syndrome, polycystic ovarian disease (an increasingly common cause of infertility in women), hirsutism (excess facial hair on women), erectile dysfunction, sleep apnea, and fatty liver disease.[20] One might even suspect that there are no individual diseases at all! I'll say it again: We all have the same chronic disease—broken biochemistry and confused signaling between our cells. This leads to having too much inflammation and strained mitochondria, largely as a result of our lifestyle choices.

What I see when I look at this picture is a very simple message: Your health and vitality are in your hands. You don't have to be a doctor or be able to diagnose yourself to start making changes in your own body at the cellular level. No matter what details we tease out of the picture as we try to diagnose and distinguish one disease from another, the truth is that dysfunction starts at the mitochondrial and cellular levels with broken biochemistry. If we arrest it there, the body can heal. If we do a better job of ensuring cells have the building blocks they need, slowly those cells will begin practicing the biology of life more correctly. Because our cells are a complex web of chemical reactions that are self-correcting, if we eat and live the way our DNA expects, our cells will slowly put our bodies back together again. If we don't—if we starve our cells for the building blocks they need—problems will occur. You are alive because your cells are self-correcting chemical factories. Your job is to facilitate that self-correction, not impede it.

As you institute the Wahls Protocol, more and more of your mitochondrial and cellular processes and chemical reactions will move toward a healthier range. As that happens, the symptoms of whatever disease your doctors have told you that you have will likely diminish. Your sense of health and vitality will slowly improve as your cells replace the broken, faulty, incorrectly built molecules with healthy, correctly built, functional molecules. After three or four years of eating and living the way your DNA expects, it is likely that you will look and feel younger, be stronger, and have more even moods. I predict you will be on fewer, if any, prescribed medications. You will begin to reclaim your body as well as your life.

You will begin to be well.

Chapter 3

GETTING FOCUSED

Y OU MIGHT BE ready to jump right into what you're supposed to eat and take and do to follow the Wahls Protocol. Change is exciting, and I know you want to start optimizing your cells, organs, and body as soon as possible. But before we get into the specific instructions for following the Wahls Protocol, it's very important to get something in order: your priorities.

This chapter's message is extremely important. Consider it a prerequisite of the Wahls Protocol. You might be thinking you can deal with the psychological and emotional aspects later. You want to get right down to business. I've found throughout the years of working with people, however, that unless they get their heads in the right place, they are much less likely to comply with the plan. To do this, I'd like you to think about a few things, including what's really important to you and whether the way you are living your life *today* truly reflects these priorities.

Think about your motivation. Maybe you want to set an example and be there for your children. Maybe a spouse or parent depends on you. Maybe you have something you still need to accomplish in this life. Whatever it is, large or small, it has to be important enough and meaningful enough to you to get you through those hard times and to strengthen your resolve so you can stay

> ## WAHLS WARRIORS SPEAK
>
> *My husband has MS. He was diagnosed four years ago, but as I look back, he has had vague symptoms for years. His mother also had MS. She died in a very debilitated state. She lived with us for the first four years of our marriage, and I never understood her anger and emotional stages until now. My husband felt a lot of shock, anger, and emotional volatility after his diagnosis. He was very weak from the drugs he was given and we were scared, knowing the decline that my mother-in-law experienced.*
>
> *I started searching for every possible avenue of healing. My husband was very resistant at first to diet change, and I was skeptical despite being a registered dietitian with a master's in nutrition because at the time I was really into low-fat/high-carbohydrate grains. However, the Wahls Diet has taken our entire family to another level of healing. No more stomach trouble, with great improvement in concentration and mood. Most of our autoimmune issues have either resolved themselves or are gradually lessening.*
>
> —Anne G., Deer Park, Illinois

strong on the Wahls Protocol. In this chapter, I want to help you define what that thing is for you and help you to get your head in a positive space for maximum success.

I know your circumstance has profound challenges that are not fair. There are no doubt many difficulties for you and your family beyond your having multiple sclerosis or some other autoimmune condition. This is an opportunity to nail down that higher purpose for your existence. A study on the impact of having a clear sense of higher purpose in life demonstrated that those with a clear higher purpose had fewer strokes, suffered fewer heart attacks, and survived longer than those without a strong sense of purpose.[1] Furthermore, having a higher sense of purpose improves a person's resiliency and personal and spiritual growth, despite declining health and increasing disability.[2] Isn't it time you figured out or articulated a higher purpose for your life? It will evolve over time, but what is it right now? I would like you to be able to articulate it.

WAHLS WARRIORS SPEAK

Having a long-term perspective on life and future goals is really important. I remember thinking that this world is so much bigger than me and what I'm experiencing now. There was an initial shock at diagnosis where I was pretty depressed and kind of numb, and I wondered why this was happening to me. Dealing with cancer was a battle on four fronts: mental, emotional, spiritual, and physical. The mental side of it means making plans for the future and for a long life, thinking about the things I want to do and why I want to live. The emotional battle is dealing with anger, fear, jealousy, resentment, bitterness, and a lack of forgiveness. Negative emotions cripple your immune system, so they definitely had to go.

—Chris W., Memphis, Tennessee

Begin Your Wahls Diary

The next thing I want you to consider—and this is something that will be a great help as you form your mission statement and work on your attitude and motivation—is to begin your own Wahls Diary. This is an important part of the process and I suggest that those in my clinic do it. It is required for those in my clinical trials. Throughout this program, you'll keep track of a lot of things, including what you eat, your stress levels, your supplements, your pain and energy levels, and how you are handling each day and the challenges of your life. This is too much to just keep track of mentally (and anybody with autoimmune-induced brain fog knows how difficult that would be!). Instead, I want you to keep a written record.

I also encourage you to take a picture of yourself and attach it to your journal. My patients and study subjects enjoy being able to look back and see how much they "youthen" as time goes by on the Wahls Protocol. Do it right now if you can. Just snap a picture of yourself. A few months—a few years—from now, that picture will be enlightening.

When you have a medical issue or a health problem, monitoring your symptoms, medication, diet, and exercise and tracking your progress is cru-

FROM MY WAHLS DIARY

Following my diagnosis in 2000, I realized my rules had changed. I had to redefine who I was and reinvent myself. I was still "Terry Wahls, doctor" and "Terry Wahls, mother," and "Terry Wahls, partner to Jackie," but the dynamics of all these relationships had changed, and I had to deal with that. The most dramatic of these was in the way I was able to parent.

I have always been a strong believer in the importance of teaching my children determination, resilience, and perseverance. I always planned to do this through athletic activities like camping, and challenges like mountain climbing. As I became more and more disabled, however, I began to realize that my plans were going to have to change. Many of the things I'd planned to do, I soon realized would never happen. We weren't going to go mountaineering. We weren't going to compete together in martial arts. They wouldn't be cheering me on to any athletic victories. No family Birkebeiner races. No Nepali treks. All those dreams I'd had seemed lost. How could I be a role model for them? How could I teach them something I couldn't even do myself? But then I realized that MS could be a tool I could use to teach my kids about resilience in a completely different way.

One morning, I saw my daughter, Zebby, who was only eight at the time, sitting and watching my every move. When I thought about it, I realized both my children, Zebby and Zach, often watched me to see how I would handle things. They were young and confused about their active, athletic mother losing her ability to do the most basic things. They wanted to know what I was going to do. They wanted to know how I would handle this new tribulation in my life. This was a wake-up call for me. I began to smile. I began to get out of bed with energy. I got into my Endless Pool, dialed up the current, and began doing the crawl stroke with the singular thought: *They are watching me.* I began to tell myself they were *always* watching me, because this changed my whole attitude and the whole way I went about doing things.

This was my motivation to keep pushing myself. I told myself that if I wanted them to learn to cope with difficult times, then I needed to show them how I was handling adversity. I realized that I could still be a role model with MS, and in some ways a more powerful role model with MS than without it. Climbing a mountain is tough, but getting up every day and going to work and staying engaged in life with multiple sclerosis is actually a hell of a lot tougher. This became my purpose and motivation to prevail over my condition rather than to lose myself to it. What can you do to give yourself purpose and motivation?

cial, not only for your own information, but for your health care team. Your Wahls Diary, however, will play an even bigger role in your life. In it, you'll also monitor how you feel, how you deal with stress, what you do, what your relationships are like—all of it. This will become a record of your life, a snapshot into you as you are right now, and—even more important—an invaluable log that tracks your steady improvement as you embark upon the Wahls Protocol.

I can't overemphasize the importance of keeping a Wahls Diary. I can't make you do it. Even if you've never kept a diary before or you don't like to write things down, this is a habit worth adopting. Your Wahls Diary will become an important, even essential part of your healing. Studies have demonstrated that people who journal have improved stress hormone levels, reduced disease activity, and higher life satisfaction scores. It's time to start writing!

What to Write

You don't have to start formally. Just tell some stories about yourself until you get used to writing. You can write about your feelings, the way you've overcome past challenges, and the positive aspects of those challenges. Make lists of what you are grateful for, whom you love, what you hope to do, even what you miss from your old life. All of this can help you find the gifts in your current circumstances, including the people and things for which you are grateful, and that can add to your resiliency.[3]

Much of the power of the Wahls Diary is in its psychological impact. You are getting things off your chest. But don't just concentrate on symptoms. This is your diary and your space to be yourself, but I would like you to use some of that space to tell the story of you. Not your entire life story. I'm not going to ask you to pen your memoir right now while you're dealing with everything else. Instead, start small. What challenges in your life come to mind first? Think about your past and what you've accomplished. Think about what you used to do that you can't do right now. Think about things you want to remember. Spend some time daydreaming about your past, and pick a story—any story. Then write it down.

Rather than trying to forget your former self, writing will help you embrace that self. Everything that has ever happened to you has become part of your story and has made you who you are today, and you have reacted to every single thing that has ever happened to you. Your Wahls Diary can lengthen and extend that space in a way that can help you to continue your personal growth, even as your chronic disease may make you feel like your growth has been stunted or arrested. Writing is your way out.

You don't have to be good at writing to do this. You don't even have to use correct grammar and spelling. If a pen is too difficult, use your computer. Using a laptop computer in bed is a fine way to keep a journal. The medium doesn't matter. What matters is that you begin to write. Don't edit your words. Just write. Let them tumble out just as they are. No critique. No editing. I'd like you to get in the habit of journaling every day, even if you only write just a few lines, a paragraph or two. Sometimes you'll want to write more, sometimes less. It's the regularity of the writing that becomes so healing. Record your progress, your feelings (good and bad), your triumphs and challenges, and all the steps you are taking to follow the Wahls Protocol.

Throughout this book, I'll have a Wahls Diary Alert whenever it will be helpful to answer a question or record something in the Wahls Diary. Use these as starting points, as inspiration, or as a way to remember what you know you'll want to remember later. These will look something like this:

WAHLS DIARY ALERT

Answer some or all of the following questions in your Wahls Diary:

1. How do you feel today? Be specific.
2. What did you do just for yourself today?
3. What did you eat today? How did it make you feel?
4. Did you exercise today? What did you do? How did it feel?
5. For whom or what are you grateful? What matters most in your life?
6. Do you have a higher purpose or driving force in your life? This will change, but think about what it is today. Describe what it is in the form of a mission statement: My mission in this life is . . .
7. How long have you been treated with conventional medicine? How is that working?
8. Do you remember the first time you ever had a symptom of your condition? Tell the story.
9. What symptoms are most troublesome to you today?
10. Do you blame yourself for things? Like what?
11. How would you describe your stress level today?
12. What could you do tomorrow to make it a better day than today?

You could start right now by choosing any of the above questions and writing your answer in your Wahls Diary. But don't limit yourself to these Wahls Diary Alerts. This is your diary. You can use it in any way you want. The point is to begin. Your diary will evolve, as will you. It will serve many purposes for you as you go through this book and begin creating health. Writing is the beginning of taking control, of finding purpose and meaning in your life as you know it now, and in guiding you to your future.

Tracking Your Symptoms

I'd also like you to use your Wahls Diary for more quantitative information. Every day, keep track of what you eat, how much you sleep, and what you do for exercise. (I'll give you a template at the end of this chapter.) Also, right at the beginning, I'd like you to do a symptom assessment.

Keeping track of your symptoms is extremely important as you embark upon the Wahls Protocol. You will still have some bad days on the Wahls Protocol, and when you do, you might feel like you haven't progressed at all. This checklist, called the Medical Symptoms Questionnaire (otherwise known as the MSQ), will remind you how far you've come. Put it in your Wahls Diary and answer the questions every few months to monitor your progress—your answers will change. Always include the date, so you can look back on your very first questionnaire and all the others you filled out, to see improvements you might not feel at the moment. This will give you strength and courage to keep going. You can point to an objective list and say to yourself, "I'm making progress!"

This medical symptoms questionnaire comes from the Institute for Functional Medicine, and I've reprinted it with their permission. This is what I use with my patients in my clinics and the people enrolled in my clinical trials, and I have them fill it out periodically to monitor their progress, just as I would like you to do. Remember, your first questionnaire will be your baseline. You might want to do it twice, first to keep track of how you've been feeling for the past thirty days, and then to track how you've been feeling for the past forty-eight hours. Check the appropriate box for each one:

MEDICAL SYMPTOMS QUESTIONNAIRE (MSQ)

Name _____ *Date* _____

Rate each of the following symptoms based upon your typical health profile for:

☐ *Past 30 days* ☐ *Past 48 hours*

Point Scale

0	*Never* or *almost never* have the symptom
1	*Occasionally* have it, effect is *not severe*
2	*Occasionally* have it, effect is *severe*
3	*Frequently* have it, effect is *not severe*
4	*Frequently* have it, effect is *severe*

Head

_____ Headaches

_____ Faintness

_____ Dizziness

_____ Insomnia

_____ *Total*

Eyes

_____ Watery or itchy eyes

_____ Swollen, reddened, or sticky eyelids

_____ Bags or dark circles under eyes

Blurred or tunnel vision (does not include near- or

_____ farsightedness)

_____ *Total*

Ears

_____ Itchy ears

_____ Earaches, ear infections

_____ Drainage from ear

_____ Ringing in ears, hearing loss

_____ *Total*

Nose

_____ Stuffy nose

_____ Sinus problems

_____ Hay fever

_____ Sneezing attacks

_____ Excessive mucus formation

_____ *Total*

Mouth/Throat

_____ Chronic coughing

_____ Gagging, frequent need to clear throat

_____ Sore throat, hoarseness, loss of voice

_____ Swollen or discolored tongue, gums, lips

_____ Canker sores

_____ *Total*

Skin

_____ Acne
_____ Hives, rashes, dry skin
_____ Hair loss
_____ Flushing, hot flashes
_____ Excessive sweating
_____ *Total*

Heart

_____ Irregular or skipped heartbeat
_____ Rapid or pounding heartbeat
_____ Chest pain
_____ *Total*

Lungs

_____ Chest congestion
_____ Asthma, bronchitis
_____ Shortness of breath
_____ Difficulty breathing
_____ *Total*

Digestive Tract

_____ Nausea, vomiting
_____ Diarrhea
_____ Constipation
_____ Bloated feeling
_____ Belching, passing gas
_____ Heartburn
_____ Intestinal/stomach pain
_____ *Total*

Joints/Muscles

_____ Pain or aches in joints

_____ Arthritis

_____ Stiffness or limitation of movement

_____ Pain or aches in muscles

_____ Feeling of weakness or tiredness

_____ *Total*

Weight

_____ Binge eating/drinking

_____ Craving certain foods

_____ Excessive weight

_____ Compulsive eating

_____ Water retention

_____ Underweight

_____ *Total*

Energy/Activity

_____ Fatigue, sluggishness

_____ Apathy, lethargy

_____ Hyperactivity

_____ Restlessness

_____ *Total*

Mind

_____ Poor memory

_____ Confusion, poor comprehension

_____ Poor concentration

_____ Poor physical coordination

_____ Difficulty in making decisions

_____ Stuttering or stammering

_____ Slurred speech

_____ Learning disabilities

_____ *Total*

Emotions

_____ Mood swings

_____ Anxiety, fear, nervousness

_____ Anger, irritability, aggressiveness

_____ Depression

_____ *Total*

Other

_____ Frequent illness

_____ Frequent or urgent urination

_____ Genital itch or discharge

_____ *Total*

_____ **Grand Total**

Note that less than 10 = optimal
More than 50 suggests the presence of significant inflammation and/or toxic load problems.
Reprinted with permission from the Toolbox, Institute for Functional Medicine

Total up your score and use this as an objective measure of how you are feeling. As the weeks progress, I expect this score to go down. On some days it may go up a bit, but it should be a relatively steady downward slope as you follow the Wahls Protocol, if you were to track your numbers on a graph. What you fill out today represents today. How will you feel next week? Next month? Next year? The MSQ will help you answer those questions and feel good about the answers.

But don't limit yourself to the MSQ when gauging your progress. Write about your progress, too: how you feel each day, as specifically or generally as you like. Or, if you prefer, make your own questionnaire tailored more specifically to your issues. Either way, later you will be able to look back and recall how you used to feel and compare it to how you feel as you advance.

Structuring Your Diary

Some of my patients buy a nice bound book to handwrite their Wahls Diary. Others use something simple: a spiral notebook or even a legal pad. Many

WAHLS DIARY ALERT

I use a number of tools in my clinics to help people assess their progress as they embark upon the Wahls Protocol. These are all publicly available, so you might want to do them all before you begin, record the results in your Wahls Diary, and then take them periodically to further gauge your progress:

- **Biologic age calculator.** There are several online. Here is one example: www.biological-age.com/index.html#. I just completed it and have a calculated age of 40 even though I'm actually 58!
- **Brain grade scale and cognitive training online.** Available from a company called Lumosity, the brain grade scale consists of a series of questions about what you eat and do, and how well your brain is working now. It took me less than two minutes to complete the test. My brain grade is A-. (When I took the test based on how I was in 2007, I had a C+.) The test also comes with a list of specific suggestions on what steps you can take to improve your brain, and there are brain training games on the Lumosity.com site. Training your brain will increase the brain growth hormones your brain needs to repair damage, build new connections, and grow more brain cells. Find it here: www.braingradetest.com.
- **Nintendo DS Brain Age games.** I also recommend these games in my clinics. You can use them to calculate your brain age and track your progress. When I first did the Brain Age game with my kids, my score said I was 85 years old. My kids howled with laughter, but I knew that my processing or thinking time was slow. Today my brain age is 40! Who's laughing now?

prefer to keep their diaries on their computers. They can then print out relevant parts to bring in to the clinic.

You may already have an idea of how your diary could look, but here is a suggestion. Each day I would like you to record any or all of the following details about your life. After that, you can add more, about whatever subject inspires you on that day, but having these details on record will be an immense help to you as you look back to see how far you've come. Your doctor may also appreciate this kind of specificity about your health.

Consider a format like this:

WAHLS DIARY DAILY TEMPLATE

Date: _____

Hours of sleep: _____

How did I feel when I woke up today? _____

Weight (at least once per week): _____

What I ate for breakfast: _____

Physical activity for the day (list all): _____

Supplements I took today, with times:

Time	Supplement

Medication I took today, with times:

Time	Medication

List all snacks:

What I ate for lunch: _____

What I ate for dinner: _____

For what or for whom am I grateful today? _____

What did I do today? _____

What helpful or happy social interactions did I have today?

_____

How would I rate my stress today on a scale of 1 to 10?   _____
(10 = lots of stress)

How would I rate my pain today on a scale of 1 to 10?   _____
(10 = lots of pain)

How would I rate my energy today on a scale of 1 to 10? _____
(10 = lots of energy)

How did I feel today, overall? _____

What else do I want to write about today? _____

List one good thing that happened today: _____

I hope you're now inspired to start tracking your life, your health, your mood, your habits, your food, your supplements, your medication, and how your day went. But don't stop there! Write about your challenges. Write about your passions. Write about the things that bother you, that upset you, that made you cry. Find your motivation and write about that, even if it changes over time. Remember why you want to live. Remember who needs you. Remember what you still need to do. And always end with one good thing. A positive note to send you off at the end of the day will reduce your stress and make you feel better. That, of course, is the end goal, and having a purpose will get you there.

Part Two

EATING FOR YOUR CELLULAR HEALTH

Chapter 4

THE WAHLS DIET 101

D IET IS WHERE it all begins. It is the one most influential element about your environment that you can control, and it is therefore your most powerful tool in healing your MS or other autoimmune or chronic disease. I didn't come to this realization right away; in fact, developing the Wahls Diet plan as it exists today has been a multistep process. Now it is refined to a great extent, and customizable, because you can choose which stage or level is right for you:

1. **Wahls Diet.** The most basic level kick-starts your system by infusing it with intense nutrition and removing dietary elements that could be contributing to your decline.
2. **Wahls Paleo.** The next level, and the level where many people choose to stay, provides more structure to further eliminate dietary elements that can compromise gut health.
3. **Wahls Paleo Plus.** This most challenging level is also the most therapeutic for those with autoimmune conditions and is particularly beneficial for anyone with neurological or psychological issues, whatever the underlying disease state, as well as for those with a history of cancer.

WHAT DOCTORS DON'T KNOW

Back in the 1980s, when I went to medical school, I received very little nutrition education, and unfortunately that hasn't changed much. Few medical schools provide a separate nutrition course to their students, and the majority of medical students receive less than twenty-five hours of nutrition instruction during their four years of medical school.[1] It's no wonder physicians don't teach their patients that the quality of diet is the main determinant of health.

While each dietary plan has very specific components, there are some underlying principles that are relevant to any and all dietary aspects of the Wahls Protocol. First and foremost, it is designed to maximize the vitamins, minerals, antioxidants, and essential fats that your brain and mitochondria need to thrive, based on what I've learned from functional medicine, my own review of the medical research, and an emulation of the diet that humans ate as hunter-gatherers. I believe it is important for you to understand why this is not only a healthful way of eating but much closer to the diet your DNA expects, so let's look at some of the background on which the Wahls Protocol dietary plans are based.

Paleolithic Nutrition

One of the basic principles behind the Wahls Diet is the Paleolithic or hunter-gatherer diet. Paleo-style diets seek to replicate the original human diet as closely as possible, considering the changes in the environment since Paleolithic times. Humans first began eating grain as a significant part of their diet approximately 10,000 years ago, and they began eating dairy and legumes approximately 8,000 years ago. This is a blip in human history. Compared to the 2.5 million years that the *Homo* genus (family) spent eating green leaves, fruits, roots, and meat, these are very recent additions. In our particular species, our direct *Homo sapiens* ancestors ate these foods for 500,000 years before the introduction of grains, dairy, and legumes.

The modern Paleolithic type of diet is a good, sound diet, in general. There are critics of this kind of diet, and also some misconceptions, but these are mostly by people who don't seem to know exactly what the modern version of a Paleolithic diet really is. Before I ask you to accept the concept, let's take a look at the arguments.

One argument is that there is no single Paleolithic diet. This is true. The original hunter-gatherers ate more than two hundred different plants and animals over a year's time. The foodstuffs our ancestors consumed were highly adapted to the specific regions they lived in, and each local society learned over hundreds of generations which plants and animals were associated with providing vitality for or bringing sickness to the clan.

Also, studies have shown that traditional diets are radically different between societies. For example, the arctic hunter-gatherers ate a pure animal product diet ten months out of the year. The Amazonian rain forest dwellers and the African hunter-gatherers ate more insects, amphibians, and lizards, and hundreds of different plants. The Native Americans ate a mix of fish, meat, and hundreds of different plants and animals unique to their environment over the course of the year. All these diets were extremely local and seasonal. Because many different cultures have existed as hunter-gatherers, there are likely thousands of diets created by humans that maximize their vitamin, mineral, essential fat, and antioxidant intake per calorie based on the food available in any given locale.

However, all these diets have some commonalities. They are all packed with many more vitamins, minerals, and essential fatty acids than the typical Westernized diets, which are filled with processed foods, like white flour, high-fructose corn syrup, and other refined sugars; contain minimal vegetables and fruits; and have far fewer vitamins and minerals in comparison.[2] Many critics of Paleo-style diets miss this point. Emulating more closely the foodstuffs of our Paleolithic ancestors is a great improvement over what most people are doing now.

Another argument against the Paleo Diet is that our world has changed and no food we currently eat resembles foods our Paleolithic ancestors ate. It's true that many of the foods we eat today have been altered through intensive plant breeding into foods that are much sweeter and richer in carbohydrates than they once were. Also, even natural, organic foods cannot escape containing some level of toxins because the world is now so polluted. Soil is also depleted, reducing nutrient content of the food grown in it. Then there is selective breeding and genetic modification aimed at producing a higher number of bushels per acre (not at improving vitamin or mineral content per bushel), and this has impacted our food, too. All of these factors result in plants that are less nutrient-dense than they once were. We can never go back to a planet as pure as it was in the Paleolithic era, but that doesn't mean we can't or shouldn't eat the best, cleanest, most nutrient-dense foods available to us. It only means we may need to eat even more vegetables and fruits to compensate for diminished nutrient levels.

Another criticism is that eliminating grains and dairy eliminates important sources of nutrition, and without them, deficiencies will result. This is simply untrue. You can get all the nutrients you need without eating grains, dairy, or legumes. A hunter-gatherer-style diet packed with natural plant foods and natural meats (from grass-fed animals, game meat, and/or wild-caught fish) contains all the nutrients you need.

Finally, a common criticism is that people didn't live very long in the Paleolithic era. This is true: Our ancient ancestors had a mean age of death in their 30s, but this is because there was a 38 to 45 percent mortality rate for those under the age of 15. Those who survived childhood actually did quite well. Gurven and Kaplan studied this question extensively and published their findings in 2007. The results might surprise you. Hunter-gatherers historically often lived past 60 years of age, and the same is true in the current hunter-gatherer societies that have not yet adopted Western lifestyles.[3] These people are physically and mentally fit without medication, and many are thriving into their 70s and even 80s. The transition from hunter-gatherer societies was associated with loss of height, increased risk for degenerative arthritis of the spine, and tuberculosis, although fertility increased, which led to an increase in population, albeit a less healthy one.[4]

Those populations that converted to Western diets continued to do worse as "progress" marched on. The next major transition came with the Industrial Revolution in 1850 with the wide availability of sugar, white flour, and a steady decline in breast-feeding. This was associated with another decline in health and an increase in chronic diseases, including heart disease, diabetes, and obesity.[5] Now, as societies move from developing economies to developed

---

WAHLS DIARY ALERT

Answer any of these questions in your Wahls Diary:

• Are you feeling ready to begin your new dietary regimen? Are you excited? Nervous? How do you feel?

• After you finish this chapter, write about which level of the diet you think will suit you best, at least for now.

• What are your expectations when you change your diet? What do you hope to feel, specifically?

Once you get started, remember to record how you react to the changes you make.

---

economies, the early mortality due to infectious disease is replaced by chronic diseases related to lifestyle—that is, diabetes, obesity, and heart disease.[6] These impact a population later, but the price is high. Consider obesity alone: According to the Centers for Disease Control, in 2010, 69 percent of Americans were overweight or obese.[7]

Put more simply, the extension in the average age of life from the Paleolithic era to the current era has occurred because of the decrease in infectious causes of death, lower childhood mortality, and increased use of medical technology—not because we as a society are enjoying more vitality and vigor.

All these criticisms overlook a simple fact: The modern Paleolithic diet concept is not meant to exactly replicate what our ancestors ate. Instead, it is meant to take the general concepts and apply them to our modern food supply as well as we can in an effort to restore human health and reverse the epidemic of chronic diseases that have plagued humans since the agricultural revolution.

Why Paleo-Type Diets Are Superior Diets for Humans

Any logical person knows that just because humans didn't do something in early history doesn't mean we shouldn't do it now. However, a hunter-gatherer type of diet isn't just good in theory. Research supports the positive effects of a hunter-gatherer-style diet. For example, when healthy volunteers adopted a hunter-gatherer diet rich in animal protein, nonstarchy vegetables, and berries, there was a significant improvement in multiple biological markers of health status with subjects experiencing improvements in blood pressure, blood cholesterol values, and improved sensitivity to insulin.[8] In another randomized crossover trial, subjects were given a standard diabetic diet or a hunter-gatherer diet for three months and then switched to the other diet. Again scientists found that the hunter-gatherer diet was associated with better blood sugar control, better blood pressure, better cholesterol values, and more weight loss than the standard diabetic diet.[9]

There are also many solid scientific reasons why a diet high in grains, dairy, starches, and sugars can be detrimental to human health, and why a diet that more closely reflects the principles of the Paleolithic diet is more conducive to good health. One of the most convincing is what starchy and sugary foods do to your microbiome (the bacterial population living in the human gut).

Most people have more than 100 trillion individual bacteria and yeasts living in their bowels that help digest both the food we eat and its collective by-products. Each of us really is our own ecosystem, and like any ecosystem we can be thrown out of balance. We rely on more than a thousand different bacterial and yeast species to help ensure that we have all of the necessary building blocks for the optimal function of our cells, but when the wrong ones take over, the biochemistry of the body can begin to malfunction.

When we eat grains, dairy, legumes, and sweeteners, all high in starches and/or sugars, our bodies are more likely to grow more sugar-loving bacteria and yeasts because we are eating the foods that feed these particular microorganisms. Consequently, we have fewer of the over a thousand different bacterial species that humans had living in their bowels for the first 2.5 million years that our ancestors existed—the ones suited to the original human diet that are part of the proper metabolism and chemistry that occur in our cells. If our collective health as a society eating the standard Westernized diet with this new ecosystem were still excellent, this might not be much of an argument. Society, however, has been progressively less well. Our new ecosystem is off. Sugar-loving bacteria, like *Pseudomonas*, and yeasts, like *Candida albicans*, cause all sorts of problems for human bodies.

One of the most dangerous conditions that the standard Westernized diet causes is called "leaky gut." Leaky gut syndrome is a condition in which holes or leaks develop in the lining between the small bowel and the blood vessels. If you have the wrong bacteria, yeasts, or parasites growing in your bowels, particularly the carbohydrate-loving yeasts like *Candida albicans*, they are more likely to create toxins that interfere with the system that regulates the cement that holds the cells lining the small bowel together (called intracellular cement).[10] Zonulin is a protein that regulates how that intracellular cement functions. When the zonulin is activated improperly, the cement that holds the cells tightly together begins to open little doors allowing the bowel contents to leak into the bloodstream, which is where the term *leaky gut* comes from. Other things can also cause or increase probability of developing a leaky gut, such as recurrent antibiotic exposure, eating a diet high in sugar and starch, development of sensitivities to specific proteins, such as gluten in grains and casein in dairy, and exposure to man-made chemicals and toxins, like tobacco smoke. Any of these things can further compromise the integrity of the gut lining.

The cement that seals the intestinal lining is the same stuff that lines all the blood vessels, so if it begins to break down, you can bet that the lining of the blood vessels—including the ones that lead to the brain—are likely breaking down as well. You could have leaky gut, leaky blood vessels, and a leaky brain! You can also develop leaky skin. With leaky blood vessels, the immune cells will be more likely to burrow into the walls, deposit cholesterol and inflammation molecules into the blood vessels, and clog and narrow veins and arteries. In the brain, the blood-brain barrier that provides an extra layer of protection for the brain against infecting bacteria will become less effective. The brain is more likely to allow overactivated immune cells in, increasing the probability of inappropriate inflammation and worsening problems with mood disorders and neurological disorders like multiple sclerosis. In the skin, you are more likely to develop all sorts of annoying rashes and skin problems that come and go. This is why leaky gut is not just about gastrointestinal issues—it's about your entire system and your health overall. This is not a situation you want happening in your body! Yet, it happens in many people, largely because of our processed, grain-based diets.

WAHLS WARRIOR SPEAKS

I was diagnosed with RRMS when I was 19 years old, but except for an episode of optic neuritis, I didn't see another symptom until I was 30. I'm 33 now, and things got really bad for me in February 2012. I discovered Dr. Wahls's work in July 2012 when my sister sent me a link to the video Minding Your Mitochondria. By the time I started the Wahls Diet in August 2012 and Copaxone in September 2012, I'd lost the ability to walk on my own after having been on multiple sports teams only three years before. In the time since starting the diet, I have noticed massive improvements in mental clarity and I have times when I can walk around without my cane, feeling like a normal person again. Those times make it so worth it. I can give up cheeseburgers if it means I can walk again! I felt so good a few weeks ago that I reintroduced bread into my diet. I won't be doing that again. I felt sluggish and the spasticity in my legs came back. To find that a doctor out there who also has MS basically experimented on herself to find an optimal diet—it was so very inspiring. Thank you, Dr. Wahls.

—Natalie S., Halifax, Nova Scotia, Canada

Is the Wahls Diet a Paleo Diet?

You may be wondering whether you even need the Wahls Diet at this point. Can't you just do one of the other Paleo-type diets? There are a lot of versions of the original human diet currently available in books right now: the Paleo Diet, the Primal Diet, the Caveman Power Diet, etc. They all have some similarities and some differences, but Dr. Cordain began the movement with his original book, *The Paleo Diet*, based upon medical anthropologic studies of people who lived more than 10,000 years ago and people who are still living as subsistence hunter-gatherers. The movement was largely popularized by Robb Wolf, co-author of *The Paleo Solution: The Original Human Diet*, as well as by Mark Sisson, the author of *The Primal Blueprint: Reprogram Your Genes for Effortless Weight Loss, Vibrant Health, and Boundless Energy*.

I am a big fan of the Paleolithic-style diet, but I also want you to understand that the Wahls Diet is not "just another Paleo diet." It provides more structure and guidance to help you maximize your nutrition, which is critical for those with any chronic disease. You need a more aggressive plan to restore your health. This was an important crux of my research as I developed the Wahls Diet. Although I was on the Paleo Diet for a long time (as originally detailed by Dr. Loren Cordain), it was not enough to heal me. Many people do well on this diet—or well enough—especially if they are already healthy. For someone with health challenges, however, you will benefit from more structure than the usual Paleo or primal or hunter-gatherer diets provide because you need to do more than just stop eating foods that may harm you. You also need to know how to maximize your nutrition for your cells and mitochondria.

Dr. Jayson Calton and Mira Calton did a micronutrient analysis of several current diets, including Diane Sanfilippo's Paleo diet as described in her book *Practical Paleo*.[11] and Mark Sisson's Primal Diet for their book *Naked Calories: The Caltons' Simple 3-Step Plan for Micronutrient Sufficiency* (revised edition), and discovered that those diets were much more nutrient-dense than the standard American diet and in fact were among the most nutrient-dense diets that they analyzed. Great news! Both the Paleo and Primal Diets, however, were still only meeting the recommended daily allowance (this is also known as the RDA) for fifteen of twenty-seven micronutrients and would have required more than 14,000 calories to meet all the RDAs. (The standard American diet would have required more than 27,000 calories!)[12] These Paleo-style diets are obviously far superior to the standard American diet, but without specific guidance to maximize the micronutrient content, anyone following these diets is still at risk for missing key brain and mitochondrial vitamins, minerals, essential fatty acids, and antioxidants. If you have an autoimmune or neurodegenerative disease (or any other major chronic disease for that matter), this is a risk you simply can't afford.

What each level of the Wahls Diet plans seeks to replicate, in an attempt to avoid or repair these detrimental processes, is to fill your plate in a very structured way with foods that will ensure you get the maximum nutrition possible using agriculturally available products. Few of us are able to actually hunt and gather our food from the wild, nor do we have the exact knowledge our ancestors had about how to get the most nutrition from the foods growing in our locale. However, if you eat a diet heavy in leafy greens, nonstarchy vegetables, and fruits like berries—as well as animal protein (without including any of those more recent troublesome dietary additions, like gluten grains, dairy products, and, at more advanced levels, legumes, all grains, and sweeter fruits)—you have the best possible chance at optimizing your health.

The main differences between the Wahls Diet plans and other Paleo-type plans are:

- **Nutrient density.** All levels of the Wahls Diet plans are rigorously and meticulously nutrient-dense. You will get a specific structure to follow to ensure maximum but not toxic vitamin, mineral, and antioxidant levels. I don't leave anything to chance, assuming you will eat enough fruits and vegetables or enough protein and/or healthy fat. You need a very specific nutrient load. Your body has been missing it. It is medicine for you.
- **A high level of fat.** The Paleo Diet recommends lean meats, but the Wahls Paleo Diet, and especially the Wahls Paleo Plus Diet, ramps up healthy fat intake in a brain-beneficial way (in the form of specific kinds of fats, like those in oily wild fish, coconut oil, and avocados). The brain is 60 to 70 percent fat. We need healthy fats to make the myelin insulation for the wiring in your brain so you won't be skimping on the healthy fats.
- **Emphasis on local.** I recommend expanding your palate and the food on your plate to include as many native/local/seasonal foods as possible. To me, this is the essence of eating Paleo—getting as close to how your Paleolithic forebears ate, living right where you live now. Locally grown foods tend to be more nutritious because you are likely to consume them shortly after harvest. The longer food is stored, the more vitamin and antioxidant levels break down. Food out of season, shipped from across the globe, has far fewer nutrients. Also, native, wild foods grow in the soil and under the conditions most natural for them, so they are likely to be healthier plants. Healthier wild soils lead to healthier plants that are more nutritious. They have built-in protections against native insects and have a much higher level of protective antioxidants and vitamins. I encourage my veteran patients to hunt, learn to forage for wild foods, and add gardens and edible plants to their yards. The food obtained and the time spent being out in nature are both quite healing.

WAHLS WARRIOR Q & A

Q: Why can't I eat eggs on the Wahls Diet? They are encouraged on the Paleo Diet, and as long as they are organic and from free-ranging chickens, they seem like they would be a healthy addition.

A: The simple answer is that the Wahls Protocol does not include eggs because I have a severe egg allergy, and for our clinical trial I was specifically required to exactly replicate what I did to effect my own recovery. One of the things I did was to remove all allergenic foods from my diet, and this included eggs.

You may not be allergic to eggs, but many people are and don't realize it. The best way to know whether you can tolerate eggs is to remove them completely from your diet for a month, then have a test meal. For example, have three or four eggs a day for two days, then see how you do. If you have an increase in any symptoms, you may be surprised to learn that you do react to the protein in eggs, and you are better off leaving them out of your diet. If you have no increase in any negative symptoms over the next two weeks, then eggs may not be a problem for you, but I would strongly recommend choosing eggs from pastured chickens that eat grass and insects and forage for their own food outdoors, because these eggs will contain many good fats, vitamins, and protein.

- **No gluten, no dairy, no eggs, few if any legumes.** Some Paleo-style diet plans allow dairy (preferably raw organic), encourage egg consumption, and even permit some legumes. (Note that legumes and gluten-free grains are necessary if you are eating Paleo-style and are a vegetarian.) I do not recommend these food items on the Wahls Diet. Gluten is completely out, but so are dairy and eggs. While legumes do contain some antinutrients, I'll show you how to reduce those antinutrients in the Wahls Paleo chapter if you need to eat legumes.

Now let's take a quick look at what differentiates each level of the diet.

Level One: The Wahls Diet

This is the most basic diet required in the Wahls Protocol. It involves just three primary elements:

1. *Nine cups of fruits and vegetables every day, broken down as follows:*

- Three cups tightly packed raw or cooked leafy greens, like kale, collards, chard, Asian greens, and lettuces (the darker, the better)
- Three cups deeply colored vegetables and fruits, such as berries, tomatoes, beets, carrots, and winter squash
- Three cups sulfur-rich vegetables, including broccoli, cabbage, asparagus, Brussels sprouts, turnips, radishes, onions, and garlic.

I recognize that 9 cups sounds like a lot, and there are two reasons for this. One, in order to get enough concentrated nutrition, you need to eat a lot of vegetables. Two, sufficient vegetable and fruit intake will fill you up so that you won't feel as much of a need to eat grains, sugar, and dairy. I want you to fill up mostly on vegetables, and this means learning to eat a lot of them. I also understand that for some people—especially those who don't often eat a lot of fruits and vegetables or who suffer from a delicate digestive system—such a leap in fiber consumption can be uncomfortable. In the next chapter, I'll give you more specific information about how to transition to eating 9 cups comfortably. You don't have to do it all at once.

2. *Gluten-Free/Dairy-Free*

The 9 cups puts nutrients into your body that you were missing, but this next step is about taking out what may be causing reactivity in your body, and that requires removing gluten and dairy from your diet. Unlike the first step, where it's okay to ease in, I recommend you go cold turkey on this one. Stop eating gluten and dairy *today*. It could be the most important thing you ever do for yourself.

People with autoimmune disease are more likely to have a leaky gut, and if you have a leaky gut, gluten and dairy are particularly damaging. When the intestine has holes in it, incompletely digested wheat (gluten) and/or milk (casein) proteins can get into the bloodstream. These undigested particles are too large to be in the bloodstream. If you are genetically vulnerable to having your immune cells be activated by gluten and/or casein, this will cause even more issues. Twenty to 30 percent of those with European ancestry have the DQ2 or DQ8 genes, which put them at risk for developing gluten sensitivity.[13] In these people, gluten and casein proteins in the bloodstream can trigger an inappropriate immune response. This can lead to a hyperreactive immune system that can then become supersensitive to other foods that weren't bothersome before, such as tree nuts, citrus, strawberries, or other vegetables and fruits.

How your body will react to a leaky gut is individual. You may not have the genetic predisposition to get into trouble or your responses may still be relatively mild. Others may have more dramatic reactions, including severe allergy or gastrointestinal symptoms that can eventually lead to more severe problems. If you have MS or another autoimmune disease, however, the likelihood that you will respond drastically to leaky gut is high.

I ask you to give up these two things with the full awareness that this is extremely difficult. The reason why gluten and dairy foods are considered

WAHLS WARRIOR Q & A

Q: Is it okay to just reduce gluten and dairy, or to give up dairy but not gluten, or to give up gluten but not dairy? Or does it have to be complete?

A: It is very hard to give up the foods you love, especially comfort foods like gluten and dairy, but you need to do it 100 percent because even a tiny amount of gluten or dairy could rev up the inappropriate immune response in your body if you have an unrecognized gluten or casein sensitivity. Do not assume you don't have a sensitivity. Even if you don't notice any particular symptoms after eating gluten or dairy, your body may still be suffering from the effects of an intolerance, limping along under the daily assault of gluten and casein. Because of an amino acid sequence that is similar in both gluten and casein, most people who are sensitive to gluten are also sensitive to dairy, so I recommend giving them both up. You don't need gluten- and casein-containing foods in your diet in order to be healthy, and you have no idea how good you could be feeling without these foods.

For at least one month, take them out completely. You can tell yourself that if you turn out not to have a sensitivity, you can add them back in. Then have a test meal, testing one thing at a time. Try a test meal eating some dairy products, preferably fermented milk products like yogurt or goat's milk—these are the most likely to be tolerated. About 80 percent of people with gluten sensitivity will cross-react with dairy, but you might be in that 20 percent. If you have any negative response, cut out dairy for good. If you don't, you may be able to work it back into your diet. If, however, you can only do one thing right now, cut out gluten first. Because gluten products are the most likely to be associated with adverse reactions and so many people experience improvement when they eliminate gluten completely from their diets, I strongly urge going off gluten immediately and staying off it forever.

"comfort foods" (think macaroni and cheese, cupcakes, and cheeseburgers) is because they actually have an opiate-like addictive effect in the body. (I'll talk more about this in chapters 6 and 8.) Giving them up can actually feel a bit like withdrawal. Once you get over the initial shock of removing gluten and dairy, however, you will start to feel better rapidly.

3. Organic, Grass-Fed, Wild-Caught

High-quality protein is the third crucial element on the Wahls Diet. While you can be a vegetarian or even a vegan at this first level—and I'll explain how in the next chapter—I don't recommend it. The next chapter also includes my detailed explanation of this controversial position. The highest-quality protein sources for humans are organic, grass-fed meat, wild-caught meat (like game meat), and fish, and I strongly recommend that you eat them. Choose organic whenever you can, but don't go without high-quality protein.

Level Two: Wahls Paleo

Wahls Paleo is similar to the Wahls Diet, but now we're going to up the ante. If you are in the throes of severe autoimmune disease or have other types of neurological or psychological problems or other chronic medical problems, I recommend starting here, or moving here as soon as you have adjusted to the Wahls Diet.

Wahls Paleo includes everything the Wahls Diet includes, with these added components:

1. Reduce all non-gluten grains (presumably you are completely gluten-free by now), legumes, and potatoes to just two servings per week.

It's preferable to eliminate grains and legumes entirely, but allowing two servings a week gives you more flexibility to be social with friends and family. That is what we have done in the second wave of our study. These servings are *not required* but they are allowed, should you feel the need. Even gluten-free whole grains, legumes like black beans and lentils, and potatoes contribute to increased carbohydrate load. You also get more lectins and phytates, which are antinutrients, in these foods. I encourage you to have more nonstarchy

WAHLS WARRIOR Q & A

Q: The Wahls Protocol sounds great, but I'm not sure what my family will think of the food. Is it okay for them to go on the diet with me? What if they don't want to do this? Will I have to prepare separate meals for myself and the rest of the family?

A: It is extremely important to have family support when you embark upon the Wahls Protocol. I know from my observations that this must be a family decision. We tell our study subjects that we expect the family to eat only study-compliant food in the presence of the subject and to purge the house of foods that don't fit with the diet. Subjects whose families buy in and eat the same way as the study subjects are nearly always successful. Those whose families are not supportive and still eat the standard American diet are nearly always doomed to fail. For this reason, it's important to have a family conversation about food. What is everyone willing to do? What can everyone live with? This might take some negotiation, but fixing two different meals is not usually sustainable. We've had families go gluten-free while the study subject is on Wahls Paleo, but they may get gluten-containing foods when away from the study subject. That can work, but being surrounded by people eating the standard American diet while you are doing the Wahls, Wahls Paleo, or Wahls Paleo Plus Diets almost certainly will not. Fortunately, the Wahls Diet is not only a healthy diet for any healthy adult, but it might even be preventive, staving off a future of chronic disease. It is also an excellent diet for children, who tend (in our culture) to eat far too many processed carbohydrate and sugar-laden foods. Knowing that better health, more energy, and the loss of excess weight will likely accompany this dietary switch could help convince other family members to jump on board with you.

vegetables than gluten-free grains and to eat more vegetables than fruit. In addition, you can eat more meat as you further reduce the carbohydrates.

2. Add seaweed or algae and organ meats to your diet.

A lot of people balk at the notion of eating seaweed and organ meats. My patients who are suspicious of vegetables in the first place have a particularly hard time with seaweed and algae, and former vegetarians often have a really hard time with the concept of eating organ meats. Adding these two foods to your diet, however, is a potent healing step. Seaweed adds critical minerals, and organ meats add coenzyme Q, both of which supply valuable nutrients for your mitochondria that can be difficult to get from more common foods. In chapter 6, I'll show you some palatable ways to try these foods.

3. Add fermented foods, soaked seeds and nuts, and more raw foods.

Enzyme-rich foods are an essential part of traditional diets, but much of our modern food is bereft of enzymes because of processing and cooking.[14] The best sources for enzymes are:

* Raw fruits and vegetables
* Fermented foods like lacto-fermented sauerkraut, pickles, kimchi, and kombucha tea

WAHLS WORDS

A ketogenic diet is extremely low in carbohydrate content (as low as 25 grams or even lower) and higher in fat to facilitate having the body burn fats instead of glucose. Functional medicine health care practitioners are using ketogenic diets to treat other progressive neurological conditions like Parkinson's disease and early memory loss.

- Soaked and sprouted nuts and seeds (Soak nuts and seeds in water for six to twenty-four hours before consuming; I'll tell you more about how to do this in chapter 9.)
- Raw animal protein such as sushi, steak tartare, and ceviche.

Level Three: Wahls Paleo Plus

This is the most extreme and most intense level. This is the diet I follow because I find that I do best on it, and I recommend it for my patients who aren't seeing enough progress at the Wahls Paleo level. This is an extremely low-carb, high-fat diet, similar to ketogenic diets already being used in a medical setting to treat epilepsy. It adds the following elements to the rules of the Wahls Diet and Wahls Paleo:

1. **Eliminate *all* grains, legumes, and potatoes.** That includes nongluten grains like rice and quinoa. This may seem difficult, but once you get in the habit of not even considering grains on the menu, it won't seem so hard.
2. **Consume at least 6 cups of vegetables, divided evenly between greens, color, and sulfur vegetables.** You won't be as hungry on Wahls Paleo Plus, so you won't be able to eat as much, so you are cutting back on your vegetable consumption somewhat but still eating enough to get dense nutrients. You still need those crucial micronutrients!
3. **Reduce cooked starchy vegetables and fruit.** Limit cooked starchy vegetables to two servings a week—no more (you may have less). If you have a

cooked starchy vegetable like winter squash or beets, you will need to add a generous amount of fat such as coconut oil. If you have your starchy vegetable raw, such as a raw beet salad, you can count it in your servings of colors for the day. Also, limit fruit to one serving per day, preferably berries. This is the time to take those white-fleshed fruits like apples, bananas, and pears off your list, as well as other sweeter fruits like grapes, peaches, pineapples, and mangoes, in favor of the deeply colored fruits only: blueberries, blackberries, raspberries, cherries, etc.

4. **Add coconut oil and full-fat coconut milk.** Wahls Paleo Plus is a high-fat diet, which, contrary to what you may have read about good health, is not harmful to your heart. In fact, a high-fat diet coupled with a relatively lower carbohydrate intake will actually provide the most intensive nutritional support for your brain and your heart. This diet is even closer to how our ancestors ran their metabolisms for 2.5 million years. The fat in the diet is converted to ketones, which are excellent sources of energy for our mitochondria, brain cells, and muscle cells. This is why our species could survive and even thrive during the winters, which are typically a time of very limited carbohydrate intake, and during famine and war.

5. **Eat just twice per day and fast twelve to sixteen hours every night.** You will not be as hungry on Wahls Paleo Plus, because eating protein and fat with relatively fewer carbohydrates will tend to suppress your appetite. During the long periods between breakfast and dinner, and between dinner and breakfast, your body can focus on processing and eliminating toxins, making hormones, and healing. If you find it uncomfortable to eat just twice a day, go ahead and keep having three meals when you really need them, but always be sure to wait twelve to sixteen hours between dinner and breakfast. This significantly increases the vigor and the number of mitochondria in your cells. Your brain will love it!

Your Transition

If you are in my clinical trial, the rules are strict: You have to implement the study diets from day one. There is no easing into it. We do a two-week test to see whether participants can adopt the diet successfully. Those who are successful continue in the study for the next three years. It is a huge change

WAHLS WARRIORS SPEAK

I do not have MS, but my son does, so I follow the Wahls Protocol, too. In the beginning, I did so as a show of support for my son. I soon found, however, that my overall health was in much better shape. My body tells me very quickly if I stray back to my old eating habits. Now, at age 68, I am 116 pounds and I have a nice flat tummy, energy to burn, and blood tests and blood pressure readings that are all normal. I've never looked or felt better! This diet is good for everyone to follow as a way of life. Stop eating processed crap! You do not want to outlive your health!

—Liz B., Halifax, Nova Scotia, Canada

in eating habits for most people, but they are highly motivated and are usually quite successful.

In my clinical practice, I am not so rigid. My practice style is to educate patients about the connection between diet and health and the three diets I advocate (the Wahls Diet, Wahls Paleo, and Wahls Paleo Plus), give them options, and then ask them what they have learned and what their goals are. I do find that some of my patients are able to make the drastic change all at once because they are highly motivated and their families are fully supportive. Most of us, myself included, come to the diet gradually, step by step. Some choose to simply ramp up the vegetables, some choose to also go gluten- and dairy-free, and others choose to go all the way to Wahls Paleo Plus to get control of their bodies and the disease process as quickly as possible. Don't be too hard on yourself and your family if it takes a few months to fully implement the Wahls Diet, Wahls Paleo, or Wahls Paleo Plus. But do begin. Then, if you still aren't achieving the health outcomes that you are looking for, advance to the next level.

Anyone can benefit from the Wahls Diet, Wahls Paleo, or Wahls Paleo Plus, but if you have MS or another autoimmune disease, the benefits will likely be dramatic. You will lose excess weight and gain energy and vitality. Take on the steps one at a time, but if you have an autoimmune disease or any type of brain disease or chronic medical problem, the most important thing you can do is to adopt at least the Wahls Diet immediately: Eat the 9 cups (or proportionately what you can) and go gluten- and dairy-free *today*. Progress from there according to the steps laid out in the next five chapters. Your journey has officially begun.

Chapter 5

MASTERING
THE WAHLS DIET

I F YOU ARE ready to change your life, improve your health, feed your cells, strengthen your mitochondria, and begin the process of reversing chronic disease in your body, begin here. The Wahls Diet is a beginning. Once you've mastered it, you may decide to move on to the next level, Wahls Paleo, or the final level, Wahls Paleo Plus, but first you need to understand how to fully implement the components of this most basic dietary adjustment.

The Wahls Diet involves two primary components, and a third optional but strongly recommended component:

1. What you will add to your diet
2. What you will take away from your diet
3. The quality of the food you eat

You will be amazed at the difference in how you feel by doing these three simple things. If you have an autoimmune disease, I recommend you begin the Wahls Diet *today*.

Before we get into the specifics of the Wahls Diet, let me explain a bit

WAHLS DIET

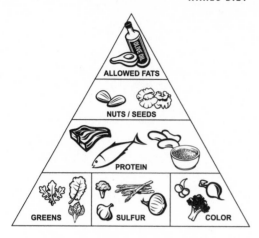

about the charts that you will see at the beginning of each diet program chapter. I show you how the three levels of the Wahls Diet stack up against the standard American diet in terms of nutrient density (based on a 1,759-calorie diet, which is the average caloric intake for my personal age and gender). The recommended daily allowance (RDA) is the amount of a specific nutrient that should meet the needs of 97 percent of the population. These values are set for every major nutrient by the Food and Nutrition Board of the National Academy of Sciences and reviewed every few years. We compared the mean intake of the nutrients identified by medical literature as being key to optimal brain health to the reported average recorded intake of a woman my age.

Dieticians and nutrition experts are reluctant to cut out major food groups like gluten-containing grains, dairy, and eggs because they supply many vitamins and minerals. For example, the average woman gets most of her B vitamins through the consumption of flours that have had synthetic B vitamins such as folate, riboflavin, thiamine, niacin, and iron added to them. Food, not synthetic supplements, should provide all the essential nutrients for optimal health.

However, you will see that the Wahls Diet gives the person 1.5 to 8 more times the supply of vitamins and minerals than the standard American diet

Wahls Diet		
Nutrient*†	U.S. Diet	Wahls Diet
Vitamin D	31%	75%
Vitamin E	55%	143%
Calcium	74%	126%
Magnesium	88%	174%
Vitamin A	100%	340%
Pyridoxine	121%	626%
Folate	122%	207%
Zinc	123%	178%
Thiamin	128%	741%
Vitamin C	133%	514%
Niacin	154%	452%
Iron	164%	235%
Riboflavin	175%	827%
Vitamin B_{12}	201%	704%

* Compared to dietary reference intakes. Recommended dietary allowances (RDA) for females 51–70 years; Wahls Diet adjusted for 1,759 calories. (National Academy of Science; Institute of Medicine; Food and Nutrition Board)

† Average nutrient intake from food for females 50–59 years. (What We Eat in America, NHANES 2009–2010, www.ars.usda.gov/SP2UserFiles/Place/12355000/pdf/0910/Table_1_NIN_GEN_09.pdf, accessed May 25, 2013.)

does, even without enriched flour. The Wahls Diet is packed with what your cells need to thrive, without relying on synthetic added vitamins.

Part One: The 9 Cups

The cornerstone of the Wahls Diet is the addition of 9 cups of vegetables and colorful fruits every day. Nine cups! It sounds like a lot, and for some people it's a daunting amount. If you are up for it, I would suggest adding in the 9 cups right away. It's the first thing you can do to start infusing your body with intense nutrition, and it will make a difference in how you feel. Although people in my study have to start in one fell swoop, people in my clinics more often work into this over a seven-day period.

Take whichever approach you and your family are willing to do. Start with

---

WAHLS DIARY ALERT

As you begin the Wahls Diet, it is important for you to begin writing down what you are eating and how you are feeling. You will begin the journey of learning what your body is telling you about your environment by tracking this information every day. The food you eat, the water you drink, the air you breathe, and what you are putting on your skin can all affect how you feel and how healthy your cells are. You will begin to notice how you respond to that environment. If you have symptoms, you will be able to look at your Wahls Diary to see what you have eaten that you might be reacting to. You will also begin to take responsibility for learning how to eat and live for maximal health and vitality. (Remember that the majority of people who are sensitive to a food will have some problem within seventy-two hours, although in a few cases it can take as long as two weeks for symptoms to show. Always look back at the last three days when you have a problem to see what the potential triggers may have been.)

---

3 cups, then gradually but persistently work your way up. This will set you on the right track and keep you from quitting the diet because you think you can't do it. Small steps are better than quitting because small steps will lead to better health, and quitting will do nothing to help you.

I don't want you to eat 9 cups of apples and iceberg lettuce, however. The 9 cups are organized in a specific way, for maximum nutrition per calorie (which the registered dieticians and nutritionists call nutrient density). You must divide them equally into three parts:

1. Three cups of leafy greens
2. Three cups of deeply colored vegetables and fruits
3. Three cups of sulfur-rich vegetables

The 9 cups are incredibly important for success on the Wahls Diet. Remember, we are trying to do two things overall to improve the health of your

WAHLS WARRIOR Q & A

Q: I'm not crazy about vegetables. Can't I just take supplements to get all those vitamins and minerals?

A: People often ask me if they can just take supplements instead of eating all these vegetables. The answer, in a word, is no! By eating 9 cups of vegetables and fruits every day, you will be effectively dosing yourself with vitamins, minerals, and phytochemicals (plant-based micronutrients) that your body has likely been missing in the most natural way your body can receive these compounds. The vitamins and antioxidants that naturally occur in food are more effective at supporting your cells when the whole family of related compounds is present. Vegetables and colorful fruits each have hundreds of related compounds in them, acting synergistically in our body to support the functions of our cells, and the vitamins and antioxidants are a far more effective support for your cells when they are taken with the hundreds of other antioxidant and phytonutrients in the whole plant. Also, the vitamins, amino acids, and antioxidant supplements you take in pill form are typically synthetic. The synthetic forms of vitamins and other compounds do not have the same shape as the naturally occurring compounds, and they are not accompanied by all of the related compounds that would exist in whole food, which contribute to the body's effective use of these compounds. As a result, synthetic vitamins do not have the same properties and are not as effective at supporting our cells' biology as the naturally occurring compounds present in food. For much more information about supplements, see chapter 10.

cells: add what they need, and take away what interferes with their function. The 9 cups accomplish that first goal. This is the primary way to provide your cells with everything they need to work at maximum efficiency, for the benefit of your health.

Let's look more closely at how to divide up the 9 cups, and what you are getting when you let yourself indulge in this cornucopia of produce.

ANCIENT NUTRITION

Our ancestors have been consuming phytonutrient-rich plants for 2.5 million years. Although science is only beginning to discover what various phytonutrients can do for us, there are thousands of articles that support the health benefits of phytonutrients for everything from antibiotic and antioxidant properties to properties that do things like keep the blood vessels more elastic, facilitate toxin removal in the body, regulate various aspects of immune system function, and improve brain function.

1. Three Cups of Leafy Greens

Leafy greens are nutritionally dense phytochemical factories. They are an excellent source of vitamins in the B group, especially folate (also called vitamin B_9), and also vitamins A, C, and K. Think Green-BACK for vitamins B, A, C, and K. These four nutrient groups (vitamins B, A, C, and K) are incredibly important for anyone suffering from MS in particular:

- **B vitamins.** Your body needs many of the B vitamins for healthy nervous system functioning. For example, you need folate (vitamin B_9) to make myelin, the fatty insulation around your nerves that is attacked and degraded when you have multiple sclerosis. Anything to shore up your myelin production is a good thing!
- **A vitamin precursors.** Greens are also rich in alpha- and beta-carotene, precursors for vitamin A, which you need for (among other things) healthy retinas, the backs of the eyes, which are stimulated by light. Many people with MS suffer from macular degeneration and other diseases involving the retina. Having more greens in the diet will improve the health of the retina and the optic nerves, lowering the risk of visual impairment. Vitamin A is also important for immune cell function. Don't be confused about autoimmunity: Your immune system may be overactive, but vitamin A won't increase harmful immune activity. Instead, it will help your body to recalibrate its immunity back to a normal, healthy state. Vitamin A also

helps improve the strength of your bones and the flexibility and elasticity of your skin, helping you "youthen" as you adopt the Wahls Diet.

- **Vitamin C.** Vitamin C is crucial for healthy immune cell function as well as healthy skin and gum tissue. Vitamin C is also a potent antioxidant that helps lower the risk of developing cancer. Although cancer may be the last worry on your list of health concerns right now, know that antioxidants work in your body to keep cell function normal, and that's important for anyone with any type of chronic disease.

- **Vitamin K.** The vitamin K in greens is converted by health-promoting bacteria in the intestine to other, more potent forms of vitamin K that can work to reduce your risk of high blood pressure and calcification (hardening) of the blood vessels and heart valves. Even more exciting, vitamin K has been linked to the prevention of the onset of MS in experimental autoimmune encephalitis in mice, an animal model of MS.[1] Scientists are increasingly aware that vitamin K is very important in brain health, including the production of myelin.[2] Vitamin K should be high on your list of important nutrients if you have MS or an autoimmune condition.

But green leaves are also so much more than "green-BACK." When you eat a big plate of kale salad, you get thousands of compounds that wouldn't be present in supplements for folate, vitamin A, vitamin C, and vitamin K. Scientists can't even name them all yet. All these substances work together in the body to give your cells what they need, but for those with MS, the potential benefits for preventing MS and/or replenishing myelin cannot be ignored. Eat your greens, raw or cooked: 3 cups a day. (Pack raw greens tightly or go by the rule that 2 cups raw equals 1 cup cooked. You could potentially eat 6 cups of raw leafy greens every day.)

Some great choices (the * indicates high in calcium):

- Arugula*
- Beet greens
- Bok choy* and other Asian greens
- Chard, all colors
- Collard greens*
- Dandelion greens*

GOOD GREENS

Greens are rich sources of powerhouse phytochemicals. Known benefits of these nutrients include:

- Anti-cancer properties
- Anti-inflammatory properties
- Better brain health
- Stronger, more elastic skin
- More balanced hormones
- Blood vessels less prone to atherosclerosis
- Better liver health
- Improved eye health

Adapted with permission from "The Phytonutrient Spectrum," Toolkit, Institute for Functional Medicine, Cardiometabolic Conference Course Materials, May 28, 2012.

- Kale, all types (curly; lacinato or "dinosaur"; red; etc.)*
- Lettuce, all types of deep-green, bright green, or red leaf lettuce (no iceberg)
- Mustard greens*
- Parsley
- Spinach*

Note: Food lists in this chapter are not necessarily complete. They are here to give you examples of types of vegetables and fruits. Find a more comprehensive food list at the back of this book if you have questions about any foods that aren't listed in this chapter.

2. Three Cups of Colors

The next 3 cups in your 9 cups should consist of brightly colored vegetables and fruits. Choose those that are brightly colored all the way through, like carrots and beets, rather than brightly colored only on the skin, like red apples. In fact, fruits that are white on the inside, like apples, pears, and bananas, do not count toward your 9 cups. You can still eat them on the

> # ANTIOXIDANT POWER
>
> Antioxidants will help protect you against more than autoimmune disease. There are hundreds of studies showing that diets rich in the antioxidants found in brightly colored vegetables and fruits are protective against cardiovascular disease, cancer, and dementia.[3] For example, studies of the consumption of beetroot juice demonstrated an association with more nitric oxide production and healthier endothelial cells (the cells that line blood vessels, directly impacting blood vessel function). You want your blood vessel lining to be elastic, resilient, and impenetrable to troublemakers like artery-hardening debris. Antioxidants do this job, and they do it well, especially if you eat a lot of them in the form of natural food. In the beetroot juice study, participants had lower blood pressure and less sticky blood cells, which naturally improves blood pressure and reduces the risk of clogging of both arteries and veins.[4]

Wahls Diet, but not until you've had your 9 cups of approved vegetables and fruits. Save that apple or banana for a treat!

The big benefit of deeply colored produce is that the color is a sign of antioxidants. When the vegetable or fruit is colored all the way through, the concentration of the health-promoting antioxidants is the highest. Free radicals cause internal damage, but antioxidants nullify those free radicals before they can cause too much trouble.

So eat your colors! Fortunately, deeply colored vegetables and fruits are some of the best-tasting of all. Aim for eating at least three different colors daily. Some great choices include:

Green

(Although they are white inside, cucumber and zucchini are permitted here if you eat the skins because they are low-starch vegetables and the skins are packed with antioxidants.)

- Asparagus
- Artichokes
- Avocados
- Beans, green
- Cabbage, green
- Celery
- Cucumbers with skin
- Grapes, green
- Green peas

- Kiwi, green
- Limes
- Melons, honeydew
- Okra
- Olives, green
- Peppers, green
- Snow peas
- Sugar snap peas
- Zucchini with skin

Red

- Beets
- Blood oranges
- Cabbage, red
- Cherries
- Cranberries (fresh or frozen without sugar)
- Grapefruits, red
- Grapes, red

- Peppers, red
- Pomegranates
- Radicchio
- Raspberries, red
- Rhubarb
- Strawberries
- Tomatoes
- Watermelons

Blue/Purple/Black

- Aronia berries (grown throughout North America and Europe)
- Blackberries
- Blueberries
- Dates
- Eggplants
- Elderberries

- Grapes, black or purple
- Figs, purple
- Kale, purple
- Olives, black
- Plums
- Prunes
- Raisins
- Raspberries, black

Yellow/Orange

- Apricots
- Carrots

- Grapefruit, yellow
- Kiwi, golden

- Lemon
- Mangos
- Muskmelons
- Nectarines
- Oranges
- Papayas
- Peaches

- Peppers, orange and yellow
- Pineapples
- Pumpkins
- Squash, summer and winter
- Sweet potatoes and yams
- Tangerines

INCREDIBLE COLOR

Different colors of vegetables and fruits indicate different properties and different combinations of phytochemicals. Here's a breakdown of just some of the benefits you're getting when you eat brightly colored vegetables:

- Anti-inflammatory properties
- Anti-cancer properties
- Stronger, more elastic blood vessels
- Healthier brain cells
- Healthier cells all over
- Improved prostate health
- DNA protection
- Antibacterial properties
- Immune system health
- Skin health
- Reproductive health
- Eye health

Adapted with permission from "The Phytonutrient Spectrum," Toolkit, Institute for Functional Medicine, Cardiometabolic Conference Course Materials, May 28, 2012.

3. Three Cups of Sulfur-Rich Vegetables

Finally, I want you to eat 3 cups of sulfur-rich vegetables, which, in addition to antioxidants, also have health-promoting sulfur compounds in them. Sul-

WAHLS WARRIORS SPEAK

I have highly active remitting multiple sclerosis with mobility impairment. Other than mild depression, I have no other symptoms. I was initially admitted to hospital with a suspected stroke with only 4/5 power in my right leg, but after three months of further tests, lesions were found in my brain and I was diagnosed with multiple sclerosis. I've been trying to follow the Wahls Diet to the letter for ten weeks. Before going on the diet, I had begun to deteriorate rapidly and my friends were noticing the decline. Almost within days, I began to feel better and now my thinking is clearer, I have less spasticity, my sleeping is better, and I feel much more positive about life and its possibilities. My friends remark how they can see a marked improvement in my well-being. I am enjoying food so much more because I can now taste the real flavors and I am better overall: I have lost weight, my hair feels healthier, I do not have dry scalp anymore, I have better libido, and I wake up refreshed every morning. I am grateful for many things in my life, and now I add Dr. Wahls to my list because she had the courage not to give up when faced with multiple sclerosis. Because of her, I now feel better equipped to deal with my own adversity.

—Richard J., London, England

fur may not get the media attention that antioxidants do, but it is an incredibly important compound for health. Sulfur-rich foods nourish cells and mitochondria, and specifically help the body to be more efficient in eliminating toxins. Sulfur is also important for synthesizing protein and for producing collagen, which makes up all your connective tissues. If you have joint issues, you need sulfur! It also helps give you strong, beautiful skin, hair, and nails. Diets containing sulfur have been associated with improvement in skin disorders and arthritis. Many arthritis sufferers take a supplement called MSM (methylsulfonylmethane) to help with joint pain, but I like to get my sulfur on my dinner plate, so it comes in its natural and complete package.

There are literally thousands of studies showing the health benefits of the compounds in the sulfur-rich family. One of the most relevant pathways for research in sulfur-rich vegetables involves their contribution to blood vessel health. This should matter a great deal to anyone with multiple sclerosis as well as those with other autoimmune problems. As I noted earlier in chapter 2, Dr. Paolo Zamboni has published studies reporting that those with multiple sclerosis are more likely to have blockages in the veins that drain the brain, which can lead to chronic cerebrospinal venous insufficiency (CCSVI). Sulfur vegetables are a natural, nonsurgical way to address this potential issue. In addition, people with systemic lupus and rheumatoid arthritis also have a higher rate of atherosclerosis than the general population, leading to narrowing of the blood vessels.[5] Sulfur-rich vegetables are crucial for them as well. Eat to keep the endothelial cells that line the blood vessels in a state of optimal health to reduce the risk of atherosclerosis.

Good sources of sulfur include the cabbage family, the onion family, and the mushroom family. All three have a long history as important medicinal foods in the Asian cultures. Let's look at these valuable vegetables more closely.

The Cabbage Family

The cruciferous, or brassica, family is also called the cabbage family and includes kale, collards, broccoli, cauliflower, Brussels sprouts, turnips, rutabaga, and radishes. The brassica family vegetables are rich in many organic sulfur compounds, including diindolylmethane (DIM), indole-3-carbinol (I3C), and sulforaphane, which in many animal studies has been shown to be beneficial in supporting detoxification processes, reducing oxidative stress, and protecting brain cells by inducing the production of glutathione, a potent intracellular antixodant.[6] Cabbage family veggies are greatly valued across many cultures and are some of the most potently nutritious of all the vegetables. They are an important key to detoxification, which is incredibly important for people with chronic disease. (I will talk more about these vegetables in the detoxification chapter.) These compounds are also potent antioxidants, which are linked to a reduction in the risk of heart disease and cancer.[7]

VARIETY IS THE SPICE OF HEALTH

It is very important to rotate the vegetables you eat for more variety. All vegetables and most fruits have some toxins in them as part of their protection against the animals that would eat them (that includes you and me). In fact, these very chemicals stimulate our cellular machinery to operate at increasing efficiency. If you eat the same plants every day, the toxins can build up and have a negative health impact; but if you rotate your foods, you get all the benefits without the risk. For example, I eat greens in rotation: kale one day, lettuce the next, then spinach, and then beet greens or chard. The wider, more diverse the foodstuffs you eat, the more health-promoting benefits and the fewer negative benefits you will experience. Our ancestors would have eaten two hundred or more different plant and animal species each year. Think about it. How many different species are you eating? Kale, as much as I love it, should not be eaten day after day. Mix it up and you will be healthier.

The Onion Family

This family includes all types of onions as well as garlic, chives, leeks, and shallots. Members of the garlic and onion family are rich in allicin sulfides (when the garlic or onion is crushed, these compounds transform into diallyl suffides), which also have a long history of medicinal use across many cultures because of their antibacterial properties and blood and blood vessel health–promoting properties. Regular consumption of these vegetables is also associated with a reduced risk for heart disease, cancer, and dementia.[8]

There are many studies showing that using aged garlic extract is associated with healthier blood vessels, less atherosclerosis, less clogging of the vessels, and greater fluidity of the blood.[9] While one could take aged garlic extract or L-arginine (the active compound in the extract), I prefer to see people rely on whole foods over extracts as a more comprehensive therapy. The extracts require processing and purification and likely lose useful elements during that process. The best and safest approach, in my view, is to eat more garlic, onions, and sulfur-rich vegetables.

STOP THE WASTE!

Buying fresh fruits and vegetables can be expensive, especially if you throw away nutritious parts or don't eat them before they spoil. Stop wasting your money and medicinal food with these strategies:

- When vegetables begin to look a bit stale, chop them and put them in a Crock-Pot on low all day with water or broth to make vegetable soup.
- Don't throw away the leaves on radishes, beets, or turnips. These can be used in smoothies or cooked and enjoyed. They are highly nutritious and count toward your daily quota of greens. The leaves on cauliflower, broccoli, and kohlrabi are also edible. Use them in smoothies and soups, and eat them steamed.
- Two easy ways to use greens: (1) Put them in a blender with fruit and/or orange juice or full-fat coconut milk and blend on high to make a green smoothie. (2) Sauté onions and mushrooms in coconut oil, add chopped greens, and stir until wilted (just a minute or two). If the greens seem bitter, add more coconut oil or some full-fat coconut milk.

The Mushroom Family

The last category of sulfur-rich vegetables consists of mushrooms, which are not only rich in sulfur but also in B vitamins. Mushrooms in particular have been used medicinally in Asia for thousands of years. We know they contain beta-D-glucan and fucogalactans, components of the cell walls of mushrooms, and that these compounds stimulate the natural killer cells that help balance the immune system and are protective against cancer[10] and autoimmune disease.[11] Mushrooms are an excellent and delicious addition to the diet, but with one caveat: Some individuals with autoimmune disorders are sensitive to mushrooms. I'll talk more about this in chapter 6 when I discuss fermented foods, but if you perceive that you have more headaches, fatigue, or worsening of any brain symptoms after consuming mushrooms, I suggest removing them from your diet, at least temporarily. You may be able to introduce mushrooms back into your diet after six months on the Wahls Diet to see if you tolerate

SUPERIOR SULFUR-RICH

Known health benefits of sulfur-rich foods include:

- Anti-cancer properties
- Anti-microbial action
- Blood vessel health
- Detoxification
- Gut health
- Heart health
- Hormone balance
- Immune cell action support
- Liver health

Adapted with permission from "The Phytonutrient Spectrum," Toolkit, Institute for Functional Medicine, Cardiometabolic Conference Course Materials, May 28, 2012.

occasional use, but don't have them more than once a week. Fortunately, you've got plenty of other sulfur-rich foods to choose from, so have 3 cups' worth each day.

Here are some choices of sulfur-rich vegetables. You will note some crossover with other lists: some foods—like kale, which is a sulfur vegetable and a leafy green—fall into multiple categories. Include these in one or the other group as you assemble your 9 cups—your choice:

- Asparagus
- Bok choy
- Broccoli
- Brussels sprouts
- Cabbage
- Cauliflower
- Chives
- Collard greens
- Daikon
- Garlic, all types
- Kale
- Leeks
- Mushrooms
- Onions: red, yellow, and white
- Radishes
- Rutabagas
- Scallions
- Shallots
- Turnips and turnip greens

WAHLS WARRIOR Q & A

Q: I can't eat FODMAP foods without digestive trouble. Can I still do the Wahls Diet?

A: FODMAPs (fermentable oligosaccharides, disaccharides, monosaccharides, and polyols) are short-chain carbohydrates such as fructose and lactose. Examples of FODMAP foods are wheat, rye, legumes, onions, garlic, mushrooms, avocados, stone fruits, and apples. These compounds are not generally absorbed in the small bowel but instead are further digested by bacteria in the small bowel through fermentation and then absorbed. In some people this will cause irritable bowel–like symptoms. In my clinical observation, the irritable bowel problems of my patients and followers are nearly always resolved by following the Wahls Paleo Diet (see chapter 6). If for some reason you still have trouble, I would advocate trying Wahls Paleo Plus (see chapter 7). The micronutrients from organ meats and natural high-quality fats at that level tend to be well tolerated by people with irritable bowel issues.

Making the Most of Your 9 Cups

It's not easy to just start eating 9 cups of vegetables and fruit every day. Where and how often should you buy them? How do you store them to keep them fresh? How should you prepare them for meals and snacks? What if all those vegetables give you a stomachache? Let's talk about these questions.

Where and How Often to Buy

Because the vitamin and antioxidant content in fresh vegetables and fruits degrades over time, the first thing to think about is buying your food as close to locally and as fresh as possible. Farmer's markets and farm stands are excellent sources for your 9 cups when it's the right season for these things. Getting your vegetables locally minimizes the time between harvest and consumption and maximizes the vitamin and mineral content of your food. Buy vegetables and fruits at least once a week. If you are able, several times a week is even better. There is nothing nicer than eating a big plate of vegetables that were picked that day.

Even better, you can grow many of your own vegetables in your backyard if you have the available space. Ideally, you walk to your deck or yard to pick your food for your supper. There is no fresher way to eat, and I believe that growing more of your own food is an important strategy for reclaiming your (and your family's) health and vitality.

Of course, becoming a backyard gardener takes some work, but perhaps less than you think. Many of your 9 cups can be easily grown in container gardens hanging from or sitting on your deck. This includes greens like spinach, kale, collards, chard, and lettuce, as well as other vegetables like onions, garlic, chives, tomatoes, and strawberries. You can also begin to add in vegetables and fruits with your existing landscape in low-maintenance ways. Berry bushes, for example, require very little care after planting.

Some people worry about the physical strain of gardening, but raised beds can put your vegetables at waist level. You won't even have to bend over to weed them. Raised beds also allow you to improve your soil quality, because you can fill up the beds with higher-quality soil and enrich it with compost and natural fertilizer. Your family might also enjoy lending a hand. Gardening is extremely rewarding and a good stress reliever—another important part of the Wahls Protocol that I'll discuss later.

If you live in an apartment, you may be able to join a community garden. Or if you can't or don't want to grow your own food, consider joining in the community-supported agriculture (CSA) movement. In a CSA, you purchase a share from a farmer in that year's crop. You then get a weekly box of freshly picked vegetables and fruit from the farmer throughout the growing season. Some CSAs are only for the summer, but an increasing number now have spring, fall, and even winter shares. It's fun to see what you will get each week and to think of ways to cook and eat all the different vegetables. It's also a great way to add more variety and rotate your vegetables. I recommend finding a CSA that is organic. Look online for CSAs in your area. You can also grow less traditional foods, like sprouts and mushrooms. Kids often enjoy growing these foods. See the Resources section at the back of this book

WAHLS WARRIOR Q & A

Q: Does juicing the 9 cups of vegetables and fruits have the same impact as consuming the whole food?

A: No. If you use a juicer that extracts and removes the fiber, the juice will have a very high glycemic index and will cause your body to manufacture more insulin in response. The juice will be rapidly absorbed along with the vitamins and enzymes. I'd rather you use a high-speed blender such as a Vitamix or HealthMaster to make a smoothie. Smoothies retain the entire fruit or vegetable including the fiber, which results in a slower rise in blood sugar. If you add a generous amount of water to liquefy the vegetables and fruits, a smoothie can seem just like juice, but it will have a much more beneficial effect in your body because you have not converted your produce into a high-glycemic form. We have had subjects in our trial who are very petite and could not eat 9 cups of vegetables. They ate 4 to 6 cups and made the rest into a smoothie using a Vitamix. This can be a good solution for those who have trouble eating the 9 cups.

for good sources to buy supplies for growing sprouts and mushrooms. Another fun family activity is looking for edible wild foods that grow throughout North America, especially in empty lots in cities and towns and along roadways. Remember, however, that you do have to be careful to identify the plants correctly, as some plants and mushrooms are poisonous. (See the Resources section for information about where to learn about foraging.)

The rank order of preference for best nutrition from your vegetables and fruits are:

- Picked from your garden and consumed the same day
- Purchased from a local farmer (or picked up from a CSA) and consumed on the same day
- Purchased fresh from a store, from a regional farmer, picked that week (You won't always be able to tell this.)

- Frozen or fermented (often preferable to fresh that is shipped from a distance)
- Purchased fresh from a store, from a farmer across the country (like from the coast if you live in the Midwest, or from one coast to another)
- Purchased fresh but from overseas
- Canned

Remember, the farther food travels and the more it is heated, the more vitamins and antioxidants it will lose. Note: If food is dried at 105 degrees or less, it is as good as fresh as long as it is kept dry and below 85 degrees.

Produce Prep

When you bring home your vegetables, consider preparing them immediately. Fill the sink with water and wash everything. You can rinse with water alone or add a tablespoon of vinegar to two quarts of water. Dry with paper towels and put vegetables and fruits into ziplock bags or clear plastic containers so everything stays clean and is easy to see. For an even easier time later, prepare your produce: Scrub and trim off ends of root vegetables, snap the ends of beans, and tear up lettuce so it is salad-ready. Break apart broccoli and cauliflower into florets. If you can open a neat crisper drawer and see all your vegetables nicely arranged and ready to eat, you will be much more likely to make a salad or stir-fry, or just snack on raw vegetables than if you know you have to start from scratch, scrubbing, trimming, peeling, coring, seeding, and chopping everything. Don't forget to reserve the outer leaves: Throw them in the Crock-Pot (or freezer) for vegetable soup stock. For your berries, it is better to wash and prep them just prior to eating. Also, berries have a shorter shelf life and are best consumed within one or two days of purchase.

If you buy or harvest too much produce to eat at once, preserve your produce for later. I recommend washing, de-seeding and coring, and freezing it in heavy ziplock freezer bags so you can defrost and enjoy good local produce all year. Canning is another option, although it is a lot of work and not everyone will enjoy it. Another great option: Learn how to use lacto-fermentation to store your food and increase its nutritional quality. You'll find some fermented

WAHLS WARRIOR Q & A

Q: Why are nightshade vegetables a problem for some people? Why do you allow them on the Wahls Diet?

A: For some genetically susceptible people, lectins, which are sugar-protein molecules, will cause excessive inflammation, increasing the risk of autoimmunity. Nightshade vegetables (potatoes, tomatoes, eggplants, and bell peppers) contain lectins, which may lead to overactivity of the immune systems. Others won't have a problem with nightshade vegetables, some of which are good sources of nutrients. The reason I do not exclude nightshade vegetables is because if I tell people to remove every foodstuff that has the potential to cause trouble for anyone, there would be very little left to eat. Some people even have food sensitivities to kale! Instead, I remove only those foods I believe are deleterious to anyone with a chronic disease (gluten and dairy) and that are most likely to cause food sensitivity issues. If you have individual food sensitivity issues beyond these general exclusions, there are many ways to determine that—first and foremost by tracking your reactions to foods in your Wahls Diary. So if you react poorly to nightshade vegetables, by all means, exclude them. If you don't react poorly to them, there is no reason to eliminate them from your diet.

recipes in the recipe section at the end of the book. (Of course, you can also buy high-quality, organic frozen or fermented fruits and vegetables in the off-season.)

When the 9 Cups Are Too Much or Upset Your Stomach

You don't think you can eat all those vegetables! I understand. I hear this all the time. First of all, your problem might be solved largely when you are implementing all parts of the Wahls Diet, including the elimination of gluten and dairy foods. (I'll talk about this later in this chapter.) Most people eat so much grain-based and dairy-based food that eliminating it leaves a lot of room in your stomach. How better to fill it than with vegetables and fruits?

I also understand, however, that this is a major dietary change. For some people, gastrointestinal distress is a problem that comes with the sudden increase in vegetable matter. You may have gas, stomach cramps, diarrhea, or even constipation as your body adjusts. If you have MS or an autoimmune disease, you may have more serious GI issues as well, such as inflammatory bowel disease, making eating all those vegetables difficult.

If you need to ease in, this is absolutely acceptable. Better to go slowly than to start suddenly and then quit. If you are having a lot of GI issues, I have two suggestions:

1. First, begin eating 1 to 3 cups of homemade bone broth (see the recipe section at the end of this book) and some coconut milk every day to help heal the lining of your gut.
2. Start eating your vegetables in the form of vegetable broth. First, add vegetables to water and simmer for twenty minutes. Strain out the vegetables and add the vegetable broth to your bone broth. Once this is going well and you've adjusted, begin pureeing the vegetables and adding them to your soup. Start with smaller amounts and work up. Your body will get used to the nutrition, but the fiber will be broken down and the vegetables will be easier to digest.

The reasons for the difference in tolerance to vegetables have to do with your digestive enzymes and which bacteria are living in your bowels. Each of us has unique DNA and therefore a unique balance of digestive and toxin-processing enzymes. I have observed that some people can't do 3 cups of greens because of diarrhea but do fine if they cook their greens instead or eat just 1 to 2 cups of salad greens a day. For people with inflammatory bowel disease or any kind of abdominal issues like irritable bowel syndrome, having vegetables as soups and stews is the easiest way to get in all the vegetables. As you advance, steamed vegetables are usually well tolerated, and then eventually you will likely do well with salads, smoothies, and raw vegetables. Take your time and increase your vegetable and fruit intake as your tolerance

WAHLS WARRIOR Q & A

Q: What is your advice for people on medications (like Coumadin) that make it hard to eat a lot of dark leafy greens and other healthy foods?

A: Coumadin thins the blood through its interference with the vitamin K_1 pathways in the liver. For this reason, it is very important to have a consistent intake of vitamin-K-rich foods like greens every day. In other words, you must eat the same amount of greens every day (such as the 3 cups specified on the Wahls Diet), so that the dose of Coumadin can be adjusted to match the daily intake. If you eat a plateful of greens once or twice a month and avoid greens all the other days, you could experience wild swings in the blood-thinning effect (also referred to as prothrombin time) of your Coumadin on the days you eat a lot of greens.

Unfortunately, many people believe that this means they have to avoid vitamin K–rich foods entirely. This is a mistake. Avoiding greens will, over time, lead to multiple vitamin and mineral deficiencies. As the micronutrient deficiencies pile up, the prothrombin time often fluctuates widely, making the management of the Coumadin dose increasingly difficult. In fact, when this happens, it's a sign that multiple nutrient deficiencies are present, and this increases the risk of developing calcium deposits on heart valves and in blood vessels, leading to aortic stenosis (often severe enough to need heart surgery) or worsening high blood pressure that requires more and more medication.[12]

My recommendation to patients on Coumadin is to talk to your prescribing doctor and explain that you want to ramp up your vegetable intake and that you will need more frequent blood checks as you do this so your dose can be appropriately adjusted. Then, eat the same amount of greens every day. This method should allow you to fully nourish your body with all the goodness greens provide while you continue to benefit safely from your medication. Another option I would recommend to only those people taking Coumadin is to take a daily dose of menaquinone-7 (vitamin K_2) so that you have a consistent intake of vitamin K, so the Coumadin dosing can be safely adjusted. This will lessen the risk of having your heart valves and bloods vessels hardened by excessive calcium depositions as a result of vitamin K depletion, but talk to your doctor before starting this supplement. You must always work with the physician who is managing your Coumadin dose so that she or he is aware that you're working to maximize your nutrition intake.

improves. Your digestive enzymes and the bacteria living in your bowels will likely adjust as your health improves, although the adjustment can be slow.

If you have a marked adverse reaction to a specific food, honor that and avoid it for three months. Practice the other aspects of the Wahls Diet, and in three months you may have healed sufficiently to tolerate a small amount of the offending food once a week. If not, continue to avoid it.

Part Two: Gluten-Free/Dairy-Free

Now that we've talked all about what you get to eat, let's talk about what's now off the list, and the reasons for that. Giving up gluten, which is the protein in wheat, rye, and barley, as well as casein, which is the protein in dairy foods, seems like a pretty tall order. You love bread! You love cheese! How can you live without these creature comforts?

Although they might not seem to be related on the surface, gluten and casein molecules have a similar amino acid sequence, and so to our immune cells they are often equivalent. When we eat these foods, our dopamine levels rise, making us feel good—even doped up and high. (Think about how you feel when you eat a gooey, cheesy pizza, an ice cream cone, or a chocolate chip cookie.) Our brains get addicted to that high, so we end up eating too many calories and not enough nutrients. Gluten (the protein in wheat, rye, and barley) and casein interact with the same receptors that are stimulated by narcotics, the opioid receptors.[13] Refined sugars and processed foods are addictive, too. They have been specifically designed to stimulate our pleasure centers, making us feel good, so we want more and more.[14] But addictions can be broken, and they must be if you want to stop suffering from the ill effects of unhealthful foods. It's time to go cold turkey. The Wahls Diet is your path!

You are now eating 9 cups of fruits and vegetables a day, markedly increasing the nutrient density of your diet. Most starchy foods—especially grains and potatoes—as well as dairy products have a lot of calories and are transformed into sugar as your body digests the food. These foods have relatively few vitamins, minerals, and other micronutrients compared to greens, colors, and sulfur-rich produce. By replacing the grains and white potatoes with vegetables, deeply colored fruits, and berries, you will get a lot more antioxidants and other phytonutrients each day and fewer empty calories.

Then there is the issue of allergies, intolerances, and sensitivities. There is a lot of buzz in the media these days about going gluten-free and/or dairy-free. There are some recognized conditions, like celiac disease and lactose intolerance, which require taking gluten and/or dairy off the menu, but what about all the other people going gluten-free and dairy-free, claiming vague symptoms and self-diagnosed "intolerances"? It's become a fad, no doubt, and some physicians have become concerned that many perfectly healthy people are removing wheat and dairy from their diets needlessly.

I would argue that many people can benefit from removing all sources of gluten and casein from their diets, whether or not they have a diagnosed allergy, reactivity, or sensitivity. The truth is that for people with chronic disease in particular, gluten and casein can be very problematic. Food allergies and sensitivities are difficult to diagnose and are much more common than is generally medically recognized, especially in people with chronic disease. You may not have any indication that you have a problem with gluten and casein, because 90 percent of the time there are no acute abdominal symptoms. Instead, the symptoms are insidious and come on gradually, and result in a wide variety of manifestations: unexplained fatigue, unexplained rashes that come and go, headaches, and mood problems. Unrecognized gluten and/or casein sensitivity has been associated with a wide variety of health problems,[15] including but not limited to:

- Allergies
- Asthma
- Autism and other brain disorders
- Chronic migraine
- Eczema and other skin disorders

- Infertility
- Inflammatory bowel disease (IBD)
- Irritable bowel syndrome (IBS)
- Psoriasis
- Psychiatric disorders
- Thyroid disease

In fact, for many with chronic, unexplained symptoms, and those with autoimmune problems, food sensitivities may be one of the root causes for many of their symptoms. In North America, no food sensitivities are more common than those to gluten and casein.[16]

Because you have been consuming grain and/or dairy most of your life, you don't know if you have sensitivity issues or not and you may not realize how many of your symptoms may be related to food sensitivity to gluten and/or dairy. Your body is in a steady state based on what you are eating now and has adapted to the damage that is being done. You are used to feeling the way you feel. Get ready to start feeling a lot better.

These are the items that contain gluten that you should avoid:

- Barley and anything containing it (including most beer, as well as barley malt and malt extract, including malt vinegar)
- Bulgur (the wheat grain in tabouli salad)
- Cereal containing wheat, barley, or rye (hot or cold)
- Couscous
- Matzo flour/meal/bread
- Panko (most breading contains gluten)
- Pasta made from semolina and/or durum (both of which are wheat)
- Rye and anything containing it
- Seitan (pure wheat gluten)
- Udon noodles
- Wheat and anything containing it, including wheat bran and wheat germ. That includes most bread, bagels, crackers, muffins, cookies, cake, and pastries.
- Wheat cousins: spelt, triticale, faro, Kamut (Khorasan wheat), einkorn

Gluten is also hidden in many things you might not think about, like deli meats, condiments, communion wafers, salad dressings, soups, soy sauce, and even medications, cosmetics, and envelope glue! If you aren't sure if something contains gluten, look on the label for a gluten-free statement, or call the company.

Now for the good news: There are still grains and starches you can eat, at least at this level of the diet! I will restrict grains and all starches much more at the next level, Wahls Paleo, but for now, in limited amounts, you may eat these gluten-free grains and starches:

Wahls Diet–Approved Grains and Starches

- Amaranth
- Arrowroot
- Buckwheat
- Chickpea flour and other legume-based flours
- Coconut flour
- Corn
- Flax meal
- Millet
- Nut flours (like almond flour)
- Oats, but only if specifically certified gluten-free (Standard oats are typically cross-contaminated with gluten.)*
- Packaged foods labeled "gluten-free"
- Potato flour
- Quinoa
- Rice, all types
- Sago
- Sorghum
- Soy flour
- Tapioca
- Teff

*A caution about oats: Up to 30 percent of those with gluten sensitivity have some symptoms when eating oatmeal, even when it is labeled gluten-free. Be cautious with oatmeal use. It may still be a problem for you.

These are the dairy foods you should eliminate from your diet:

- Cheese made from cow's, goat's, or sheep's milk
- Cream (heavy cream, whipping cream)
- Dairy ice cream
- Dairy yogurt
- Half-and-half
- Milk chocolate and many other forms of chocolate and candy (Read the label: Many dark chocolate varieties still contain milk.)
- Milk that comes from cows, goats, sheep, or mares. (Once you have been weaned, I don't recommend consuming milk products again, with the exception of ghee, or clarified butter, which has the milk proteins removed.)
- Nondairy creamer (Although it is labeled "nondairy," it does contain milk derivatives.)
- Nondairy "whipped topping"
- Packaged food with milk, casein, whey, caseinates, or hydrosylates in the ingredients list
- Vegetarian "cheeses" that contain some milk solids (Read the label.)
- Whey

WAHLS WARRIOR Q & A

Q: I know there are a lot of problems with dairy products, but what about raw milk? Many diets similar to yours recommend raw milk products.

A: When milk is pasteurized and homogenized, the shape and availability of the protein and fat molecules are slightly changed. That is why some people report that milk has many more health benefits when it is raw. I do agree that raw milk may be better nutritionally than pasteurized and/or homogenized milk, but it still has casein, which increases the risk of food allergy and sensitivity and has the potential to transmit infection if the milk is from an unhealthy cow. For this reason, milk, cheese, yogurt, ice cream, whey (as in whey protein powder), and all other dairy products (except for clarified butter, also called ghee, which has the milk proteins removed) are not part of the Wahls Diet, Wahls Paleo, or Wahls Paleo Plus.

Wahls Diet–Approved Milk Substitutes

Fortunately, there are many dairy substitutes that are just fine on the Wahls Diet. Read the labels to see what has been added, and minimize exposure to high-fructose corn syrup, sugars, and other foodlike compounds that are added to the product (often to give it a better "feel" in the mouth). The exception is the addition of calcium citrate for the additional calcium content; this is fine. I suggest unsweetened varieties with short lists of basic ingredients you recognize, or make your own by combining nuts or seeds and water in a high-speed blender and straining the liquid.

Enjoy any of these:

- Almond milk
- Coconut milk (full-fat is just fine)
- Hazelnut milk
- Hemp milk
- Rice milk (organic preferred)
- Soy, almond, or coconut-based coffee creamer (marked "vegan")
- Soy, almond, or coconut yogurt
- Soy, almond, or coconut frozen desserts (ice cream substitutes) with unrefined sweeteners
- Soy milk (organic only)
- Soy or other nondairy cheeses that are labeled "vegan"

You may also enjoy dark chocolate if it doesn't contain any milk products. For the best nutritional benefit and an intense chocolate taste, choose 75 percent or higher cacao content.

VEGETARIAN ADVICE

You can be a vegetarian on the Wahls Diet, although you cannot progress to the next two levels if you remain a vegetarian. If you are at an ideal body weight and enjoy excellent health, then you can simply stay at the Wahls-

Diet and you will still reap immense benefits. I urge you, however, to read the Wahls Paleo chapter to learn about the benefits of seaweed and soaking grains, legumes, and nuts even if you do not plan to begin to eat meat. If you experience a decline in health, however, I urge you to consider Wahls Paleo. I do not recommend vegetarianism, and the next chapter will also offer my arguments, if you care to consider them. However, your diet is your choice, and that's why I give you three dietary levels for the Wahls Protocol.

I understand that some people have strong beliefs that necessitate vegetarianism, and I respect that. If this is you, then in order to get sufficient protein and calories, you will need to eat more grains and legumes than I would regularly recommend. The amounts below are based on a 2,000-kcal diet and USDA dietary guidelines:

- Protein foods, 5.5 ounces per day (a one-ounce-equivalent portion would be 1 tablespoon of peanut butter, ½ ounce nuts and seeds, ¼ cup cooked dried beans or peas, ¼ cup tofu, or 1 ounce veggie meat). I recommended rotating your protein sources for more variety and less concentration on any one item.
- Grains (choose gluten-free varieties), 6 ounces per day
- Calcium-fortified vegan "dairy" products, 3 cups per day (such as calcium-fortified soy, rice, or almond milk; calcium-fortified soy yogurt; or tofu made with calcium sulfate.

Because of this higher grain and legume consumption, I also strongly recommend that all vegetarians soak their grains and legumes before eating. There are some very important reasons for this, which I will talk about in the next chapter, but in brief: Germination decreases the activity of antinutrients like phytates, lectins, and trypsin inhibitors that occur naturally in grains and legumes. Soak your grains and legumes in water, in a bowl or jar, for twenty-four hours before preparing. Drain and rinse well. This causes the grains and legumes to produce phytase, which neutralizes some of the antinutrient action. An added perk: Soaking decreases cooking time.

Part Three: Organic, Grass-Fed, and Wild-Caught

The last component of the Wahls Diet isn't about what you can and can't eat but about the quality of the foods you choose. I understand that it isn't always affordable or even available, but whenever possible I want you to choose organic vegetables and fruits, organic grass-fed meat, wild game, and wild-caught fish.

Some people believe that terms like *organic*, *grass-fed*, and *wild-caught* are purely marketing ploys that drive up cost without any real benefit. While it's true that fruits and vegetables as well as animals and fish raised without chemical intervention are more expensive, there is good reason for this. While all vegetables, fruits, meat, and fish may be healthy in essence, what conventionally raised food also contains is not so healthy after all.

Organic produce is easy: Most grocery stores now carry it. Even Walmart carries it. You can grow it in your yard or buy it at the farmer's market. If you can't afford it all the time, go organic, where it really matters. The Environmental Working Group (www.ewg.org) has several food guides to help identify which produce items have the most pesticides applied to them and which have the least, so that you can prioritize your shopping. (Look for their current list of the Dirty Dozen and the Clean Fifteen, updated yearly.)

Aside from the Dirty Dozen, there is one area where reducing chemicals matters more: meat and fish. This is because of something called bio-concentration. The chemicals in an animal's feed are concentrated in the meat of the animals you eat. This happens in nature, too, because of the pollution on our planet. A very small fish, for example, will eat plant matter and may absorb a tiny bit of mercury and other chemicals from a polluted environment. When a larger fish eats that fish, it not only gets mercury and chemicals from living in a polluted environment but gets all the mercury and chemicals concentrated in the smaller fish it eats. As you work your way up the food chain, with successively bigger fish dining on other fish, the concentration grows. This is why the largest fish have the highest rates of mercury and other chemicals in their flesh.

And guess who is at the top of the food chain? Us, of course. If you eat conventionally grown meat and aquaculture ("farmed") fish, you will be ex-

---

WAHLS WARRIOR Q & A

Q: How do people who are allergic to fish get omega-3 fats in their diet?
A: If you do not tolerate even fish oil, then see if you can tolerate algae DHA oil. If you can't take that, either, then it is important to take 2 table-spoons of flax oil daily. It will also be even more important for you to have grass-fed meat. Another option is getting checked for an egg allergy and/or sensitivity. If you are not sensitive to eggs, you may be able to eat eggs that are DHA-enriched.

---

posing yourself and your family to the growth hormones, antibiotics, and pesticides used to grow that animal. The highest bioconcentration of toxins are in your fat, and remember that your brain is 60 to 70 percent fat.

The meat our Paleolithic ancestors ate was very different from the meat we eat today. Animals did not contain much saturated fat until late summer and fall, in preparation for winter. Throughout the rest of the year, the animal was very lean and more of the fat contained unsaturated omega-3 fatty acids. The fall animals were valued for the increased fat. Coastal communities ate much more seafood from much cleaner waters. The result was a diet higher in both protein and omega-3 fatty acids in comparison to the modern Westernized diet, and containing far fewer toxins. When I was growing up on the family farm, most of the farms in this country were run by families like ours. The average farm size was 170 acres. These farms were typically diversified into several crops. People had small herds of dairy cattle, beef cattle, and hogs. Crops included corn, soybeans, alfalfa, and oats. We had a huge garden and picked wild plums, grapes, and berries that grew around the yard, in the farm along the fencerows, along streams, and in the local woodlands. We also raised flocks of chickens, ducks, and a couple of turkeys each year. But we were also beginning to use chemical fertilizers, herbicides, and pesticides that were becoming popular because they increased production.

I remember that my dad had a sprayer that he used to spray atrazine over the corn and a broadleaf herbicide over the thistles in the pastures. He also used antibiotics for the livestock to combat infections, and he dewormed all of the animals annually. He fed corn to the hogs, to fatten them for sale to the slaughterhouse. My father sold beef calves in the fall to other people who then fattened them with corn on a confinement lot somewhere else. The dairy herd was milked twice a day. The cows ate from lush pastures in the spring and summer and had corn and hay during the winter. It was a farm experience on the cusp of modern technology—one foot in the old ways, the other foot in the new ways.

Today, farming is much different. There are far fewer small family farms, with the average size of the corporate farm steadily rising. Meat is produced efficiently and relatively inexpensively. Most of the meat you see in the supermarket comes from animals grown in large confinement systems. The animals are often kept indoors or in crowded outdoor pens, and fed rations to maximize growth in the shortest number of days. These rations often contain antibiotics and growth-promoting hormones.

The result is that nonorganic, conventionally raised meats and farmed fish almost always contain chemical toxins that you will have to process and eliminate via your liver and kidneys. A healthy body may be able to tolerate the chemicals for a while, but eventually the harmful substances in conventionally raised animal and fish products are likely to begin wreaking havoc in your cells, leading to a variety of diseases. Which particular disease you get depends on your particular genetic vulnerability and which toxins are accumulating and which hormonal imbalances are occurring in your body. If you suffer from an autoimmune condition like MS, your body is already clearly imbalanced, so you of all people should be particularly careful about what's in your meat.

This is why you want to eat the healthiest, most vigorous, least polluted animals. If you were a Paleolithic human, you would be getting your meat and fish from the unpolluted wild, but this is a lot more difficult today. However, you can definitely increase the purity and nutrient density of your animal protein if you select it from the right sources:

- **Do you hunt, fish, or know a hunter or fisherman?** These practices can make people squeamish, but they are how our ancestors survived, and there is no fresher, more natural way for acquiring your animal protein.

WHERE TO GET YOUR MEAT

Ideally, all of your animal protein will be organic, grass-fed, and/or wild-caught. Here are explanations of various sources for animal protein:

Conventional. Conventionally raised animals are grain-fed, often with genetically modified corn; typically confined to small living spaces; and usually given hormones to make them grow faster and antibiotics to fight illnesses caused by living in close quarters.

Farmed fish. Farmed fish are raised in netted cages in coastal waters. They are sometimes fed grain products, which make their omega-6 levels higher, and they are more likely to contain contaminants like neurotoxic polychlorinated biphenyls (PCBs) and hormone-disrupting polybrominated diphenyl ethers (PBDEs); antibiotics; and pesticides that are used to control infestations of sea lice.

Grass-fed. Grass-fed animals are fed only grass and forage from weaning to harvest. Look for meat from animals that are both grass-fed and grass-finished. (Note: Some game and bison are grown on tall grass prairie, which provides more nutrients than grass.)

Grass-fed, grain-finished. These animals ate grass after weaning but were fed grain, typically corn, the last six weeks before slaughter. This is enough time to change the fatty acid composition of the animal to increase the amount of omega-6 fatty acids and decrease the amount of desirable omega-3 fatty acids, losing much of the benefit of grass feeding.

Organic. Organic meat is raised without hormones and antibiotics, but these animals may still be fed grain and have too much omega-6. Some small family farms that do not have USDA organic certification nevertheless choose to raise grass-fed, free-range animals without hormones and antibiotics. Talk to the farmer.

Wild. Wild game and fish are not domesticated or contained by humans and they find their own food sources. Try to find a friend who hunts and you can often get all the venison or elk that your freezer can hold.

- **Do you have access to products from a game farm that lets their animals forage?** Bison farms, deer farms, and elk farms all sell delicious meat with minimal toxic residue and a higher concentration of healthy nutrients like omega-3 fatty acids. Be sure to confirm that the animals are not being fattened or finished on grain.
- **Do you have access to a farm that raises grass-fed, free-ranging, organic, domesticated animals?** Organic animals cannot be fed any hormones or antibiotics, and their feed must also be organic. Grass-fed organic farms are more common and easier to find than ever before, especially since you can mail-order some of these products if they aren't available near you.
- **Can you find meat from grain-finished animals that is organic?** This is still superior to conventional meat.
- **Can you find wild-caught fish, shrimp, and other seafood?** Choose smaller fish to stay lower down on the food chain, ideally from small family fisheries bringing in small catches from cold waters. These will be the least contaminated and most natural fish options.
- **Unless you have no other option, avoid conventionally raised meat from feedlots, confined poultry, and farm-raised fish.** These are the most polluted sources of animal protein.

It can be difficult to find these foods, and if they are out of your budget, please know that getting your 9 cups and going gluten-free and dairy-free are the essential elements of the Wahls Diet. You can do this without going organic, or going organic according to what your budget will allow. Priority number one with the Wahls Diet is to get those nutrients into you *now* and to stop causing an attack response in your body with gluten and dairy. These two steps alone have effected dramatic changes in hundreds of people following the Wahls Diet, and you can expect dramatic changes, too.

Additional Prescriptions

Although adding the 9 cups and avoiding gluten and dairy are the keys, I would also like you to consider eliminating a few more things at the Wahls Diet level that will help reduce the chances of food sensitivity reactions:

- Eggs. As I've mentioned before, give your body a break from eggs to see if you are sensitive. Many people are but don't realize it until they remove eggs from their diets.
- Nonorganic soy (which can lead to excess inflammation)
- Nonorganic soy or rice milk
- High-fructose corn syrup
- Refined sugar (like white and brown sugar)
- Artificial sweeteners and monosodium glutamate (which can lead to excitotoxicity, overstimulation of brain cells, which leads to strained brain cells, and an unfavorable gut bacteria balance, like that on a sugar and high-carbohydrate diet)
- All trans-fat, hydrogenated, or partially hydrogenated oil
- Any vegetable oil, especially corn, soybean, canola, grape seed, and palm kernel (We'll discuss oils and fats more in chapter 7.)
- Any soda, including diet soda

In addition, I prefer that you not eat food that has been irradiated or microwaved. My preference is to have food that is in as natural a state as possible. Treating food with either microwave energy or ionizing radiation reacts with the food at the molecular level to either heat it (microwave) or kill microbes (ionizing radiation). I'd rather eat food that is fresh, local, and handled and prepared in ways that food has been prepared (raw, cooked, or fermented) for hundreds of generations. Personally, I also believe microwaved food tastes strange.

WAHLS DIET AT A GLANCE

Note: Eat to satiety. You may increase or decrease the amount of vegetables, fruit, and meat you eat according to your size, but make sure to do so in proportion.

- Consume 9 cups of vegetables and fruits daily, divided as follows (or proportionately to what you can consume without feeling gorged):

- 3 cups green leaves
- 3 cups sulfur-rich (cabbage family, onion family, and/or mushrooms)
- 3 cups bright color (yellow-orange, red, or purple-blue-black)
- Eat grass-fed or wild-caught meats and fish (6 to 12 ounces per serving, depending on your size and gender). I recommend minimizing processed meats like sausage, ham, bacon, or salami, but if you like them, look for gluten- and nitrite-free and monosodium-glutamate-free products.
- If you are a vegetarian, consume adequate calories and eat a varied diet including vegetables, grains, legumes, nuts, seeds, beans, and soy. You should take 2 tablespoons of flax, hemp, or walnut oil. You may include soy in your diet, but it should be organic, non-GMO (i.e., not a genetically modified organism—the package should state that it is non-GMO), and if you are a vegetarian and consuming soy frequently, I recommend you eat fermented soy, like pickled tofu, tempeh, natto, or miso. (More information about why fermenting is important if consuming soy regularly is in chapter 6.)
- You may eat gluten-free starch, like gluten-free grains or potatoes, but try not to overdo it. Ideally, you won't have them every day. Vegetarians, however, will need to eat more gluten-free grains to ensure complete protein.

What you can enjoy in moderation:

- Apples, bananas, and pears, although they do not count toward the 9 cups and should be eaten only after meeting the 9 cups goal.
- Nuts and seeds (including raw almond butter, tahini, and sunflower seed butter), up to 4 ounces per day
- Non-grain-based alcohol (like wine, preferably organic, or gluten-free beer), up to 1 serving per day (optional)
- Sweeteners, up to 1 teaspoon per day (honey, molasses, real maple syrup, and raw sugar or natural evaporated cane juice)
- Omega-3 oils (flax, hemp, walnut), cold only (do not cook with these!),

and no more than 2 tablespoons per day (unless directed otherwise by your physician)

- Other oils (olive oil; rarely use sesame oil, avocado oil), cold-pressed only (Make sure these products are organic and non-GMO.)

Forbidden foods:

- All gluten-containing foods
- All dairy-containing foods
- Eggs
- Non-organic soy or rice milk
- White sugar, high-fructose corn syrup, and artificial sweeteners, including soda and diet soda
- All trans-fat, hydrogenated oil, and omega-6-rich vegetable oils (corn, soybean, canola, and cottonseed oils)
- Preservatives and flavor-enhancers, including monosodium glutamate
- No microwaved or irradiated foods!

Wahls Diet Rules and Meal Plan

Now you know the reasons. Let's get to the method. Practicing the Wahls Diet is simple. The following chart summarizes the key components of what you should eat on the Wahls Diet, including amounts, with guidance on how often to eat certain allowed foods. Afterward, find a seven-day meal plan to launch you successfully into the Wahls Diet.

Helpful hint: Breakfast is going to change. You will be dropping the emphasis on grains. Instead, you will be focusing on vegetables, fruit, and high-quality protein.

Note to vegetarians: Even if you are vegetarian and therefore do not plan to progress beyond the Wahls Diet level, please read the other diet plans in the next two chapters; there is still a great deal of information there that is highly relevant to you.

Wahls Diet Week

All foods that have corresponding recipes at the end of this book are marked with an asterisk (*). Also note that I sometimes recommend almond milk, soy milk, or coconut milk. This is for the sake of variety but feel free to substitute any of these for any other at this stage of the diet.

	Breakfast	*Lunch*	*Dinner*
Day 1	Smoothie: • 1 cup kale • 1 small orange • 1 cup pineapple • 1 cup unsweetened organic soy milk • 1 tablespoon nutritional yeast 1 serving Rosemary Chicken* (prepared the night before)	Salad: • 2 cups kale • 1 cup bok choy • 1 small tomato • 2 teaspoons extra virgin olive oil • rice vinegar to taste 4 ounces sardines in tomato sauce 1 cup raw turnips 1 medium peach	1 serving Red Chili with Beans* 1 cup brown rice ¼ Hass avocado Salad: • 3 cups romaine lettuce • 1 medium stalk celery • ½ cup mushrooms • 1 clove garlic • dried basil to taste • 2 teaspoons extra virgin olive oil • rice vinegar to taste 6 ounces plain coconut milk yogurt ¾ cup blackberries Tension Tamer® herbal tea
Day 2	Smoothie: • 1 cup parsley • 1 cup green grapes • 1 kiwi • 1 tablespoon nutritional yeast • water/ice 1 cup oatmeal or brown rice hot cereal • 1 teaspoon blackstrap molasses • ⅓ cup raisins • 2 tablespoons chopped walnuts ½ cup unsweetened organic soy milk	1 serving Basic Skillet Recipe* (Ham and Collards) 1 cup chopped baked sweet potato • 1 teaspoon extra virgin olive oil • ⅛ teaspoon cinnamon 1 cup raspberries 1½ cups unsweetened organic soy milk	1 serving Basic Skillet Recipe* (Lamb Chops with Broccoli) Salad: • 4 cups spinach • ½ cup orange sections • ¼ cup sliced assorted mushrooms • ¼ cup chopped onions • 1 tablespoon extra virgin olive oil • vinegar to taste 1 medium apple with skin 1 serving Wahls Fudge* peppermint herbal tea

	Breakfast	Lunch	Dinner
Day 3	Smoothie: • 1 cup spinach • 1 cup honeydew melon • 1 kiwi • 1 cup unsweetened almond milk • 1 tablespoon nutritional yeast 1 serving leftover Basic Skillet Recipe* (Lamb Chops with Broccoli) ½ cup sliced carrots 6 dates	1 serving Salmon Salad* 8 gluten-free rice crackers Salad: • 3½ cups spinach • ½ cup raspberries • ½ cup raw zucchini slices • 2 teaspoons extra virgin olive oil • balsamic vinegar to taste Fruit cup: • 1 cup watermelon • 1 cup honeydew melon 1 cup unsweetened almond milk	1 serving Basic Skillet Recipe* (Steak and Mustard Greens) 1 serving Quinoa and Red Peppers* 1 cup cubed winter squash 2 teaspoons clarified butter 1 serving Wahls Fudge* 1 medium pear 1 cup unsweetened organic soy milk Detox herbal tea
Day 4	Smoothie: • 1 cup kale • 1 small orange (1 cup) • 1 cup unsweetened organic soy milk • 1 tablespoon nutritional yeast 1½ ounces raw almonds 6 dried apricot halves 4 dried prunes	1 serving Wahls Pizza* 1 medium raw carrot 1 cup black grapes 2 cup unsweetened organic almond milk	1 serving Seafood-Tomato Soup* ½ cup boiled potato with skin Salad: • 3½ cups romaine lettuce • ½ cup cilantro • 1 garlic clove • ¼ cup green peas • 2 teaspoons extra virgin olive oil • lime juice to taste 6 ounces almond milk yogurt 1 cup strawberries ½ cup banana Throat Coat™ herbal tea

	Breakfast	*Lunch*	*Dinner*
Day 5	Smoothie: • ½ cup raw beets • ½ cup mango • ½ cup blueberries • 1 cup unsweetened organic soy milk • ½ teaspoon grated gingerroot • 1 tablespoon nutritional yeast 3–4 ounces sardines canned in oil 2 slices gluten-free bread ½ cup celery	• Wahls Spaghetti: • 1 cup cooked spaghetti squash • ¾ cup marinara sauce • 3 ounces ground beef • ¼ cup mushrooms • 2 tablespoons Rawmesan* 1 cup green beans Salad: • 3 cups bok choy • ½ cup summer squash • 1 clove garlic • 2 teaspoons extra virgin olive oil • lime juice to taste 2 medium plums 1 cup unsweetened organic soy milk	1 serving Algerian Vegetarian* 1 serving Quinoa and Red Peppers* 1 cup cooked butternut squash Salad: • 3 cups bok choy • ½ cup tomato • ½ cup cucumber with peel • ½ cup grapes • 1 clove garlic • 3 teaspoons sunflower butter • lime juice to taste 8 ounces coconut milk yogurt 1 cup peaches 2 tablespoons almonds chamomile herbal tea
Day 6	Smoothie: • 1 cup cilantro • 1 small orange • 1 cup pineapple • 1 tablespoon nutritional yeast • water/ice 1 cup grits ½ cup pink grapefruit sections 1 cup unsweetened organic soy milk	Salad: • 3 cups bok choy • 2 cups romaine lettuce • ¼ Hass avocado • ½ cup tomato • ½ cup sweet red peppers • ½ cup mushrooms • 2 tablespoons almonds • 2 teaspoons extra virgin olive oil • lime juice to taste 1 medium chicken breast without the skin Fruit Cup: • 1 medium banana • ½ cup grapes	1 serving Basic Skillet Recipe* (Salmon and Mustard Greens) 1 serving Mashed Turnips* 1 teaspoon extra virgin olive oil 1 cup green peas Fruit Cup: • 1 medium peach • ½ cup unsweetened cherries 1 cup unsweetened organic soy milk rooibos herbal tea

	Breakfast	Lunch	Dinner
Day 7	Smoothie: • 1 cup collards • ½ cup watermelon • ½ cup muskmelon • 1 cup unsweetened organic soy milk • 1 tablespoon nutritional yeast 6 ounces almond milk yogurt • ½ cup unsweetened cherries • 4 tablespoons chopped walnuts	1 serving Vegetarian Kale Soup* 15 gluten-free rice crackers Salad: • 2 cups spinach • 2 cups kale • 4 florets cauliflower (½ cup) • 1 clove garlic • ½ cup raw mushrooms • 2 tablespoons chopped almonds • 2 teaspoons flax oil • Bragg apple cider vinegar to taste (lime juice would work as well) 1 cup pineapple	1 serving Basic Skillet Recipe* (Pork Chops and Red Cabbage) 1 small (2-inch diameter) baked potato with skin 1 teaspoon extra virgin olive oil 6 medium spears asparagus 1 cup blueberries herbal tea

SNACK IDEAS

- Dried raisins and nuts
- Fresh raw walnuts, almonds, or sunflower seeds
- Sliced apples (after your 9 cups are in!) dipped in organic almond butter
- Dried mango slices
- Dehydrated kale chips
- Pickled herring and gluten-free crackers
- Guacamole and sliced raw vegetables
- Eggplant dip (roasted eggplant and crushed garlic and olive oil blended in a food processor) with raw vegetable slices (turnip, rutabaga, kohlrabi, celery)
- Fresh fruit
- Nitrite-free deli meat rolled up with a lettuce leaf, pickle, and mustard
- Green tea sweetened with fruit juice
- Green tea with coconut milk

Chapter 6

WAHLS PALEO

Now that you are on the Wahls Diet, you are likely already experiencing some benefits. Maybe you feel a change in your energy, or your mental clarity, or maybe you are already noticing some mobility differences. If you are feeling good, you may decide it is time to take it to the next level. Or maybe you have decided to start here because you want to see faster results. Either way, welcome to Wahls Paleo, my most popular diet plan!

I would estimate that most of my patients end up at the Wahls Paleo Diet. They want a more powerful plan than the Wahls Diet, but they aren't quite ready for the extremes of Wahls Paleo Plus (see chapter 7). If you stay here, at the level of Wahls Paleo, rest assured you will be getting powerful medicine in the form of food, and your body will be free of many of the toxins that have hindered your healing in the past.

Wahls Paleo contains all the elements of the Wahls Diet, but with the addition of a few more elements. You will still eat your 9 cups of fruits and vegetables a day, keep gluten and dairy out of your diet, and consume high-quality protein. Now you'll also be doing these four things:

WAHLS PALEO DIET

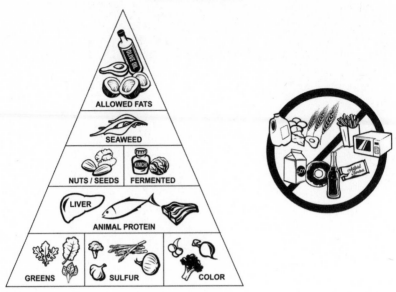

1. Reduce all remaining grains, legumes, and potatoes in your diet to just two servings per week.

2. Eat animal protein every day. You'll be eating more at this level than on the Wahls Diet. Shoot for between 9 and 21 ounces per day to get your protein intake high enough. (Adjust that according to your weight and gender: Small women may eat closer to 9 ounces, larger men may eat closer to 21 ounces.) Sixteen ounces per week of this allowance should be wild, cold-water fish.

3. Add seaweed and organ meat to your diet: ¼ teaspoon powdered kelp or 1 teaspoon dulse flakes per day, and 12 ounces of organ meat per week. (Organ meat is also included as part of your animal protein allowance.)

4. Add fermented foods, seeds and nuts (preferably soaked), and more raw foods to your diet. (I'll explain in this chapter how soaking can reduce the antinutrients in grains and legumes for those who are committed to the vegetarian diet for ethical or spiritual reasons.)

Let's look at each one of these items in turn. As in the last chapter, I have compared the average American diet to the mean intake on the Wahls Paleo,

Wahls Paleo		
Nutrient*†	U.S. Diet	Wahls Paleo
Vitamin D	31%	52%
Vitamin E	55%	108%
Calcium	74%	70%
Magnesium	88%	138%
Vitamin A	100%	523%
Pyridoxine	121%	638%
Folate	122%	251%
Zinc	123%	351%
Thiamin	128%	703%
Vitamin C	133%	661%
Niacin	154%	531%
Iron	164%	303%
Riboflavin	175%	781%
Vitamin B$_{12}$	201%	850%

* *Compared to dietary reference intakes, recommended dietary allowances (RDA) for females 51–70 years; Wahls Diet adjusted for 1,759 calories. (National Academy of Science; Institute of Medicine; Food and Nutrition Board)*

† *Average nutrient intake from food for females 50–59 years. (What We Eat in America, NHANES 2009–2010, www.ars.usda.gov/SP2UserFiles/Place/12355000/pdf/0910/Table_1_NIN_GEN_09.pdf, accessed 5/25/13)*

and once again, you can see that Wahls Paleo has markedly more nutrition for your cells!

Part One: Reducing Grains, Legumes, and Potatoes

At the Wahls Diet level, you eliminated gluten and dairy because of their potential for causing food sensitivities. Now it's time to cut the carbs down further. In our study, we allow people to have two servings of starchy non-gluten grains like brown rice, starchy vegetables like potatoes, or legumes like lentils or chickpeas each week, but acknowledge that going entirely grain-, legume-, and potato-free is ideal. (I'll encourage you to do that at the Wahls Paleo Plus level, but it's never required. I understand how life can be in the

WAHLS DIARY ALERT

If you decide to transition from the Wahls Diet to Wahls Paleo, be sure to track exactly what you change in your diet and report how you feel. Do you notice any improvements in your symptoms? Any side effects? This can help you pinpoint which foods work best for you and also inspire you to stick with your new level of dietary commitment. Stay inspired!

real world!) Many of our subjects are mostly grain-, legume-, and potato-free but have these foods only very occasionally, usually when social situations make it difficult to say no. Feel free to be similarly strict if you are so inspired.

This limit sometimes baffles people because they believe that foods like brown rice, lentils, and potatoes are healthy foods. In some ways, they are. They contain vitamins, minerals, and protein, and they are gluten-free. Even gluten-free whole grains, legumes like black beans and lentils, and potatoes, however, contribute to increased insulin demand because they are also high in carbohydrates. Your pancreas still needs to manufacture and dump insulin into your bloodstream to keep your blood sugar stable as your body digests those carbohydrates, making you more likely to develop insulin resistance (more on this later in the book), which may increase your risk of early cognitive decline, depending on your genetics and other environmental risk factors. When you are battling chronic disease, especially one with brain symptoms, you don't need to do anything to diminish your brain's capacity for healthy functioning, and one of the primary goals of the Wahls Protocol is to maximize, not compromise, your brain function. Reducing your carbohydrate intake will also help reduce inflammation and improve your gastrointestinal health. Too many high-carbohydrate foods, even those that don't contain gluten, can also be detrimental to the balance of your microbiome (the bacteria in your gut) because the carbohydrates can act as fertilizer to sugar-loving bacteria and yeasts, and that can lead to many other health problems.

Nonstarchy vegetables and colorful vegetables and fruits like winter squash, beets, and berries also have carbohydrates, but they have far fewer carbs than grains, legumes, or potatoes, and often have more vitamins and minerals per calorie, which gives them a higher nutrient density than grains, potatoes, or legumes. For this reason, you may keep enjoying these vegetables and fruits at the Wahls Paleo level. They can increase insulin demand, but at a much more moderate level. We're working the worst things out of your diet a little at a time.

Even so, I encourage you to enjoy more nonstarchy vegetables (like green vegetables) than starchier choices like cooked beets and squash, and to enjoy those starchy vegetables raw or gently boiled or steamed, so that the food doesn't become completely soft and mushy. When starchy vegetables remain a bit crunchy, the starch in the vegetable is not so readily converted to sugar in the bloodstream. I also encourage you to begin eating a much greater percentage of vegetables than fruit at this level of the diet. To really ramp up the positive effects of Wahls Paleo, you are best off getting most of your nutrients from lower-carbohydrate, less insulin-demanding sources.

Part Two: Eat Animal Protein Every Day

If you aren't a vegetarian, you might already be doing this, but now I want to be sure that you're not only getting animal protein but getting *enough* animal protein. Animal protein is an incredibly important component of Wahls Paleo. You should eat 9 to 21 ounces of meat each day, according to your size and gender. Remember to choose organic, grass-fed, and wild-caught whenever possible.

Meat and fish are an essential part of the Wahls Paleo plan because of their unique nutrient profiles, yet I have found that even regular meat eaters tend to feel like they probably shouldn't be eating meat. They feel guilty. We have been indoctrinated to believe that a vegetarian diet is healthier, so I want to talk in a little more depth about meat as well as about vegetarianism.

For more than a decade I did not eat any meat, poultry, or fish, but I am now a firm believer in the importance of animal protein, especially for people suffering from chronic health issues. I recognize this is a controversial position, so I want to give you my reasons. Let's start by looking at the great benefits you will receive from eating animal protein.

Animal Protein Perk #1: Complete Protein

Our bodies need to manufacture proteins to conduct the business of life and make our cellular structures, many of which require complicated protein molecules. Those proteins are all manufactured from amino acids, which are classified in three ways: essential, conditionally essential, or nonessential. We must get the essential ones in our diets because we lack the machinery or enzymes to manufacture them internally. *Conditionally essential* means that we can manufacture the amino acids ourselves under the right conditions. Our body can manufacture nonessential amino acids, so we needn't get them through food.

Because there are so many amino acids we need, our bodies will go to drastic measures to get them if we don't provide them. For example, if we don't have the correct amino acids to make the proteins needed by the body, we will resort to autophagy ("eating of self"), meaning that we begin "eating" or cannibalizing and digesting some of our own muscle and organ cells. The

AFFORDING QUALITY ANIMAL PROTEIN

I prefer to spend my money in my community. Buying meat from a local farmer and paying a local butcher to process it keeps the money local and is often cheaper than buying meat in a supermarket because you can buy in bulk. In order to find farmers who are growing grass-fed, hormone-free meats in your area, contact your local county extension office. Many of the farmers who practice community-supported agriculture (CSA) for vegetable produce are also producing eggs and meat. If not, they will likely be aware of the farmers in the community who are and can give you recommendations about local farmers. You can even go out to the farm and see the operation itself to know that the farm animals are being raised humanely. I buy the majority of my meat directly from farmers I know. That way I know the animal was fed organic rations; lived outside, eating grasses and prairie plants; and, most important, was healthy. In addition, I make sure the animals have not been given antibiotics or hormones. In addition, organic organ meats are often much less expensive than the organic muscle meat.

body takes what it needs for its most essential tasks, even if it means sacrificing parts of itself that it deems less essential. This may be beneficial to us as in short-term fasting, in times when food is scarce, or in cases of famine, but it is obviously very harmful in the long term, compromising our ability to maintain our own muscle and organ integrity, leading to muscle wasting, weakness, and internal organ damage. High-quality proteins are essential for optimal health and function!

The great thing about meat is that it contains all of the essential amino acids. You get everything you need. Plants, however, do not contain all the amino acids necessary for your body. Grains are limited in their supply of lysine and/or threonine, and legumes are limited in the sulfur-containing amino acid methionine. That is why vegetarians need to eat a combination of grains and legumes to have all of the essential amino acids necessary to make complete proteins. You can do it, but it's trickier. If vegetarians eat only grains or only legumes, they are not consuming a complete protein and will need to digest some portion of their own bodies to get the missing amino acids (usually methionine, lysine, or threonine) to manufacture the proteins necessary for life.

Animal Protein Perk #2: Essential Fatty Acids

Essential fatty acids are the fats that our cells need but cannot make themselves. We must consume them or we can become deficient, to the detriment of our own health. These include alpha-linolenic acid (ALA), an omega-3 fatty acid, and linoleic acid (LA), an omega-6 fatty acid. In addition, there are two conditionally essential fats: docosahexaenoic acid (DHA), an omega-3 fatty acid, and gamma-linolenic acid (GLA), an omega-6 fatty acid. The conditionally essential fatty acids, DHA and GLA, are more likely to be required if the person has developed a brain problem, autoimmune problem, or disease involving too much inflammation.

For the first 2.5 million years of the human genus, *Homo*, and the first 500,000 years of our species, *Homo sapiens*, humans ate these omega-6 and omega-3 fatty acids at roughly a 1:1 ratio. We ate things like plants and seeds that had omega-6, but we also ate a lot of wild animals that foraged for grasses, other greens, and wild fish, all of which contain omega-3 fatty acids. This provided us with that 1:1 balance[1] associated with a lower risk of both neurological and cardiovascular diseases.[2]

Today, life, and the human diet, is much different. That ratio has been dramatically skewed in favor of omega-6 fatty acids, and the amount of omega-3 fatty acid has dramatically declined.[3] The introduction to the human diet of seed oils such as corn oil, soybean oil, and canola oil—which were originally considered waste products until World War II—as well as an increase in feeding animals grain rather than grass (reducing the omega-3 fatty acid content in their meat) led to the dramatic increase in omega-6 consumption. The current omega-6-to-omega-3 ratio for some Americans is as high as 15:1 or even 45:1!

When the ratio shifts so far toward omega-6 fatty acids, many of our chemical pathways tilt toward inflammation and the development of chronic disease.[4] As a result, we are much more likely to develop excessive inflammation in our blood vessels, leading to higher rates of autoimmune problems, atherosclerosis, heart disease, and mental health problems.[5] This can easily be reversed, however, by ramping up the amount of grass-fed meat and wild-caught fish in your diet (while simultaneously eliminating or markedly decreasing the amount of vegetable oil). On a vegetarian diet, it is especially difficult to achieve a 1:1 balance. (I'll explain this in more detail momentarily.)

Fish Sources of Omega-3 Fatty Acids	
(Adapted from the "Toolbox for Clinicians" from the 2013 International Symposium for Functional Medicine, June 1, 2013, held by the Institute for Functional Medicine)	
Fish (4-ounce serving)	*Omega-3 fatty acids*
Chinook salmon	2.1 g
Herring, pickled	1.9 g
Scallops	1.1 g
Halibut	0.6 g
Shrimp	0.4 g
Snapper	0.4 g
Tuna, yellowfin	0.3 g
Cod	0.3 g

Animal Protein Perk #3:
Bone and Joint Benefits

When traditional societies ate meat, they used the entire animal to maximize the health of the clan. Today we tend to focus on muscle meat only, but many other parts of an animal, such as chicken feet, contain beneficial nutrients that aren't contained in the muscle.

Bones, sinews, gristle, and cartilage were staples in the diets of traditional societies. These people typically made soups and stews from the bones, cartilage, and connective tissue of animals. This nourished the bones and joints of the people who drank that broth by providing collagen and compounds from the glucosamine/glycan family of molecules. I remember both of my grandmothers gnawing on the cartilage on the end of chicken bones. They told me that they needed that gristle for their joints. Unfortunately, I didn't value

> ## WAHLS WARRIOR Q & A
>
> **Q: Are there specific beneficial effects of the Wahls Protocol for neuropathy?**
>
> A: I believe it is quite artificial to consider damage to the peripheral nerves as distinct and very different from diseases that damage the spinal cord and brain. The peripheral nerves need the same important vitamins, minerals, antioxidants, and essential fats. They are also damaged by the same toxins and excessive inappropriate inflammation. In my clinics, I have seen several individuals with diabetic neuropathy and others with neuropathies in which we could not find the cause (idiopathic) respond quite favorably to adopting the Wahls Diet or Wahls Paleo Diet.

their wisdom at the time because I thought the whole practice a little bit disgusting. Now, however, I realize that they were doing what should come naturally to humans: taking advantage of a potent source of joint-healing compounds. I'm happy to say I now chew on that gristle and include those gnarly parts in soups and stews.

Bone broth is savory, comforting, and delicious, and although we don't know exactly how it happens, the glucosamine in bone broth tends to go straight to the joints, where it is most needed.[6] Nature's magic! Bone broth is also filled with all the minerals that our skeletons need, in addition to glutamine and other amino acids that are especially healing for someone suffering from a "leaky gut." Our intestinal cells prefer to use the amino acid glutamine (instead of blood sugar or glucose) as their primary fuel for operating their cellular machinery, so when they get enough, they heal internal damage more efficiently. A daily cup or two of bone broth is an excellent start to healing leaky gut.[7] The intestinal cells' preference for glutamine also explains why you suffer from body aches when you have the flu. Your body pulls glutamine from your muscles, leading to that deep muscle ache that accompanies many fever-related illnesses. Eating bone broth the next time you have a fever will likely reduce that achy feeling because you won't be pulling as much glutamine from your muscles. It's the secret to that old-fashioned chicken soup remedy—as long as you cook that soup broth with the chicken bones. Our great-grandmothers were very wise! (See the recipe section at the end of the book for an easy bone broth recipe.) There is no vegetarian substitute for bone broth.

The Potential Harm of Vegetarianism

I hope I've convinced you that meat has a lot of great benefits for your health, but maybe you don't care. You're a vegetarian and you plan to stay that way. I understand. You can be a vegetarian and still practice the Wahls Diet, but once you proceed to Wahls Paleo, vegetarianism is no longer an option. This surprises some people. Isn't vegetarianism the healthiest diet? Don't doctors say it's the best diet for your heart? Isn't meat bad for you? Since this is the level of the diet in which you can no longer be a vegetarian, I would like to take a moment to explain my reasons.

As a physician and researcher, I do not agree that a vegetarian diet is the healthiest diet for humans—and in fact I believe it can actually be harmful, particularly if it is not practiced carefully. Furthermore, I believe that my many years as a vegetarian could have helped trigger or at a minimum accelerate my multiple sclerosis. But I also understand that some people have strong religious, moral, or ethical reasons for not eating meat. I will not try to convince you that those beliefs are wrong.

However, as my own research has led me further and further down the path of eating for health, I have become a complete convert. I will never be a vegetarian again. Wahls Paleo combines the most healthful aspects of vegetarianism (the 9 cups of fruits and vegetables each day) with the best aspects of the traditional Paleo Diet (natural animal protein sources), and this is what I believe to be the best diet for human health.

Too many people become vegetarian and stop eating meat but continue eating a lot of highly processed foods, few vegetables, and no sources of complete protein, leading to increasingly severe deficiencies in essential fats, protein, vitamin, mineral, and antioxidant intake. Such diets put them at serious risk. Even for those vegetarians who are eating plenty of vegetables and protein, however, there are other compelling reasons why I believe a vegetarian diet can be harmful to your health.

Vegetarian Danger #1:
Skewing Your Fatty Acid Ratios

You know you need a better omega-6-to-omega-3 ratio, but what you may not know is that you probably won't get it eating only a vegetarian diet. There are many plant foods that are commonly advertised as being rich sources of omega-3 fatty acids, like flaxseeds, walnuts, and hempseeds. These foods are nutritious, and I eat them myself. These foods, however, not only contain high levels of omega-6 fatty acids (not something you typically hear about), they don't actually contain omega-3 fatty acids in the form our bodies need: docosahexaenoic acid (DHA) and eicosapentaenoic acid (EPA). Instead, they contain alpha-linolenic acid (ALA), which our bodies must convert to a more usable form. ALA is a shorter chain of molecules, and your cells need to lengthen the ALA through several steps to make the form of omega-3 fats that our cells most need: EPA and DHA. It is an inefficient process. Only about 5 percent (7 to 10 percent if you are pregnant) of the ALA you eat will get converted to DHA. You need to eat ten to twenty times the amount of ALA to get the equivalent amount of DHA made for your brain.

In studies comparing the effectiveness of high doses of olive oil, flaxseed oil, and fish oil in patients with ADHD, only those receiving the fish oil changed the ratio of omega-6 to omega-3 in the red cell membranes.[8] This is just one of many studies that show the superiority of fish oil to plant-based oils when it comes to improving the omega-6-to-omega-3 ratio. There is no question that the body benefits from the omega-3s in fish oil much more than it benefits from the omega-3 ALAs in plant foods.

Vegetarian Danger #2: Vegetable Oil

As long as we're on the subject of an ideal omega-6-to-omega-3 ratio, let's talk about vegetable oils, which are made by extracting the oils from seeds like corn, sunflower, or rapeseed (often using solvents like hexane, which is quite toxic). I already told you in the last chapter that I want you to limit consumption of these oils to a few specific types and eliminate most others, but let's look more closely at why.

Vegetable oil sounds healthy, but it is one of the richest sources of omega-6 fatty acids. As I explained earlier in this chapter, you need omega-6 fatty acids, but they should be in balance with omega-3 fatty acids, and most people today get much more omega-6 than omega-3. Eating vegetable oils only exacerbates this problem.

But this isn't just a matter of getting a slightly better fatty acid balance. For people with autoimmune conditions, too much omega-6 can actually be dangerous. Corn oil and soybean oil are the worst offenders. They drive the ratio of omega-6 to omega-3 way out of balance. For that reason I tell my patients never to eat any corn oil or soybean oil. Canola oil is often promoted as a source of omega-3 fatty acids, and it does contain more of these than some other vegetable oils. However, when you heat the canola oil, you break down the omega-3 fats so they become useless to your body. In addition, canola oil has more trans fat in it and can more easily generate trans fat as it is heated. Furthermore, most soybean, corn, and canola oils are made from GMOs, which I don't recommend for anyone with an autoimmune disease. I suggest you avoid all of them.

You may think olive oil is still a good choice, and yes, it is, on one condition: *that you never heat it!* The double bonds in olive oil are more likely to be damaged (oxidized) by heat, destroying much of the benefit. Also, the more than twenty different health-promoting polyphenols (antioxidants) that olive oil contains are destroyed when it is heated.[9] I'd rather you use it cold as part of a salad dressing so you can keep all those healthful antioxidants. Don't cook with olive oil! The best fats for cooking—the fats that remain most stable—are rendered animal fats like lard, tallow, or chicken fat. If you must use a plant-based oil, use coconut oil, which does not denature at high temperatures.

More bad news about vegetable oil: I bet you thought that trans fats were found only in processed foods, but you make them in your own kitchen and eat them unwittingly if you heat polyunsaturated oils. When vegetable oils are used for frying, especially deep-fat frying, the high heat will oxidize (damage) some of the bonds, increasing the risk of trans-fat formation. The higher the heat, the more trans fats are made, and the more vitamins and antioxidants are lost in the oil (and the foods you are frying)! The more often oil is reheated, the more trans fats will be created, which is why you should never reuse frying oil. This is just one more good reason to avoid fried foods in fast-

THE DANGERS OF TRANS FATS

Scientists first made trans fats back in the 1890s by adding hydrogen to fats (hydrogenation), which made them solid at room temperature. But these new fats didn't really enter the food supply until after World War II. One of the advantages of this new fat was that it was "spreadable" even under refrigeration. Also, a lot of money was spent on promoting the new cholesterol theory of heart disease, which emphasized replacing saturated fat with polyunsaturated fat (vegetable oil). The vegetable oil industry convinced the American public to replace butter with margarine (made of partially hydrogenated fats, which include trans fats) because the partially hydrogenated fats were believed healthier than the saturated fats contained in butter. How wrong they were!

Now we know trans fats are disease promoting. There is much solid research to confirm this. The trans-fat molecules are inserted into our cell membranes, making the membranes stiff, and interfering with the messaging between our cells. Trans fat confuses our cell biology as well, increasing the inflammation in our blood vessels and our brains and disrupting our hormone signaling.[10] The result is more rapid development of atherosclerosis (clogging of the arteries) and shrinking brains that have more difficulty communicating between the brain cells. Trans fats in the diet also increase the probability of developing obesity and diabetes. In a study by Bowman[11] I've mentioned previously in which scientists measured the thinking ability and brain sizes of older adults (average age 87), they also measured brain levels of vitamins, minerals, essential fatty acids and antioxidants, and the level of hydrogenated or trans fats in the blood. The more trans fats the study participants had, the more impaired their thinking ability and the smaller their brains.[12]

food restaurants. They certainly don't change out that french fry oil after every batch, and you can bet they use cheap vegetable oil, not lard, like they once did.

Vegetarian Danger #3:
Grains and Legumes

If you are a vegetarian, you likely eat a lot of grains and legumes. It's the easiest way to get your protein. Even if you go gluten-free based on the damage gluten may do to you when you have an autoimmune disease, you will still need to combine other nongluten grains (including whole grains) with legumes to get a sufficient amount of all the essential amino acids to make a complete protein. (You may have heard that it's not true that you must combine grains and legumes at the same meal, as long as you get enough variety over the course of a few days; but the truth is that combining grains and legumes at the same meal is probably still the easiest way to be certain you get all the amino acids you need at every meal.) But there are problems with even nongluten grains as well as with legumes. Grains and legumes contain several antinutrients that you'll get more of as a vegetarian, even if they're gluten-free. These antinutrients are phytates, lectins, and trypsin inhibitors. Phytate, or phytic acid, is inositol and phosphorous locked together, and it will chelate, or bind, minerals like zinc, iron, calcium, and magnesium, carrying them unused out of the body. In other words, phytates block the body's absorption of magnesium, calcium, and especially zinc, which can lead to mineral deficiencies.[13] Lectin is a type of sugar-protein molecule that can markedly increase inflammation in those with autoimmune problems and in the genetically vulnerable individual.[14] Trypsin inhibitors, which primarily exist in legumes, block the digestion of the proteins crucial to maintaining your health.[15] Your efforts to eat more protein by eating legumes may be foiled by the protein source itself!

There is a way to get around some of these inhibitors, however. Germination decreases the harm from the phytates and the lectins.[16] If you soak grains, legumes, seeds, and/or nuts to begin the germination process, the plant food will produce phytase, which reduces the activity of phytates, lectins, and trypsin inhibitors. That is why I advise vegetarians to soak their grains and legumes for twenty-four hours prior to eating and wash them carefully before cooking. This also decreases the cooking time for grains and legumes. It may seem like a time-consuming or unnecessary step, but it can make a big difference in how well your body absorbs protein and hangs on to valuable minerals!

WAHLS WARRIORS SPEAK

After being diagnosed with stage 3 colon cancer and choosing radical life changes over chemotherapy, I adopted a raw vegan diet, eating only fruits, vegetables, seeds, and nuts, and I drank eight glasses of vegetable juice every day (usually carrot, celery, beet, and gingerroot). I focused on eating cancer-fighting foods every day, especially vegetables from the cruciferous and allium families: broccoli, cauliflower, cabbage, kale, onions, and garlic. I ate giant salads for lunch and dinner. I also drank fruit smoothies every day with fresh young coconut, blueberries, raspberries, blackberries, straw-berries, and a banana.

However, I was not maintaining a healthy weight. After ninety days, at the recommendation of my naturopath, I added some clean meats back into my diet, including organic free-range chicken and eggs, wild-caught Alaskan salmon, and grass-fed beef and lamb. The addition of clean meats helped me gain and maintain a healthy weight, which I was not able to do as a raw vegan. When I discovered Dr. Wahls in 2012 through her TEDx talk, I was excited to see her success in using the healing power of nutrition and her mission to share it with others. The principles of her diet are iden-tical to the ones I followed to heal myself. I continue to follow the principles of the Wahls Diet and now I'm cancer-free. Whole foods from the earth support the body's ability to function at optimal levels: to detoxify, repair, and regenerate. They promote a healthy weight, give you energy, and make you feel good!

—*Chris W., Memphis, Tennessee*

Vegetarian Danger #4: Soy

Soy is one of the most popular forms of protein for people who don't eat ani-mal products, and vegetarians, especially in the United States, tend to be heavily reliant on soy products. If you are a vegetarian, it is likely that you consume a large amount of soy because so many easy-to-make vegetarian products like veggie burgers and veggie hot dogs are made from it, and many popular vegetarian dishes contain soy foods like tofu and tempeh. Then there is soy milk, soy cheese, soy ice cream . . . Soy is the only vegetarian protein that is considered complete by the USDA. Although some studies show some benefit to some soy products, especially for women nearing menopause, over-all soy is bad news when it is consumed in large amounts, particularly when it's not fermented.

My first concern is that 95 percent of soy products in the United States are genetically modified and do not have to be labeled as such. These geneti-cally modified crops are grown with many applications of glyphosate, a com-pound found in the herbicide Roundup that food giant Monsanto produces to control weeds in fields of genetically modified corn and soybeans. Glypho-sate has been shown to be toxic to human cells grown in the lab and also to confuse hormone signaling[17] and interfere with some of the enzymes used for processing and eliminating toxins.[18] The increased use of pesti-cides with all GMOs (genetically modified organisms) and the uncertain effects of genetic modifications are reason enough for me to avoid eating them. You now have to assume that everything not labeled organic is likely a GMO.[19]

Another concern is that soy, like other legumes, also contains phytic acid, which binds to minerals, especially magnesium, calcium, and zinc, so your cells can't readily use them; lectins, which can increase inflammation in the genetically vulnerable individual;[20] and trypsin inhibitors, which can inter-fere with digestion. Soy also contains phytoestrogens, which are plant-based compounds that can interact with the estrogen receptors in your body. These include isoflavones, genistein, and daidzein. In traditional cultures, soy was fermented, which helped to neutralize all of these things; but most of the soy we eat in this country is not fermented, so many of these antinutrients are still present in soy products like soy milk and tofu. Eating fermented soy prod-ucts like tempeh and miso, as has been done in traditional Asian societies, has far fewer health risks. If you're eating a lot of soy, it is better to have it be both labeled specifically as non-GMO and also in a fermented form such as tempeh, miso, or natto.

Just in case that's not enough evidence for why vegetarianism is a nutri-

---

LOVE YOUR SOY PROTEIN SMOOTHIE?

Do you make your smoothie with soy protein powder? Soy in the form of isolated protein powder is a very recent addition to the human diet. These highly processed products are often manufactured at temperatures that denature (change the shape of) the proteins, making them harder to digest.[21] We also have no historical way to predict how these fake-food meal replacement products will impact human health in the long term. Remember, scientists once told us that trans fats were better for us than butter and therefore health promoting. It took years to discover that trans fats are in fact harmful. Keep drinking those smoothies, but instead of using processed soy protein powder, just mix fresh or frozen berries and a big handful of leafy greens with some nuts or nut butter and coconut milk. Add ice or not, a little cinnamon if you like it, and enjoy, protein-powder-free!

---

tionally inferior diet, consider these additional facts relevant to what you are or are not getting if you eat a vegetarian diet:

- Animal products are the only true sources of premade vitamins A (retinol) and D (cholecalciferol). Vegetables contain beta-carotene, which the body can convert to vitamin A, but the efficiency of this varies with the individual and some people can't do this very well.[22] Having some preformed vitamin A in the diet is helpful. Vitamin A is necessary for vision, bone health, reproductive health, and immune health. The best source of vitamin D is the sun, but you can also get vitamin D from fish and ghee (clarified butter). Vitamin D is important to brain health, bone health, immune cell health, and the proper reading of your DNA. Liver and cod-liver oil are both good sources of premade vitamin A and vitamin D. Our wise grandmothers knew to give cod-liver oil to children each day.
- To absorb cobalamin (vitamin B_{12}), your body will link intrinsic factor (made in the stomach) to the cobalamin molecule (obtained through diet). Because intrinsic factor only attaches well to the animal form of cobalamin, your gut cannot readily absorb cobalamin from bacterial and

algal sources. The richest source of cobalamin is liver and other organ meats. Nutritional yeast has cobalamin added to it in a form that can be absorbed, so use this liberally if you are a vegetarian. I also recommend supplementing with sublingual (under the tongue) methyl B_{12}. Methyl B_{12} is the form our brains need, and taking it sublingually means you don't need intrinsic factor in order to absorb it.

- If you've followed a vegetarian and/or vegan diet for years, there is a greater risk of developing low stomach acid, which makes you less efficient at absorbing vitamin B_{12} (in addition to the intrinsic-factor issue mentioned above) and many minerals.[23] This can lead to a higher risk of brain and heart problems, osteoporosis, and an unhealthy balance of bacteria in the bowels, which in turn can lead to leaky gut syndrome and greater risk of autoimmune problems.

In closing this argument, I want to emphasize that I am not trying to "bash" vegetarians or vegans. I am only telling you what I believe is the optimal diet for those suffering from autoimmune or other chronic health conditions. You need every possible avenue to heal and maximize your health. I believe that includes animal protein, but the choice is yours.

WAHLS WARRIORS SPEAK

In August 2012, I was diagnosed with multiple sclerosis. The symptoms came on suddenly: tingling and numbness in my right arm and right and left hands, bladder urgency, cognitive issues and brain fog, lower back pain, and right-foot drop. One Saturday, I was playing golf, and by the next Friday, I was using a cane to walk. I was scared and I did not know what was happening. I was started on a five-day treatment of IV steroids. I began physical and occupational therapy, and speech therapy to assist with my word-finding issues.

Desperate, I searched the Internet and read as much as I could about multiple sclerosis. I tried to discuss diet with my neurologist because I read that people with autoimmune diseases may benefit from going gluten-free.

My neurologist recommended that I stick with my "balanced" diet because gluten-free may be a fad and it was difficult to do. In October 2012, I went to a holistic practitioner who recommended that I eliminate gluten, dairy, and eggs from my diet and then take an allergy test. About that time, I discovered Dr. Wahls, whose story provided me hope. I began to incorporate the 9 cups of produce and to eat organic lean meat, lots of wild fish, seaweed, and some organ meat (though I still struggle with that). My allergy tests came back and, sure enough, I was highly sensitive to gluten, dairy, eggs, soy, and almonds. This test further validated Dr. Wahls's work.

By eliminating highly inflammatory foods and replacing them with vegetables, lean meat, and seaweed, your body can heal. It's been four months since I started the Wahls Diet, and I've increased my vitamin D levels from 17 to 52, my medicine has been reduced, and I have lost 14 pounds. I now exercise and run two miles several times per week, walk three miles a day, bike, swim, strength train, meditate, and stretch daily. I prepare smoothies and real meals in my kitchen. Gone are the days of eating out or ordering takeout three to four times a week. By eating this way, my energy levels have increased, my brain fog and stumbling over words has been eliminated, my skin looks great, and I am more alert and present. It is not easy eating this way, and my family has also had to make some adjustments, but, in the end, I choose health. I am more in tune with my body and I feed it the fuel it needs to thrive.

—*Michelle M., Baltimore, Maryland*

Part Three: Add Seaweed and Organ Meat

Our ancient ancestors were scavengers and hunters on African savannas millions of years ago. Food was precious, so if we killed a small animal, we ate the liver, heart, kidney, and brain, in addition to the muscle meat. We also benefited from the kills of larger predators, like lions. When lions killed their prey, they smartly ate the organ meats first. The hyenas and jackals ate the muscle meat. Our ancestors, however, were able to use early tools to break open the remaining skulls and long bones and eat the brains and marrow, which are rich sources of DHA, a key nutrient for brain growth.

We also waded in coastal waters and ate whole shellfish, again using our early tools to pry open the clams and mussels we found. Seaweed and sea vegetables, rich with iodine and dense concentrations of minerals, were also on the menu. These adaptations are widely believed to be what gave us the competitive advantage to survive and grow larger, more complex brains.[24] If we want to keep those big brains, we need to feed ourselves and our children more parts of the animals we eat and more vegetables from the sea, packing our diets even more full of vitamins, minerals, and antioxidants.

You: Sea Creature?

Life began more than 3 billion years ago in mineral-rich seas. Our bloodstream mineral content reflects those ancient seas: We still have a little of the ocean within us. I believe this is why the human body responds so favorably to the plant foods that grow in the oceans. Seaweed contains intense mineral nutrition as well as beneficial vitamins. Eat romaine lettuce and kale all day if you like, but adding seaweed will take your nutrition to a whole new level.

Seaweed has been used medicinally, in spas, and in food, for thousands of years.[25] Traditional peoples traveled great distances or traded to ensure access to seaweed. They may not have known that seaweed provides a rich supply of minerals, but somehow they knew the value of this important food source. Traditional coastal communities in particular have naturally consumed seaweed as part of their diets, and historically Japanese and Okinawans have had 10 to 15 percent of their diet come from seaweed. These cultures have a much lower rate of heart disease, diabetes, and autoimmune problems, even though the rate of smoking and salt consumption is higher in the Japanese and Okinawans. However, as the young people abandon the traditional diets in favor of Westernized diets high in simple sugars and refined carbohydrates, we have seen the incidence of those chronic diseases steadily climb.

Sea vegetables contain nutrient profiles you can't get anywhere else. In particular, they are rich sources for iodine, which has many important functions in the body.[26] The thyroid gland, the gland that directs the metabolism and energy level of the body, is highly dependent upon iodine. In addition, the white blood cells use iodine as part of their arsenal in attacking and killing invading viruses, bacteria, and cancer cells. Iodine also helps the body properly process and then eliminate heavy metals like lead and mercury. If your diet has been low in minerals, vitamins, and antioxidants, and you or someone in your family has a history of brain or heart problems, it is more likely that you have stored some toxins such as lead and mercury in your fat, which includes the fat in your brain. When you are low in iodine, you are more likely to have problems with an enlarged thyroid or goiter and underactive thyroid gland (hypothyroidism). You are also more likely to have problems clearing infections like Lyme disease.

Iodine and trace mineral intake has steadily declined in the United States over the course of the last half century, in part because physicians have been telling patients to cut back on salt. Iodized salt has been the primary source of iodine for most Americans. To make matters worse, we've been steadily adding to our diets halogen compounds that interfere with the iodine receptors in our cells, primarily through the addition of fluoride and chlorine to the water supply and bromine to the food supply. Because these halogens are chemically similar to iodine, they compete for the iodine receptors. (Some foods—including soy, flax, and the cabbage family vegetables, if consumed raw—can also slightly interfere with iodine uptake, but the benefits of these foods, as long as they are not consumed excessively, outweigh this consideration.)

Thus, our daily requirement for iodine has increased at the same time that our intake has fallen. It is true we are taking in far more salt and that doctors advise against this trend, but the salt we tend to eat the most is the kind in processed foods, and that salt is generally not the iodized kind. Americans cook less at home, so they use less iodized salt or choose other types of salt. In response to falling iodine levels, hypothyroidism levels have steadily climbed, with some estimates putting the level of American women affected at 10 to 25 percent, all largely a result of iodine insufficiency.[27] Fortunately for you, you needn't add more salt to your diet to get more iodine. Seaweed is a rich natural source of iodine.

Seaweed also contains many valuable minerals, including calcium, copper,

WAHLS WARNING

Because of the radiation release following the Japanese earthquake and subsequent tsunami in 2011, and the partial meltdown of the nuclear reactors that followed, many wonder about the safety of seaweed from Japan and China. These days, I am purchasing my seaweed from companies located in Canada and Maine. For convenience, I look for powdered kelp and dulse flakes that have been harvested from clean waters, are sustainably harvested and labeled organic, and have been tested for radioactivity, heavy metals, and pesticide content to provide added safety. You can also purchase dried seaweed from the companies listed in the Resources section.

chromium, iron, iodine, lithium, manganese, magnesium, potassium, selenium, silicon, sulfur, vanadium, and zinc. You'll also get vitamins in the vitamin B group (B_1, B_2, B_3, B_5, B_6, B_9) and vitamins A, C, E, and K. Other useful compounds include alginates, which are very helpful in increasing the elimination of solvents, plastics, heavy metals, and even radioactivity in the body,[28] and U-fucoidans, which improve the effectiveness of the white blood cells in fighting chronic viral infections.[29]

There are thousands of different seaweeds, which are categorized into three groups: green, brown, and red. The colors indicate which type of chlorophyll is present in the plant. The green seaweeds, such as sea lettuce, must grow in shallow water near the shore. The brown seaweeds can grow a hundred feet below the surface, and the red seaweeds can grow four hundred feet below the surface. Ideally, we should be consuming all colors of seaweed for optimal benefit.

This isn't as difficult as it sounds. You might not have noticed, but your local supermarket may carry some sea vegetables and your natural foods store almost certainly has at least a few packaged varieties to choose from. Seaweed comes in various forms, including fresh, reconstituted, flakes, and powdered. The supplement section may also include powdered versions. If you go to

IF YOU ARE ON THYROID MEDICATION, READ THIS FIRST

If you are being treated for an under- or overactive thyroid, adding seaweed to the diet will likely change the amount of thyroid medication that you require. Check in with your physician for guidance. Slowly add seaweed to the diet, starting with once a week, adding seaweed to the foods you are cooking. Gradually increase the frequency and amount of seaweed you are adding, and check in with your physician to monitor your thyroid levels. You may find that your medication needs to be adjusted downward (very rarely upward). Go gradually and work with your personal physician.

Asian food markets, you will be able to find large bags of a wide variety of seaweeds.

If you are not being treated with thyroid medication, I suggest you start with a small amount of seaweed every other day for a month. I'd also mix up the types of seaweeds you eat. The simplest is to alternate between kelp powder and dulse flakes. Start with ¼ teaspoon every other day for a month. If that is going well, then you can go to the equivalent of ¼ teaspoon every day for a month. It is best if you are adding seaweed to what you are cooking and eating. That way your taste for the food will help guide how much you are consuming. Alternatively, if you can find fresh seaweed or dried seaweed, you can add that to your cooking. The point is to gradually increase the seaweed and to use a variety of seaweeds.

Here's how much seaweed I would like you to work up to eating every day on Wahls Paleo. Choose one of the following each day:

- **Fresh (or soaked and reconstituted):** 2.5 ounces. One ounce of dried seaweed will reconstitute to about 1 cup of fresh seaweed.
- **Dried flakes:** 1 teaspoon in the form of flakes
- **Powdered:** ¼ teaspoon

Organ-ize Yourself

I get even more resistance from my patients about eating organ meats than I do about eating seaweed. I'm not sure why, because just a few generations ago, organ meats were a common part of Western diets. I have my great-grandmother's cookbook, an 1890 edition of *Compendium of Cookery and Book of Knowledge*, and my grandmother's 1939 *Fanny Farmer Cookbook*. Both cookbooks include many recipes for a wide variety of organ meats. My great-grandmother had recipes for boiled calf's head, sweetbreads, brains, tongue, tripe, heart, and liver, all of which were designed for cooking over a fire or a woodstove. I remember my own mother making liver and onions at least once a week, and we kids all ate a good helping. For some reason, however, Americans have become squeamish about this healthful habit.

Weston A. Price, in his studies of the diets of traditional societies around the globe, analyzed organ meats and found them full of what he called "powerful activators" (the term *vitamins* had not yet been adopted).[30] Animal proteins, particularly the organ meats, concentrate fat-soluble and water-soluble vitamins. Liver is the richest source of the whole family of B vitamins and is the best source of vitamin B_{12}. The organ meats, liver in particular, are rich sources of vitamin A (retinol), which is critical for many functions in our cells. Liver also contains premade vitamin D (cholecalciferol). The organ meats are excellent sources of easily absorbed zinc, magnesium, phosphorous, and other minerals.

The liver, heart, kidneys, and other organ meats are potent sources of both the fat-soluble vitamins, D, A, E, and K, as well as potent sources of B vitamins and in an organic, grass-fed animal, good sources of the essential fatty acids, including desirable omega-3s. Organ meats are also excellent sources of creatine, carnitine, alpha-lipoic acid, and ubiquinone (which is coenzyme Q), all of which are needed for optimal functioning of the mitochondria. Although we can manufacture coenzyme Q when we are young, by the time we are 50 years old, our capacity for doing so slowly declines (rapidly with some medications, especially the statin family of medications, which are used to treat elevated cholesterol).

Organ meats have a more intense taste than muscle meats, so they might take some getting used to, but there are good ways to prepare them. Here are some key points:

- **Eat organ meats several times each week, for a total of 12 ounces per week.** Leave the organ meats as rare as you are comfortable eating them. Well-done organ meats will be dry, tough, and less pleasant to eat. Gently cooked organ meats will be juicier and tastier, and retain more vitamins.
- **Start with heart.** Heart may the easiest to start with because you will think you are having a good steak. Note that heart is the best source of coenzyme Q that we have.
- **Cut up the liver into small chunks and then blend the chunks with water to make a liver slurry.** This could be added to the next soup or chili as another way to "hide" the organ meat. Or try making pâté.
- **Add kelp or dulse to organ meat recipes to enrich your recipes with more trace minerals.** Add this to a recipe along with the liver slurry and you've got seaweed and organ meat in one dish!

For recipe ideas, see the recipe section at the end of this book.

WAHLS WARRIORS SPEAK

I was diagnosed with MS in July 2012 and, honestly, I was not sure what to expect with it. Since my diagnosis, and thanks to my sister, I jumped rather quickly on trying to fix it and immediately started doing extensive research on the Wahls Diet. I have always been very active and fit, and I thought my diet was always good, but now I know I was consuming hormones and chemicals. I now eat only organic, hormone-free food. I make a smoothie every morning consisting of about 3 cups of kale; parsley; sprouted sesame, sunflower, and pumpkin seeds; sprouted walnuts; ginger; sea salt; spirulina powder; BioKefir immunity; and a few different fruits. This makes almost 64 ounces for my breakfast and lunch smoothies. I try to eat organ meat once per week, and I also eat wild-caught fish several times a week, California sushi rolls, and seaweed salad. I stay clear of the foods tests have shown I'm allergic to, one of which is dairy, and I had all six of my fillings that had mercury in them replaced. I am working hard to follow Dr. Wahls's recommendations in full and I am happy with my health.

—DeLeia A., Indianapolis, Indiana

Part Four: Add More Raw, Soaked, and Fermented Foods

Enzymes are catalysts that make it easier for your body to do its work. They facilitate chemical reactions like those necessary for digestion and the absorption of nutrients. As we age, our effectiveness at manufacturing enzymes declines. In the presence of a nutritionally inadequate diet, the situation gets worse. By supplying some of the digestive enzymes we need in the foods we eat, we can ensure more effective digestion and absorption of nutrients.[31] There are three good ways to do this:

1. Eat more raw foods.
2. Eat more soaked foods.
3. Eat more fermented foods.

Let's consider these one at a time.

Raw Deal

In the beginning, our ancestors ate all of their food raw. Even when we began cooking our foods approximately 500,000 years ago, we still consumed a large proportion of it raw, including meat. Cooking foods breaks down cell walls, making some of the digestive processes easier and allowing for more absorption of the minerals and vitamins, but all raw plant- and animal-based foods are loaded with enzymes that trigger the digestion process for that food. However, once the food is heated above 117 degrees Fahrenheit, all those helpful digestive enzymes are denatured (i.e., the shapes change), which means they are no longer biologically active and have been, in essence, destroyed. Considering how much potent nutritional power animal protein has, it would be a shame not to absorb it all; yet, that's what many people do when they cook—and especially when they overcook—their meat and vegetables.

Here's an interesting example of this principle in action: The first explorers of the Arctic region, who carted along their Westernized cooked rations, all died. The explorers who followed them and chose to eat according to Inuit traditions (raw meat) survived and even put on weight during their extreme experience, even though they were not native to that area or climate. Many hunter-gatherer and traditional diets include not just raw vegetables and fruits, nuts and seeds, but raw meats and fish in their diets, as well as fermented meat and pickled meat, which is only "cooked" via the fermentation or pickling solution rather than heat.[32]

WAHLS WARNING

If you choose to eat raw meats, be sure to store the meat in a deep freeze for at least two weeks before consuming, then marinate the meat in vinegar and salt for twenty-four hours prior to consumption. This will decrease the probability of bacteria and parasitic contamination but does not take it down to zero, so be aware of the very real risk of infection if you choose to do this. This risk is especially high with factory-farmed and feedlot meat.

WAHLS WARRIORS SPEAK

Since changing my eating habits, I have not had an MS symptom in more than four weeks. My skin has cleared up, I sleep better, I have stopped taking my acid-reflux medicine, and my dizziness and balance issues have been significantly reduced. I am on the Wahls Paleo Diet, and I don't eat anything prepackaged unless it is grass-fed meats. I am grain-free, sugar-free, soy-free, and chemical-free; I go organic as much as possible; and I eat plenty of veggies and colors. I like that I am discovering new and colorful foods that taste good! Everything is so much fresher now, and I also thoroughly enjoy the fact that I don't have the daily muscle spasms in my chest that felt like a heart attack! I exercise three to four times a week with biking, swimming, running, calisthenics, and a weekly yoga class. Dr. Wahls has been an inspiration and a great source of encouragement. If I had not seen her video on feeding your mitochondrias, I may not have even considered that what I eat could save me from pain and suffering.

—Jodi M., Thornton, Denver, Colorado

Today, unfortunately, there are health risks to eating raw meat, because when food is processed in massive amounts—mixing meat from hundreds of animals, as it is done at the large meat processing plants—contamination of meat from unhealthy animals is more likely. Because of the health risk of contaminated meat, particularly in conventionally raised animals housed in massive operations, I generally don't recommend raw meat. There are times and situations where it could be appropriate: a well-prepared steak tartare from a trustworthy source, for example, or sushi from a responsible restaurant. However, one needs to be very cautious about where you are getting your meat if you elect to eat raw meats.

A much safer route is to include plenty of raw fruits and vegetables in your diet and to use low-temperature cooking, for as brief a time as possible, of clean, preferably organ meat obtained directly from a farmer you trust. Order your meat rare when you can, or at least as rare as possible for you to eat it happily, and enjoy pickled meat and fish when you can get them.

Raw fruits and vegetables are, of course, easy to find and eat. I like to include raw plant food with every meal, whether a big salad or fruit for dessert, or the mixture of fruits and greens I put into my smoothie. If raw food upsets your stomach, start slowly and eat small amounts as your system adjusts. Even a little raw food is better than no raw food.

Soaking and Sprouting

Another great way to generate more enzymes in the foods you eat is to soak and sprout them. Soaking seeds in water begins the sprouting (germination) process and helps neutralize some of the antinutrients in cereal grains and legumes. You can accomplish this by soaking these foods for twelve to twenty-four hours. Sprouting adds another level. When grains and legumes begin to sprout, enzymes are generated that aid in digestion and nutrient absorption. Soaking and sprouting helps you to get the nutritional benefits from these foods without the potential harm.

Although you will only be eating nongluten grains, legumes, and starchy vegetables twice a week on Wahls Paleo, choose soaked grains and legumes when you have the choice, for maximum benefit. Likewise, if you are consuming nuts and seeds, soak them first if you have the time. Nuts and seeds contain antinutrients, although at lower levels than grains and legumes. Still, soaking them helps to generate more healthful enzymatic activity.

But how do you do it? The first step to easy sprouting is soaking.[33] Put your grains, legumes, nuts, or seeds in a glass jar or bowl; cover them with water; and soak them for six to twenty-four hours to initiate the germination process. This will increase the enzyme phytase, which eliminates those nasty mineral-binding phytates, trypsin inhibitors, and toxic lectins. Nuts will also begin to manufacture other enzymes, including trypsin, which will aid in their easy digestion. If the foodstuff has been irradiated, then they won't sprout, but soaking will still reduce the antinutrients.

After the initial soaking period, you can continue the germination process by rinsing the nuts, seeds, grains, or legumes three times a day and leaving them inverted in a jar so the water can drain away until they sprout (though you may not see any visible change). The enzymes produced rapidly climb in the first three days. Since that is what I am most interested in, I

GO NUTS!

Forget roasted nuts. Raw nuts are important to include in your diet because they provide some key nutrients. I advocate eating raw soaked or sprouted nuts in particular, especially almonds, walnuts, sunflower seeds, and hazelnuts. Walnuts are a good source of health-promoting omega-3 fatty acids. Almonds and sunflower seeds are excellent sources of vitamin E, a group of eight fat-soluble compounds (tocopherols and tocotrienols) that are potent antioxidants and provide key protection to myelin in the brain. They also protect cell membranes from free radical damage. I recommend eating up to 4 ounces of soaked nuts every day. Cold-pressed nut oils such as walnut and almond oil also make excellent additions to salad dressings and smoothies. (Never heat nut oils over 117 degrees or you will destroy the essential oils and their associated antioxidants.)

Some people have food allergies or sensitivities to tree nuts and will not be able to tolerate them. If you perceive that you have a problem with headache, fatigue, or any troubling symptom that is worse when eating tree nuts, stay away from tree nuts. Instead, try soaked or sprouted sunflower or pumpkin seeds as an alternative. If those both bother you, then you will need to find other sources of vitamin E, such as avocado or olive oil. Always check with your doctor for guidance if you have severe food allergies.

generally stop by the third day and either use the food item by cooking or eating it raw,[34] or I dehydrate at temperatures below 117 degrees Fahrenheit for future use. (Soaked nuts and seeds tend to be a bit chewy, but dehydrating them restores their crunchy texture.)

At a minimum, soak grains, legumes, nuts, and seeds for twenty-four hours, but you can continue to the sprouting phase, even beyond three days, until you see sprouts and leaves. When this happens, eat the food right away. Sprouts are fragile and easily contaminated with bacteria that can cause diarrhea, so fresh is best. (This is another reason why I generally don't sprout food for longer than three days: This minimizes the chances of bacterial contamination.) After you are done soaking, do one final rinse. You could take your soaked nuts and blend them with water and ice in a high-powered blender such as a Vitamix to make your own homemade nut milk. You could use the nuts combined with an avocado as a base for a pudding. Or you could put the soaked nuts or seeds in a dehydrator at the lowest temperature overnight and have a lovely crunchy snack that is packed with minerals, enzymes, and essential fatty acids.

Fermented Foods

Each of us is an ecosystem. We have 1 trillion body cells and 100 trillion yeasts, bacteria, and even, in some cases, parasites living on and in us. Every moment, trillions of chemical reactions are being driven by them, and many of those by-products will eventually get into our bloodstreams, where they will either facilitate health or the development of disease.[35] We have coevolved with the 100 trillion microbes over thousands of generations and selected over time the most health-promoting mix to have in our ecosystems. I call this healthy mix of bacteria, yeasts, and parasites our "old friends." They will help digest the foods we eat and their by-products, so we can either efficiently use or safely excrete them.

Scientists continue to deepen our understanding of how these bacteria and yeasts influence our health, but we do know this much: What we eat has everything to do with that bowel population of critters. Are you creating an unruly mob in there, or a well-behaved, health-promoting population of good bacteria citizens?

Thousands of years ago, our ancestors learned how to harness the power of lacto-fermentation to help store the plentiful food they had available during the growing season. The combination of fresh food, salt, and sealing the food from air created fermentation, which happens when oxygen is not present. The initial fermentations humans probably undertook involved fermenting honey to make mead and then eventually beer and wine. Next, they likely began to ferment roots and greens. Fermentation not only added more vitamins and antioxidants to these foods but made it possible to store food over the winter, when fresh vegetables and fruits were not available.

But we don't eat the way our ancestors ate, and our dietary changes have

SHOULD YOU TAKE A PROBIOTIC SUPPLEMENT?

Taking probiotics without changing your diet will be of little consequence. Probiotic supplements can add 5 billion to 15 billion live cultures per capsule to our bowels, but even these seemingly high numbers will not have much chance of making an impact in the midst of the 100 trillion bacteria and yeasts living in and on your body. Adding fermented foods—especially those you make yourself—is a much more effective way to add the friendly bacteria back into your system, along with feeding that good bacteria with soluble fiber (from vegetables, seeds, and fruits, especially psyllium seed husks, ground flax- or chia seeds, prunes, berries, almonds, legumes, cabbages, onions, and mushrooms; hunter-gatherer societies typically had 80 grams of dietary fiber a day, mostly from nonstarchy greens and roots[36]). If you are constantly feeding the "bad guys" with too much sugar and starch, those good bacteria won't get a foothold. Once your gut is doing well, however, probiotic supplements have a better chance of flourishing in a friendly environment. If you do use probiotics, rotate the kinds you use, to increase the variety of species to which you are exposed.

also affected the populations in our guts. By shifting our diet as our culture has in the last hundred years by adding many more carbohydrate-rich foods like sugar, white flour, and white potatoes, unfamiliar species are thriving in there, and our old reliable friends are dying off. Antibiotics kill off many more beneficial bacteria and yeasts, giving the bad guys an even greater advantage.

By removing processed foods and replacing them with greens, sulfur, and color (the 9 cups), you will provide the good bacteria in your bowels with the fiber they need to thrive, but eating more fermented foods with live cultures will bring more of the friendly, health-promoting lacto-bacillus species to your gut, returning your bowels to a healthier condition. That is why fermented foods are often called lacto-fermented foods. Traditional cultures would have a live-culture fermented food with every meal. You can, too. (I do.)

Fermented Choices

Not sure what fermented foods to eat? These are the ones I recommend:

- **Yogurt.** This is probably the most common fermented food in the American diet, but because I have you avoid dairy, you should still avoid milk-based yogurt and kefir. Instead, there are lacto-fermented almond and coconut milk yogurts, which are delicious with fresh berries. Choose unsweetened varieties.
- **Kombucha tea.** This is a delicious combination of yeast and bacteria. Kombucha is made by adding a kombucha mother (a pancake-shaped symbiotic colony of bacteria and yeast) to green or black tea along with some sugar, which is digested by the bacteria. You can buy it in health food stores or possibly in your regular supermarket. You can also make it at home. (See the recipe at the back of this book.)
- **Lacto-fermented cabbage, sauerkraut, kimchi, and pickles.** See the recipes and resource section at the back of this book.
- **Nutritional yeast (*Saccharomyces cerevisiae*).** It is grown on sugarcane or beet molasses for several days and is then killed by heat and dried, typically forming into light yellow flakes. It is rich in B vitamins, RNA (ribonucleic acid), minerals, and protein. Additional B vitamins, including cobalamin (vitamin B_{12}), are often added, making it a very useful foodstuff for vegetarians. However, nutritional yeast has naturally occurring free glutamate, which may act as an excitotoxin for some, leading to headache and irritability.

  Nutritional yeast will not increase the growth of *Candida* (a harmful, troublemaking yeast) and it has a rich, cheeselike flavor that can make the transition to dairy-free easier, so if it agrees with you, then by all means enjoy it. If you have any sense of headache or problems with it, however, do not use it. Brewer's yeast is also made from *Saccharomyces cerevisiae*, but it does not have the B_{12} added, which is why I prefer nutritional yeast.
- **Non-grain-based spirits.** Because beer and many distilled spirits are made from grain, I suggest avoiding those unless they are specifically labeled gluten-free. However, non-grain-based spirits such as rum, wine, and

WHY SOME FERMENTED FOODS MIGHT GIVE YOU TROUBLE (AND WHAT TO DO ABOUT IT)

Some people with MS have evidence of an overgrowth of *Candida albicans*, a harmful yeast, in their bowels.[37] The *Candida* species releases by-products that diffuse into the bloodstream and can be toxic to brain cells and mitochondria, leading to severe fatigue and brain fog.[38] This can occur because of antibiotic use as a child or an adult and/or because of a sugar/carb-intensive diet. It could also occur because of acid-lowering medication.[39]

Some people who have trouble with *Candida* may find that they cannot tolerate nutritional yeast or even any kind of mushroom. Some with MS and autoimmune problems cannot tolerate products made through yeast fermentation, either, like kombucha, vinegar, and wine. I did not eliminate such foods from my diet, and most of my clinic patients and study patients have done well with nutritional yeast, but I do acknowledge that the occasional person will do better removing all yeast products and mushrooms. There will be some MS patients who do better if they avoid all products of yeast fermentation, including wine and vinegars. This is an individual matter, so if you eat these foods, pay attention to how well you tolerate them.

gluten-free beer are permissible, and fermented. (Have no more than one small glass of wine or beer or one shot of spirits a day for women and two for men.)

That is the essence of Wahls Paleo: Cut back on your carbs, eat more meat, gradually add seaweed and organ meat as your taste buds adjust, and eat more raw, soaked, and fermented foods every day. It won't take long before you'll be noticing a distinct and wonderful difference in your health. You're eating more like your ancestors now, and that ancient, natural, healthy glow is going to creep back in. Keep going, stay strong, and if you make a mistake or eat something you shouldn't, forgive yourself and get back on track. Wahls Paleo is your path to healing, and the healing has already begun.

Below is a box containing all the basic rules for Wahls Paleo, followed by one week of Wahls Paleo meals.

LEVEL 2: WAHLS PALEO

For Wahls Paleo, you will follow all the rules for the Wahls Diet (the 9 cups, gluten-free, dairy-free, and all other foods and processes forbidden or limited, including eggs, nonorganic soy, refined sweeteners, and microwaving). You will also add these additional rules. Continue to eat to satiety. You may increase or decrease the amount of vegetables, fruit, and meat you eat according to your size, but make sure to do so in proportion:

- Increase grass-fed, wild-caught meat and fish intake to 9 to 21 ounces per day, according to your size and gender. Include 16 ounces per week of wild-caught, cold-water fish (herring, sardines, salmon) as part of your total animal protein allowance.
- Work up to 2.5 ounces of fresh or reconstituted seaweed, 1 teaspoon dried flakes, or ¼ teaspoon powdered seaweed daily.
- Eat 12 ounces of organ meat per week as part of your total animal protein allowance.
- Have lacto-fermented food daily.
- Have up to 4 ounces daily of nuts and seeds, either raw or soaked for six to twenty-four hours.
- Limit white potatoes, gluten-free grains, and legumes to two servings per week. (This is a maximum: Complete elimination is preferred.)
- Fats permissible for heating are ghee, coconut oil, lard, and other rendered animal fats, such as duck fat and chicken fat. Do not cook with any vegetable oils other than coconut oil.
- Eliminate all nonfermented soy products. (Tempeh and miso are still okay, but tempeh is often made with grain, so be sure it is gluten-free—and it counts as one of your two weekly grain servings.)

Wahls Paleo Meal Plan

	Breakfast	Lunch	Dinner
Day 1	Smoothie: • 1 cup bok choy • 1 cup orange sections (2 small) • 1 cup pineapple • 1 tablespoon nutritional yeast • water/ice 2 medium chicken breasts without skin (6 ounces)	1 serving Basic Skillet Recipe* (Pork Chops and Red Cabbage) Salad: • 3 cups bok choy • 1 small tomato (½ cup) • ½ cup sweet red pepper • ½ cup daikon radish • 1 tablespoon sliced almonds • 1 tablespoon extra virgin olive oil • balsamic vinegar to taste Fruit cup: • 1½ cups strawberries • 1 kiwi ½ cup Kombucha Tea*	1 serving Liver, Onions, and Mushrooms* 1 cup cooked carrots Salad: • 2 cups bok choy • 1 tablespoon sunflower seeds • ½ cup summer squash • ½ cup raw celery • dried basil to taste • 1 tablespoon extra virgin olive oil • balsamic vinegar to taste ¼ cup fermented beets 1½ cups fresh pineapple Throat Coat™ herbal tea
Day 2	Smoothie: • 1 cup parsley • 2 cups green grapes • 1 tablespoon nutritional yeast • water/ice 1 serving Liver Pâté* 2 ounces raw turnip slices (about ½ cup) 1 medium stalk celery	1½ servings Salmon Salad* 2 cups raw collards (wrap) 4 scallions or spring onions 4 medium radishes ½ cup cubed cantaloupe ½ cup Beet Kvass* mixed with ½ cup water	2 medium chicken breasts without skin (about 6 ounces) 1 cup chopped sweet potato 2 teaspoons extra virgin olive oil ⅛ teaspoon cinnamon Salad: • 3 cups spinach • ¼ cup sliced onion • 1 clove garlic • 1 tablespoon sunflower seed butter • lime juice to taste ¼ cup fermented red cabbage ¾ cup fresh blueberries Tension Tamer® herbal tea

	Breakfast	*Lunch*	*Dinner*
Day 3	Smoothie: • 1 cup bok choy • 1 cup kiwi • 1 cup strawberries • 1 tablespoon nutritional yeast • water/ice 3–4 ounces canned sardines in tomato sauce 1 medium celery stalk ½ cup raw turnip slices	2 servings Basic Skillet Recipe* (Pork Chops and Red Cabbage) Salad: • 3 cups romaine lettuce • 2 cups spinach • ½ cup red peppers • 2 teaspoons flax oil • balsamic vinegar to taste 1 cup raw kiwi ½ cup Kombucha Tea*	6 ounces beef rump roast 1 medium potato with skin 1 teaspoon extra virgin olive oil 1 medium cooked carrot ½ cup lacto-fermented okra 1 cup strawberries chamomile vanilla herbal tea
Day 4	Smoothie: • 1 cup cilantro • 1 small orange (~½ cup) • 1 cup pineapple • 1 tablespoon nutritional yeast • water/ice 7 ounces turkey breast without skin 6 medium spears asparagus 1 teaspoon extra virgin olive oil	1 serving Basic Skillet Recipe* (Collards and Ham Skillet) 1 cup chopped baked sweet potato • 2 teaspoons extra virgin olive oil Fruit Cup: • 1 cup pineapple • 1 cup raspberries • 2 tablespoons raw almonds ½ cup Beet Kvass* plus ½ cup water	2 servings Chicken Salad* Salad: • 2 cups bok choy • 2 cups spinach • lime juice to taste • 1 tablespoon flax oil • ½ cup tomato • 2 tablespoons soaked sunflower seeds ¼ cup lacto-fermented carrots 1 cup grapes mint herbal tea
Day 5	Smoothie: • 1 cup spinach • 1 cup strawberries • 1 cup peaches (~1 medium) • 1 tablespoon nutritional yeast • water/ice 1 serving Basic Skillet Recipe* (Salmon and Kale Skillet)	2 servings Basic Skillet Recipe* (Lamb Chops with Broccoli) 1 cup cooked beets Salad: • 3 cups bok choy • 2 cloves garlic • ½ cup cilantro • ½ cup green pepper • ½ cup fresh grapes • 1 tablespoon sunflower butter • lime juice to taste ½ cup Kombucha Tea*	2 servings Algerian Chicken with Asparagus* ¼ cup kimchi 1 medium peach herbal tea

	Breakfast	Lunch	Dinner
Day 6	Smoothie: • ½ cup raw beets • 1 small orange (~½ cup) • 1 cup cherries • ¼-inch piece fresh gingerroot grated • 1 tablespoon nutritional yeast • water/ice 1 serving Basic Skillet Recipe* (Heart and Mustard Greens) 1 cup cantaloupe	4 ounces sardines in tomato sauce ½ cup daikon radishes 1 medium celery stalk ½ cup zucchini 1 cup chopped baked sweet potato Salad: • 2 cups spinach • 2 cups kale • ½ cup strawberries • 4 medium spears asparagus • 2 teaspoons extra virgin olive oil • lime juice to taste 1 medium orange ½ cup Beet Kvass* plus ½ cup water	1 medium turkey drumstick with skin removed (~6.6 ounces) 1 serving Mashed Turnips* 2 teaspoons extra virgin olive oil ½ cup parsley 1 cup cooked carrots ¼ cup lacto-fermented pickles 1½ cups cherries chamomile herbal tea
Day 7	Smoothie: • 1 cup parsley • 1 cup green grapes • 1 kiwi (about ⅓ cup) • 1 tablespoon nutritional yeast • water/ice 6 ounces beef steak, topped with the following (to be cooked together): • ¼ cup onions • ¼ cup mushrooms • ¼ cup green peppers • 2 teaspoons ghee	2 servings Rosemary Chicken* 1 cup acorn squash 2 teaspoons extra virgin olive oil 6 medium asparagus spears, topped with 1 teaspoon extra virgin olive oil ½ cup Beet Kvass plus ½ cup water	1 serving Seafood Stew (Paleo version)* Salad: • 3 cups bok choy • 2 cups spinach • ½ cup cilantro • ½ cup tomato • 1 tablespoon extra virgin olive oil • lime juice to taste ½ cup organic raw cultured carrots Fruit Cup: • ½ cup muskmelon • ½ cup watermelon • ½ cup blueberries herbal tea

Chapter 7

WAHLS PALEO PLUS

YOU MAY NEVER need to do Wahls Paleo Plus, but I hope you will read this chapter anyway. This is the diet level I practice. After progressing through every level of the Wahls Protocol and experimenting with every aspect of the nutrition program, I settled here because I have the most mental and physical energy eating this way. Some will enjoy so much improvement at the Wahls Paleo level that they don't feel the need to move on to Wahls Paleo Plus. However, I recommend it for those who aren't seeing as much progress as they were hoping for at the Wahls Paleo level.

Wahls Paleo Plus includes everything you were doing at Wahls Paleo, with a few additional considerations:

- **Eat more fat!** I want you to add at least 5 tablespoons of coconut oil or ¾ can (or more) of full-fat coconut milk. (You may also use unheated olive oil or ghee to get some of your fat calories.)
- **Reduce the daily 9 cups of fruits and vegetables to 6 to 9 cups, depending on your gender and size (or even 4 to 6 cups for very petite women).** Fruit is limited to 1 cup per day with a preference for berries. All dried fruits are excluded, as are canned fruits and commercial fruit juices.

WAHLS PALEO PLUS

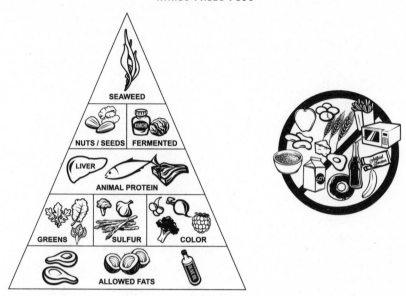

- **Eliminate all grains, legumes, and white potatoes.** This includes rice milk (use coconut milk instead) and all forms of soy, including organic and fermented.
- **Limit starchy vegetables, like cooked beets or winter squash, to a maximum of twice per week, always with at least 1 tablespoon of fat and some protein to lower their glycemic index.** I'll talk more about what this is later in this chapter. If you want more starchy vegetables, you may eat them raw, but also with at least 1 tablespoon of fat.
- **Reduce your meat intake back to 6 to 12 ounces.**

Are you surprised? This diet sounds crazy to a lot of people, and I understand why. How can you possibly eat that much fat for health? That little fruit? No grains or potatoes at all? I have very good reasons for prescribing this diet, and as I mentioned, it is the diet I follow myself, with great results. I believe you will be more likely to get behind the diet if you understand how it evolved.

Once again I have laid out the comparison of the average diet compared to my program, this time the Wahls Paleo Plus. What is noteworthy is that

Wahls Paleo Plus		
Nutrient*†	U.S. Diet	Wahls Paleo Plus
Vitamin D	31%	59%
Vitamin E	55%	97%
Calcium	74%	54%
Magnesium	88%	122%
Vitamin A	100%	411%
Pyridoxine	121%	226%
Folate	122%	191%
Zinc	123%	200%
Thiamin	128%	215%
Vitamin C	133%	393%
Niacin	154%	239%
Iron	164%	238%
Riboflavin	175%	301%
Cobolamin	201%	524%

* Compared to dietary reference intakes, recommended dietary allowances (RDA) for females 51–70 years; Wahls Paleo Plus Diet adjusted for 1,759 calories. (National Academy of Science; Institute of Medicine; Food and Nutrition Board)

† Average nutrient intake from food for females 50–59 years. (What We Eat in America, NHANES 2009–2010, www.ars.usda.gov/SP2UserFiles/Place/12355000/pdf/0910/Table_1_NIN_GEN_09.pdf, accessed May 25, 2013.)

Wahls Paleo Plus is still much more nutrient-dense than the standard American diet, even though I have increased the fat consumption so drastically. Most ketogenic diets (I'll define this term momentarily) require the addition of vitamins and other supplements because the nutrient density becomes so poor due to the severe restriction on carbohydrates. Wahls Paleo Plus is much more balanced than the traditional ketogenic diets in use because it has a somewhat higher carbohydrate intake from nonstarchy vegetables.

Wahls Paleo Plus is a modified version of what doctors call a "ketogenic diet." In a ketogenic diet, fat is high and carbohydrates are low, so that the body begins to burn fat as fuel instead of sugar from carbohydrates. (I'll explain how later in this chapter.) This has traditionally been a diet prescribed for people with certain health issues like seizure disorders, but in my research I have found it to be of extreme benefit to people with other types of brain problems, not just seizures, in the modified form you will find in this chapter.

Ketogenic diets are nothing new, but they continue to evolve. In order for you to accept the unconventional dietary characteristics of Wahls Paleo Plus, I want you to understand what a ketogenic diet is and why it is so good for your brain, especially if you have an autoimmune disease with neurological symptoms. Let's first look at what a ketogenic diet is.

Ketogenic Diets and MCTs

In the simplest terms, ketosis means you are burning fat, rather than sugar, as your primary fuel source. Specifically, when your body is in a state of nutritional ketosis, the liver begins producing ketone bodies—acetoacetate, acetone, and beta-hydroxybutyrate. The brain cannot burn long-chain fats because long-chain fats can't cross the blood-brain barrier. Instead, the brain uses for fuel what *can* cross the blood-brain barrier: ketone bodies. Thus, your liver will burn fat and produce these small molecules known as ketone bodies as a by-product of burning the fat. These then proceed to cross the blood-brain barrier to be burned as fuel in your brain cells' mitochondria. The longer you are in nutritional ketosis, the more enzymes for burning the ketones will be upregulated—that is, increased—making it increasingly easy for your body to utilize the ketones.

You may have heard that ketosis is dangerous, and there are forms of ketosis that can be damaging to you, but nutritional ketosis is *not harmful*. In fact, it is healing, and has long been a mechanism for human survival. In human history, depending on environment and season, fat was often an easier fuel source to find than carbohydrates. In winter, the food supply declined and our metabolism switched to burning fat because simple carbohydrates were less available as food. Our bodies are very good at burning fat, but our cells do not choose to burn fat when they have an easy supply of simple sugars. The splitting of the sugar molecule (glycolysis) occurs outside of the mitochondria in the cell cytoplasm. That is what yeast and bacteria do, and it is called fermentation. When oxygen first appeared, it was toxic, killing off 90 percent of the bacterial species. But some tiny bacteria were able to use oxy-

> ## WAHLS WORDS
>
> Fatty acids are considered long-chain if they have more than twelve carbon atoms, medium-chain if they have between twelve and six carbon atoms, and short-chain if they have fewer than six carbon atoms. The medium-chain fats found in coconut oil and short-chain fats found in ghee can enter the bloodstream directly from the small bowel. The long-chain fats, by contrast, are absorbed into the bloodstream through a longer, more complex process. That difference is just one of the reasons why consuming coconut oil and ghee is more desirable while practicing Wahls Paleo Plus.

gen as the bacteria burned sugar. Those small oxygen-using, sugar-burning bacteria were engulfed by larger bacteria and made the larger bacteria much more efficient. These tiny bacteria were the precursors to the modern-day mitochondria living in each of our cells. That made us far more efficient at extracting energy from our food than the fermentation process that occurs in yeasts and bacteria. It is because of mitochondria that those ancient bacteria were able to evolve into multicellular organisms!

When starchy foods became plentiful with the advent of agriculture, and even more so with industrialization and modernization, however, humans didn't go into ketosis as often. Modern industrialized societies have diets packed with carbohydrates year-round. We burn sugar for fuel, but that isn't ideal, especially if you have a problem with your brain. Sugary, starchy diets promote inflammation. We have lost touch with the benefits of the metabolic state of ketosis, and we have paid the price.

However, ketogenic diets haven't disappeared. In 1911, a clinical study showed that water diets, also called fasting, benefited treatments for epilepsy.[1] Although scientists didn't fully understand why, the reason was that in a state of fasting, no simple sugars are coming in, so the body switches into nutritional ketosis, burning fat stores. In 1921, Dr. R. M. Wilder at the Mayo Clinic developed a diet that would allow patients to eat some food but have the same benefits as they would enjoy from fasting. This diet was very high in fat, included some protein, and almost zero carbohydrates. He reported success with his epilepsy patients.[2] Dr. M. G. Peterman, also at Mayo, described the first ketogenic diet that was used with success with children suffering from epilepsy.[3]

Some of this research fell out of favor when Dilantin, the first effective anticonvulsant drug, became available in 1938. (Anticonvulsants continue to be a popular treatment for epilepsy, even though these drugs are not effective for up to 30 percent of individuals with seizures.) But scientists continued to explore the notion that a diet that promoted fat burning instead of sugar burning could improve seizure disorders. In 1971, it was discovered that consuming medium-chain triglyceride (MCT) oil, extracted from coconut oil and palm kernel oil, generated more ketones per calorie than other fats.[4] Because a ketogenic diet depends on the manufacture of a certain level of ketones, this meant that diets using MCT oil as the sole fat source could include carbohydrates at a slightly higher level than was used in the 1920s and still generate ketones. That discovery made it possible to modify the original ketogenic diet into what became known as an MCT ketogenic diet, which was much easier to follow because it allowed a wider variety of food. Wahls Paleo Plus is actually a modified MCT ketogenic diet, because it relies heavily on coconut oil and full-fat coconut milk.

The public interest in ketogenic diets increased when, in 1994, two-year-old Charlie Abrahams, son of Hollywood director and writer Jim Abrahams, became seizure-free on a ketogenic diet after previously having uncontrolled seizures. This led to the development of the Charlie Foundation to promote the diet and fund research. In 2011, there were more than seventy-five centers that used a ketogenic diet to treat refractory epilepsy. Additionally, physicians are now studying whether ketogenic diets can treat a much wider array of health problems: Parkinson's disease, dementia, Lou Gehrig's disease, chronic migraine, autism, stroke, and psychiatric diseases.[5] There is also exciting research indicating that ketogenic diets are an excellent way to fight an active, even advanced cancer.[6]

My own research, as well as self-experimentation, has centered on an exploration of how a diet rich in MCT fats and low in carbohydrates might impact multiple sclerosis and other neurological conditions. This is how

WAHLS WORDS

Glycemic index is a measure of how much a food causes a rise in blood sugar. The highest number on the glycemic index is 100, which indicates how much pure glucose raises the blood sugar over a two-hour period. Every food is rated in comparison to this number. (Glycemic index values for foods can be found at this website, from the University of Sydney: www.glycemicindex.com.) The glycemic index varies depending on many different food factors, such as amount and types of sugars and starches, fat, protein, and fiber content of food; physical structure; food processing; and type and amount of cooking. Other factors, such as how well the food is chewed and what foods were eaten at prior meals, can also impact blood sugar levels. Foods that contain carbohydrates—starches and sugars—will have glycemic index numbers, while foods containing only proteins and/or fats, such as meat and vegetable oil, are assumed to be zero. Vegetables and fruits vary dramatically, depending on variety as well as other factors, like whether they are cooked or raw, ripe or unripe. You can also lower the glycemic index of a food by combining it with fiber, fat, and protein, which slows down the absorption rate of the carbohydrate.

Glycemic load predicts the blood sugar response when a specific amount of a particular food is consumed. It considers both the glycemic index of a food and the amount of available carbohydrate in the portion eaten. A high glycemic index food could potentially have a low glycemic load if the amount of carbohydrate in the food is low and/or if the amount eaten is small. This can also be influenced by ripeness and how long the food was cooked.

Wahls Paleo Plus evolved. This diet, if followed strictly, will put you into a mild state of nutritional ketosis, but it contains more carbohydrates than the traditional ketogenic diets because of the importance of including a rich supply of nonstarchy vegetables for nutrient density. Vegetables contain carbohydrates, but these and a small amount of berries (a relatively low-carb fruit) are the only carbohydrate sources. To me, this is the best of both worlds: The diet has the benefits of ketosis and high fat for brain health and low carbohydrates to reduce inflammation and stabilize blood sugar, but is also nutrient-dense beyond other ketogenic diets. To some, Wahls Paleo Plus may seem extreme, but I want you to understand that it is far less extreme than standard ketogenic diets that require supplementation because they are so nutrient-poor. Wahls Paleo Plus is designed to be workable in the real world. It's challenging, but it's certainly not impossible. I do it, and so do many other Wahls Warriors, with great results.

Are You in Ketosis?

When you embark upon Wahls Paleo Plus, adding fats and reducing carbohydrates further, you may want to know whether you are actually in nutritional ketosis. When I developed Wahls Paleo Plus, I began by choosing low-glycemic foods and eating them in a way that would give them a low glycemic load, reducing cooked starchy vegetables like sweet potatoes, reducing fruit to 1 cup of berries only, and consuming an entire can of full-fat coconut milk every day.

To see how well this was all working, I began checking my urine for the presence of ketones using a urine dipstick. If you want to know whether you are in ketosis, you can do this, too. Buy urine ketone test strips at your local pharmacy and follow the package instructions for measuring your urine ketones. I recommend checking your urine ketones at the same time each day, such as first thing in the morning or just before bed, in order to get the most consistent look at them. Another more accurate, but also more expensive, method is to purchase a meter for measuring blood sugar that also measures blood ketones.

If your cells are still burning sugar (carbohydrates), you will have zero ketones in the urine. My goal was to have some ketones in the urine—not a high number, just some. Any sign of ketones means you are in ketosis, and more isn't necessarily better. I didn't need the level to be high, but I wanted to see if I could induce at least a low level of ketosis while still consuming my green, colorful, and sulfur-rich vegetables.

WAHLS WARNING

In some studies, medium-chain triglyceride diets, upon which Wahls Paleo Plus is based, have been associated with side effects such as diarrhea, vomiting, bloating, and cramps. Other studies have found that these side effects can be reduced by more slowly increasing the amount of medium-chain triglycerides (like coconut oil) in the diet. This means you may want to ease gradually into Wahls Paleo Plus rather than leaping in with both feet. There is also the theoretical risk of having a higher cholesterol value. We tell our study patients that diets high in coconut fat and low in carbohydrates may increase the total cholesterol and your HDL (high-density lipoprotein), or "good cholesterol," but would also likely at the same time reduce the number of oxidized cholesterols that are the most damaging of all the cholesterol particles. (The oxidized cholesterol is a different number from the LDL, or low-density lipoprotein. See the Resources section at the end of the book.) With my patients, whose brains need healing, I don't worry as much about this increase in cholesterol. With the reduced inflammation typical of being in nutritional ketosis, vascular health is likely to remain strong. One real danger for children and young adults up to the early 20s: Neither the medium-chain-triglyceride diet nor Wahls Paleo Plus should be used by people in this age group who take valproate, as there have been some reports that the combination causes liver failure.

When I tried this, I found that within forty-eight hours on Wahls Paleo Plus, my urine was showing trace to small levels of ketones (5 to 40 mg/dl). As I continued to check my urine ketones and further restrict fruit, I found that the ketone levels would fluctuate between moderate to large (80 and 160 mg/dl). I was eating 3 cups of greens, 1 or 2 cups of sulfur vegetables, and 1 to 2 cups of color. I thought I was doing great, but to be sure the test was accurate, I decided to measure my blood ketones: Sure enough, I found that the blood ketones ranged from 0.4 micromoles/L to 3.0 micromoles/L. Nutritional ketosis begins at level 0.5 micromoles/L. I was often, though not always, in nutritional ketosis. I was ecstatic. I could still eat a very nutrient-dense diet that would give me the nutrition my brain cells needed while maintaining nutritional ketosis! Now, with more time and experience, I am consistently in ketosis.

Because I was also consuming 500 to 700 calories either as coconut oil or as full-fat coconut milk, I was only consuming around 6 ounces of meat per day instead of my usual 9 to 12 ounces, and 6 to 9 cups of vegetables and berries, but it was working and I was still getting plenty of antioxidants. When we did an analysis of the micronutrient content of my diet, I was still well over the RDAs for vitamins and most minerals, but I was a bit low on calcium. I would, therefore have to pay special attention to eating high-calcium foods to be sure I was still getting sufficient calcium and plenty of vitamin D.

Follow the urine ketones to get feedback on whether you are likely in nutritional ketosis. If you have zero ketones, you need to reduce the carbohydrates further and increase the coconut milk, coconut oil, and/or ghee until you see small to moderate ketones on the urine strips. You may have to eliminate starchy vegetables entirely, even the raw ones, or you may be able to tolerate small amounts now and then. If you pay attention to your urine ketones, it will help guide your diet.

Also remember that medium-chain-triglyceride-rich coconut fat will allow you to eat slightly more carbohydrates while still maintaining a state of ketosis, so keep the coconut fat coming in!

In our current study, we are using Wahls Paleo Plus and studying its impact on patients' quality of life, fatigue level, and walking ability. In order to more effectively isolate the dietary effects, we are not employing the other aspects of the Wahls Protocol, such as meditation, massage, and neuromuscular stimulation. (Find out more about all of these in the final section of the book.) Instead, we are comparing the Wahls Diet, Wahls Paleo Plus, and "usual care" (no dietary intervention). Subjects are using a daily food log to guide their selection of food to meet the food plan goals and are testing their urine daily and their blood weekly for ketones. We don't yet know if our subjects will be as successful at maintaining nutritional ketosis as I am, though I expect them to be! Nor do I know if the Wahls Diet will be just as good as Wahls Paleo Plus, though we expect Wahls Paleo Plus to show greater benefit. (Of course, this is why one does research: for proof.)

WAHLS WARRIORS SPEAK

I learned about Dr. Wahls from my dentist, who told me that someone close to him was using diet to turn around their MS and having significant results. I have primary-progressive MS, spine and hip arthritis, ankylosing spondylitis, mitral valve prolapse, situational depression, epilepsy, and neuropathy. When PPMS spread to my speech centers, it was a shock, more so than the physical limits.

Over the initial three months on this diet, and on targeted supplements, my speech gradually made gains from severe disfluency; my tremors lessened; and I went from unintelligible speech attempts and gasping for breath to speaking coherently again. I still need to use a wheelchair to travel any distances, but I am doing more of the tasks that I had given up for more than a decade, such as cooking once or twice a week. I can clean and chop vegetables, something that used to wear me out, and I don't fall asleep in the midst of tasks anymore. My husband and daughter used to tell me that they'd shared things with me in conversation and I wouldn't remember what they'd said. Those days are over. I used to have days, even weeks, where I slept for hours after very little activity. Now I have much more energy and am able to engage in life more. I seldom nap these days, and my family is so touched by how far I have come, as am I! Thanks to Dr. Wahls, I have hope and fight in me!

—Yolanda M., Hercules, California

Once a month, the study subjects come into the clinic for blood work. We test their blood levels of glucose and insulin as well as their ketone levels. At three months, we test their thinking, walking, and quality-of-life measures and a more extensive list of vitamin markers. Soon after the publication of this book, I will have a more objective analysis of the effects of Wahls Paleo Plus and what the potential mechanisms are for the improvements in function that we will hopefully find.

I want you to be able to have a chance at getting the benefits of this diet right now, however. Do work with your personal physician if you elect to try Wahls Paleo Plus to monitor how both you and your blood work respond to this new way of eating.

Is Wahls Paleo Plus Right for You?

You may be convinced that the Wahls Way is your way, but at which level should you settle? For my clinical trials, participants must follow specific parameters, strictly adhering to the study diet; but in my clinics, patients have a choice. Do they want to try the Wahls Diet, or jump right into Wahls Paleo? Or do I think they could benefit from trying Wahls Paleo Plus? I educate my patients about exactly what we know and what we don't know about these various levels of diet, and I let them decide which diet plan will work for them. I make recommendations, but in the end it is their choice, just as it is yours.

In general, however, I do tailor my recommendation to a person's health issues and what they and their families are open to doing. The more ill the person is, the more strongly I encourage them to try Wahls Paleo, and as they adopt the diet and adjust to the changes, I encourage self-reflection. Is the person satisfied with their health, or could they improve more? We talk about what dietary changes they'd like to tackle next. Once they have been successful in fully adopting Wahls Paleo, if the person is still not as well as she or he wants to be, then I may discuss Wahls Paleo Plus, particularly if the person has issues despite fully implementing Wahls Paleo. Some of these issues might include:

1. Persistent brain fog
2. Neuro-behavior symptoms that persist following a traumatic brain injury
3. Neurodegenerative diseases (such as Parkinson's, Lou Gehrig's, and Huntington's diseases)
4. Neurological problems (such as chronic headaches, seizures, and movement disorders)
5. Psychiatric diseases that have not shown satisfactory improvement on Wahls Paleo

WAHLS WARRIORS SPEAK

My diagnosis with multiple sclerosis was a true wake-up call. Seeing my own decline at a prime time in my life altered me. At the time of my diagnosis in November 2006, I weighed more than 280 pounds. By the end of the year, I needed to use a walker. That's when I started my quest to research MS and how various factors, like nutrition and exercise, affect it. I started slowly incorporating my various findings into my daily life and progressed to only using a cane for my instability issues. In spring 2011, I gave up the cane, was more than 130 pounds lighter, and have been going strong ever since! I was determined not to be in a nursing home at 50 years old without any future. I could not bear that, so I made a decision and I continue to fight my battle with MS every day. I strongly believe in moving forward! I have had to learn to do some things differently, but that is okay. MS is not a death sentence—it just means that you will have struggles and challenges, but you can also have some wonderful rewards if you allow them into your life.

—Pam J., Pecatonica, Illinois

6. A strong family history (or personal history) of cancer
7. Fatigue that persists
8. Autoimmune brain-related problems that are not showing improvement with Wahls Paleo
9. Obesity, particularly if not losing weight on Wahls Paleo

You may be surprised to see obesity on this list. This is a new area of study for me. In the first three months of my first study, I noticed rapid weight loss in our participants who were overweight or obese and didn't report being hungry.

I am now in the preliminary stages of planning a clinical trial to study the effects of Wahls Paleo Plus on obesity. We are working on the study design and plan to propose a pilot study to the University of Iowa Institutional Review Board to collect initial pilot data. We plan to use Wahls Paleo Plus, monitoring the level of hunger and satiety that people experience; quality of life changes; medical symptoms; and changes in blood markers such as lipids, glucose, insulin, and hemoglobin A1C, and inflammation markers like highly sensitive C-reactive protein (CRP), homocysteine, and cytokines. We plan to compare Wahls Paleo Plus to the USDA's My Healthy Plate diet portion control plan that is typical of most weight-loss programs. Stay tuned for more news on this front!

In the meantime, if you do decide to try Wahls Paleo Plus, it's okay to ease into it. In fact, I prefer that you do. In our clinical trial, we ease people in over a three-week period. I find that it's easier for people to adapt if they allow their fat-burning enzymes to gradually upregulate (increase) so it is easier for their mitochondria to burn more fat. I suggest you do the same and come to this over one to three weeks (or longer) if you are coming from the standard American diet. If you have been practicing Wahls Paleo, you will likely be able to transition more quickly.

Remember that I have evolved my eating patterns over the last eleven years, adapting how I ate as I learned more about the needs of my brain and understood more and more about nutrition. I suggest you work with your family and begin making the changes at a pace your family accepts. No diet works if you don't stick to it, and it is much easier to adopt these big changes if you implement them gradually and the entire family joins you on the journey.

What to Do

Now that you understand what Wahls Paleo Plus is, let's look more closely at how to follow the guidelines. This final version of the diet takes the principles all the way. You will be incorporating every aspect of the Wahls Diet and Wahls Paleo unless they contradict the rules of Wahls Paleo Plus, which supersedes the others. You will maximize the vitamins, minerals, antioxidants, and fatty acids that are so critical for your brain while minimizing the sugars that can cause problems in your gut. You will still eat a lot of greens, sulfur-rich vegetables, and brightly colored produce, though it may be closer to 6 cups (or maybe 4 if you are a petite woman) and not the 9 cups recommended at the Wahls Diet and Wahls Paleo levels. You will still eat organic and/or wild-caught meat, including organ meat. You will still incorporate seaweed and fermented foods. The difference is that you'll tweak your ratios to add more fat and fewer carbs and you'll eat less often. As you get into nutritional ketosis, your body will begin to efficiently burn fat. I predict that you won't be as hungry on Wahls Paleo Plus, and you'll find eating just twice a day not so difficult. Here are your specifics:

Part One: Add More Fat, Especially Coconut Oil and Full-Fat Coconut Milk

Now it's time to really ramp up your fat intake, mostly through coconut oil or full-fat coconut milk (which, as I explained before, has properties that will keep you in ketosis even with vegetables and some fruit). I want the majority of your calories to come from fat. You should eat sufficient protein to meet the dietary needs of your body, but not more. Fat with minimal carbohydrates is converted to ketones, which are excellent sources of energy for our mitochondria, our brain cells, and our muscle cells. Your goal is to have a source of medium-chain fats at each eating occasion. You will get the most ketones from coconut oil as opposed to other kinds of fats. On a 2,000-calorie diet, that would be 144 grams of fat for approximately 1,300 calories. For the average woman eating 1,790 calories, that would be 129 grams of fat at 1,160 calories. Remember, if you are still not showing small to moderate ketones in your urine after fully committing to Wahls Paleo Plus for one week, you need to increase your fat intake with more coconut oil, coconut butter, or full-fat coconut milk and further reduce the carbohydrates.

You might think it will be hard to include this much coconut fat in your diet, but coconut oil can be added to smoothies and used in salad dressing and for cooking meats and vegetables. Coconut milk can be added to smoothies, soups, and other recipes, used in coffee and tea, or consumed plain. The amount of medium-chain fats in 1 tablespoon of coconut oil is equivalent to about 5 tablespoons (approximately ⅓ cup) of coconut milk. Take care not to confuse coconut water with coconut milk. Coconut water is the clear liquid from inside a coconut and it is fat-free. Also be sure you have the full-fat milk, not the "light" variety. Full-fat coconut milk provides 11 grams total fat per 0.33-cup serving compared to 4.5 grams total fat for the light version. Other coconut products that could be included in the diet include coconut cream and coconut butter. Coconut cream contains more medium-chain fat than coconut milk and is thicker. Coconut butter, sometimes called coconut cream concentrate, is finely ground dried coconut meat. Avoid "cream of coconut," because it is sweetened with sugar.

FAT FACTS

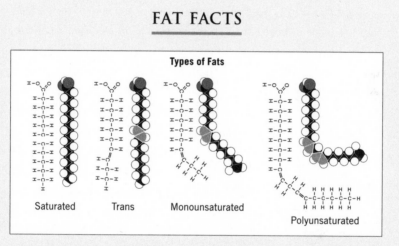

Types of Fats

Saturated   Trans   Monounsaturated   Polyunsaturated

Let's learn a little more about fats, because they are so important at this level.

Fats are chains of carbon and hydrogen atoms with two oxygen atoms at one end. In three dimensions, the carbon backbone makes a gentle zigzag pattern. In the drawings above, you see the long line of C's. These are the carbon atoms, or the black line with the zigzag white line in the drawing with balls. The hydrogen atoms are the H's and are the white balls. The dark-gray balls are the oxygen atoms. The light-gray balls represent the double bonds. A double bond is when a carbon atom does not have two hydrogen atoms attached to it, instead having only one attached. Those double bonds are fragile, and are more at risk of being oxidized and converted to a toxic fat that is very damaging to our blood vessels. Those double bonds change the shape of the fat that our cells use to conduct the biology of life. Remember, fats can be long-chain, medium-chain, or short-chain, depending on how many carbons have been strung together.

Saturated fat. Saturated fat has a hydrogen atom at every available spot on the fat. It is very stable to heat and does not convert to dangerous oxidized fats, which can be very damaging. Animal fats and coconut oil are primarily saturated fats. Their stability makes them the best choice for cooking.

Trans fat. Usually the double bonds in mono- and polyunsaturated fats have the single hydrogen atom on the same side of the chain. When they are on opposite sides of the carbon chain, it is in the "trans" position and is a trans saturated fat, often shortened to *trans fat*. The trans position puts a kink in the fat, changing its shape and increasing the likelihood that it will be oxidized and therefore become extremely damaging to your blood vessels.

Monounsaturated fat (MUFA). A monounsaturated fat is a fat with one double bond with the H's on the same side of the carbon chain. This changes the shape of the fat and is a useful fat to our cells. However, the double bond is more vulnerable to being oxidized by heat and becoming a damaging trans fat. Examples of foods rich with MUFAs include olive oil and walnuts, but both also contain PUFAs.

Polyunsaturated fat (PUFA). A polyunsaturated fat (PUFA) has more than one double bond and has more kinks and turns in its shape. As the number of double bonds increases, the fat becomes more vulnerable to heat, which will break the double bonds, creating oxidized fats, including damaging trans fats. This is why I recommend you not heat or cook with any plant oil. (Even olive oil is a combination of MUFAs and PUFAs.) Heating these oils will increase the likelihood that the double bonds will be broken and an oxidized, damaging molecule will be made. Instead, use the olive oil cold on your salads, and avoid plant oils completely if they contain primarily omega-6 PUFAs (corn, soybean, sunflower, most commercial "vegetable" oils, etc.) so that you can improve your ratio of omega-6 to omega-3 fats.

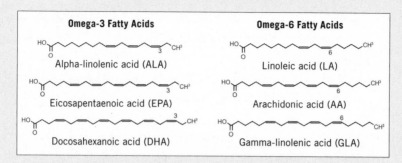

Omega-3 Fatty Acids

Alpha-linolenic acid (ALA)

Eicosapentaenoic acid (EPA)

Docosahexanoic acid (DHA)

Omega-6 Fatty Acids

Linoleic acid (LA)

Arachidonic acid (AA)

Gamma-linolenic acid (GLA)

Omega-3 fatty acids. I introduced you to the concept of essential fatty acids in the last chapter, but perhaps you would like to see how they look. As you can see from the illustration, there are three types of omega-3 fatty acids: ALA, EPA, and DHA. All the omega-3 fatty acids have a 3 on the chain on the right side; this refers to the third carbon from the distal end. As you may remember, ALA must be converted in the body to EPA and DHA, making it a less efficient source for omega-3 fatty acids. (This is the plant source, in foods like flaxseeds and walnuts.)

If you have an autoimmune problem, heart problem, and/or brain problems, it will likely be harder for you to manufacture sufficient EPA and DHA from ALA. For this reason, you are better off getting your EPA and DHA straight from animal sources like grass-fed wild game and other grass-fed meats, eggs from grass-eating chickens (but only if you are able to confirm that you do not have a food sensitivity to eggs), and wild fish, especially from cold-water climates. This is one of the reasons why I mentioned in the last chapter that I do not recommend vegetarianism.

Omega-6 fatty acids. You need omega-6 fatty acids, but most people get far too many. Ideally, you should get a ratio of omega-6 to omega-3 fatty acids of between 1:1 and 3:1, but most people get far more omega-6s. The number 6 in the term *omega-6* refers to the double bond at the sixth carbon from the end.

Linoleic acid (LA) is an essential omega-6 fatty acid, meaning your body cannot make it, and it is an important precursor to arachidonic acid (AA), which is used to make many signaling molecules in the body. Food sources for LA are nut and seed oils. Our bodies can easily make AA from

LA, though animal fats are a good direct source of AA. When the ratio of AA to DHA is shifted too strongly toward AA, the body begins producing too many inflammation molecules, leading to excessive inflammation. The typical American diet is strongly tilted toward LA because of the seed oils that were introduced seventy-five years ago.

Gamma-linolenic acid (GLA) is unusual for an omega-6 fatty acid in that it reduces inappropriate inflammation. Food sources include borage oil, primrose oil, black currant oil, and hemp oil.

Part Two: Cut Back to 6 Cups (or Even 4)

With limits on higher-carb plant foods in Wahls Paleo Plus, will you still be able to get your 9 cups of vegetables and fruits? Some people find this much more challenging, because the plant foods they like the best are the starchy ones. When I was eating Wahls Paleo, I was eating 9 to 12 cups of vegetables and fruits per day. Now that I am on Wahls Paleo Plus, depending on the day, I actually eat closer to 6 to 9 cups per day (of which 3 cups are still greens because of the emphasis on nonstarchy vegetables). If you are a petite woman, you may be down to just 4 cups. If that's the case, eat 2 cups of greens, 1 cup of sulfur-rich vegetables, and 1 cup of colorful vegetables.

Part Three: Eliminate All Grains, Legumes, and Potatoes

On Wahls Paleo, you cut down your nongluten grains, legumes, and potato servings to twice per week. Now it's time to eliminate them completely. This seems counterintuitive to those who have always heard how healthy these starchy plant foods are. While nongluten grains like brown rice and quinoa, legumes like lentils and black beans, and potatoes (including sweet potatoes) do contain many valuable vitamins and minerals, they are not part of Wahls Paleo Plus. This means ditching soy and rice milk for good (you are drinking full-fat coconut milk now), as well as all sources of soy, even those that are organic or fermented. Focus on animal protein and nonstarchy vegetables.

When your symptoms are severe and you want to create the most healing environment for your brain cells and your mitochondria, it is extremely important to drastically lower your carbohydrate intake, and these foods simply contain too many carbs. There are many other nutrient-dense plant foods to choose from on Wahls Paleo Plus. You might be eliminating the ones you are more accustomed to eating, but this is your chance to branch out and explore new foods. See the food lists at the end of this book and the menu ideas at the end of this chapter for help.

Part Four: Limit Starchy Vegetables to Two Servings per Week

Starchy vegetables have a lot of carbs, but not as many as grains, legumes, and potatoes. Still, it's time to limit these foods—like cooked winter squash, carrots, and beets—to twice per week. When you do have cooked starchy vegetables, you will need to eat them in a particular way: with more added fat and some protein. Adding a generous amount of fat, such as coconut oil or ghee (clarified butter without the milk solids), to a cooked starchy vegetable will help keep your body in a state of mild ketosis. Fortunately, cooked vegetables taste great with added fat, and the fat actually helps your body absorb more of the nutrients. Don't forget to have some protein with that cooked vegetable as well.

Another way I prefer that you eat your starchy vegetables is raw. Try a raw beet salad with cold-pressed olive oil and freshly squeezed lemon juice, or get a kitchen tool that can cut raw winter squash or carrots into thin "spaghetti noodles" and enjoy those with a raw marinara sauce (blending fresh tomatoes, herbs, and olive oil). Be sure there is fat such as olive oil with those raw salads or raw "noodles." Bonus: If you have your starchy vegetable raw, you can have as many cups as you like! The carbohydrates are not so readily absorbed, so you'll be able to maintain the nutritional ketosis. However, if you don't show ketones on the urine strips after one to two weeks, you may need to increase the coconut milk. If you're still not showing ketones, then you may need to cut out cooked starchy vegetables entirely. If that doesn't work, you may need to reduce or even eliminate raw starchy vegetables to achieve nutritional ketosis.

Part Five: Reduce Protein

You'll also have to cut your protein back to 6 to 12 ounces per day, according to your size and gender. Your cells can take amino acids from protein and convert them into sugar to burn in your mitochondria. (The scientific/technical term for this is gluconeogensis.) For this reason, if you eat too much protein, you will not get into nutritional ketosis. You need enough protein to do the work of living, but not so much that you are converting protein into sugar!

Part Six: Limit Fruit to
One Serving per Day, Preferably Berries

Fruit has a lot of carbohydrates, but the lowest-carb fruits are also the most nutritionally dense. It's time to cut out the apples, bananas, and pears because of their high carb content. (Even though they are nutritious and fine for the Wahls Diet and Wahls Paleo, they didn't count toward your 9 cups anyway.) Also, limit other orchard fruits, tropical fruits, and melons. Instead, focus on berries. You'll still get your "color," but you won't get all the carbs. If you eat your berries with a couple of tablespoons of full-fat coconut milk, you will slow down the release of sugar into your bloodstream even more, which will be more helpful for keeping you in nutritional ketosis. (This also tastes great!)

Some people find it very hard to cut down fruit to this level, and I admit that I do have an occasional orange and remain in ketosis as long as I also have my healthy fats with it. In particular, I want you to avoid dried fruit, canned fruit, and fruit juices because of their higher glycemic index and high carbohydrate content.

WHAT IF YOU ARE LOSING TOO MUCH WEIGHT?

Some people on the Wahls Diet, Wahls Paleo, or Wahls Paleo Plus, while enjoying great benefits, lose too much weight. The appetite-suppressing effects of the diets coupled with low-carbohydrate intake can cause this to happen, especially in people who already tend to be on the thin side. If you or your doctor feel that you are losing too much weight, it is fine to reintroduce more carbohydrates by eating more fruits and starchy vegetables, even at the Wahls Paleo Plus level, in amounts that stall weight loss or even help you to gain some weight back. Add a few fruits or starchy vegetables at a time until your weight stabilizes. It's okay to go out of nutritional ketosis temporarily in order to reach a healthy weight. I highly recommend making Wahls Fudge (see the recipe at the end of this book) and eating as much of it as you like until you get back up to a healthy weight. Continue to eat it at the quantity you need to maintain your weight. Again, if this takes you out of ketosis, that is fine. We don't want you underweight. Once your weight has stabilized, you can reduce the amount of fudge you're eating to get back into ketosis as long as you maintain your weight. Our study patients who have lost more weight than we wanted have all found this to be a very effective and tasty way to maintain a desired weight. This fudge is delicious and energy-dense, but still fits into the parameters of the Wahls Protocol. It is also a terrific end-of-the-meal treat to serve to your guests and still be completely compliant with the Wahls Protocol. Eat fudge! (How's that for a prescription?)

Part Seven: Eat Just Twice a Day and Fast Every Night for at Least Twelve Hours

Your mitochondria will thrive if you eat just twice a day and fast every evening for twelve to sixteen hours between your evening meal and your morning meal. Daily fasting, like the long fasting associated with winter, leads to increased efficiency in your mitochondria and encourages your cells to produce more mitochondria per cell.[7] Our bodies are primed to expect long periods of nutritional ketosis—every winter, in fact!

Although fasting is controversial and I don't recommend long fasting periods (you are not a hibernating bear), there is some evidence that caloric restriction or intermittent fasting reverses age-related decline in animal models and may also reverse progressive brain disorders. This likely occurs through improved efficiency in the mitochondria, the increase in the number of mitochondria in each cell, and the additional nerve growth hormones generated by fasting, which stimulate brain cell growth and additional brain cell connections.[8] You can achieve this effect by fasting every other day, but you don't have to go that far. Instead, just fast twelve to sixteen hours every day, which can be overnight while you are sleeping.

Eating only twice a day is not that difficult once you adjust to Wahls Paleo Plus, because nutritional ketosis diets tend to suppress the appetite (whereas high-carb diets tend to stimulate the appetite). When blood sugar is kept very stable, you will likely find that you are hungry only when your body genuinely needs food, and that is probably only twice per day for most people who adhere strictly to Wahls Paleo Plus.

It is helpful to extend the time between your meals at this level of the diet, because when your body isn't digesting, it can focus its energy on healing, eliminating toxins, and recalibrating your biochemistry in line with your new level of nutrition. It is very important to go at least twelve hours between dinner and breakfast so your body can accomplish this important work. If you find it uncomfortable to eat only twice a day, go ahead and keep having three meals until you feel ready to make this change. If you do eat three meals, try making one of your three meals a smoothie only, which is easier for your body to digest quickly. This is also a good way to pack in a good portion of your vegetables and fruit. (Don't forget to add full-fat coconut milk!)

Note: I would prefer you completely eliminate alcohol at this stage, or at least reserve it for special occasions only. If you do have a drink, choose a low-carb drink like vodka or very dry wine. The main reason to minimize alcohol is that your body will metabolize the calories in the alcohol first, before any other energy sources, including fat. Also, your liver has to work hard to process alcohol, and you don't want to tax your liver needlessly when you are trying to heal.

The longer you stick with Wahls Paleo Plus, the easier it gets. I find it's not difficult to follow at all anymore. I do suggest that you monitor at least your urine ketones once you've reached a state of equilibrium on the diet. It will give you feedback on your dietary choices and help keep you on track. Results will also keep you motivated, so as you progress with Wahls Paleo Plus, pay attention to how you feel and write down your physical and emotional reactions to the diet in your Wahls Diary. If you feel great and notice improvement in your symptoms, keep going! If it's too difficult for you at this stage in your life because of family or personal reasons, it's okay to go back to Wahls Paleo for now. This is a much preferable alternative to giving up completely. Stay strong so that your Wahls Diet, at whichever level you choose, can work.

On the following pages, find a summary of the Wahls Paleo Plus rules, and a seven-day meal plan.

LEVEL 3: WAHLS PALEO PLUS

At the Wahls Paleo Plus level, you will continue to follow all the parameters of Wahls Paleo, with the exceptions below. Eat to satiety, but remember that the goal is to consume few carbohydrates, moderate protein, and plenty of fat. Eating a diet that is approximately 65 percent fat with liberal use of medium-chain fat sources like coconut oil and full-fat coconut milk will maintain nutritional ketosis.

Eat at least 68 grams or more of coconut fat, either through 4 to 6 tablespoons of coconut oil or ¾ to 1 can (about 1¾ cups) or even more of full-fat coconut milk. At each meal or snack throughout the day, you may use both coconut oil and full-fat coconut milk, as well as unheated olive oil or ghee, as desired. If you weigh more than 150 pounds, you will probably need 700 or more calories of coconut oil/coconut milk. If you are not in nutritional ketosis after one to two weeks, you may need to increase the coconut oil and full-fat coconut milk. NOTE: You can now buy "coconut milk" in cartons in the store, but this is *not* the same as canned coconut milk. It is much lower in fat and contains fillers and additives, and often sugar. This is not the kind of coconut milk I recommend. Look for the full-fat kind in cans. There are also a few brands in cartons at Indian or Asian groceries, but the coconut milk you buy shouldn't have more than two to three ingredients. Unsweetened varieties in cartons are okay for a dairy substitute at the Wahls Diet and Wahls Paleo levels, but not for Wahls Paleo Plus.

- The 9 cups of vegetables and fruits daily may be reduced to 6 cups (even 4 cups for petite women). No white potatoes, legumes (including any soy, such as soy milk), or any grains (including gluten-free grains and rice milk). If you still need some milk, stick to unsweetened full-fat coconut milk.
- Limit starchy vegetables, like cooked beets and winter squash, to a maximum of twice per week, always accompanied by at least 1 table-spoon of fat and some protein. If you are not in nutritional ketosis after two weeks, you may need to further limit starchy vegetables.
- Limit fruit to 1 cup per day, preferably berries. Always eat these with fat, such as coconut milk. Do not consume dried or canned fruit or fruit juices, which are higher in sugar.
- Reduce protein to 6 to 12 ounces according to size and gender.
- Reduce meals to two per day, with twelve to sixteen hours between dinner and breakfast. If you must eat three meals, be sure to maintain that twelve- to sixteen-hour fast.
- Save alcohol for rare, special-occasion events.

Wahls Paleo Plus Meal Plan		
Day	*Breakfast*	*Dinner*
Day 1	Smoothie: • 1 cup spinach • 1 cup blueberries • 1 cup full-fat coconut milk • 1 teaspoon ground cinnamon • 1 tablespoon nutritional yeast • ½ cup ice 1 serving Salmon Salad* wrapped in collard leaf (1 cup) 1 serving Beet and Cranberry Mixture* ¼ cup fermented pickles	1 serving Liver, Onions, and Mushrooms* ½ cup cooked broccoli 1 teaspoon extra virgin olive oil Salad: • 2 cups romaine lettuce • 2 cups bok choy • ½ cup tomatoes • ½ cup green pepper • 2 cloves garlic • 1 tablespoon extra virgin olive oil • balsamic vinegar to taste • dried basil to taste • 1 tablespoon sunflower seeds ¼ cup kimchi Throat Coat™ herbal tea ½ cup full-fat coconut milk (add to tea if desired)
Day 2	Smoothie: • 1 cup kale • 1 teaspoon green tea powder • 1 teaspoon ground cardamom • ¾ cup full-fat coconut milk • ½ cup ice 1 serving Liver Pâté* ½ cup raw turnip slices 1 medium stalk celery ½ cup Kombucha Tea*	1 serving Basic Skillet Recipe* (Lamb Chops and Broccoli) 1 tablespoon horseradish Salad: • 3 cups spinach • 2 cups kale • 5 medium radishes • ¼ cup sliced carrots • ¼ cup cucumber slices with peel • dried basil to taste • 1½ tablespoons chopped walnuts • 2 tablespoons extra virgin olive oil • balsamic vinegar to taste ¼ cup fermented sauerkraut ¾ cup strawberry halves • 1 tablespoon full-fat coconut milk 2 cups Tension Tamer® herbal tea • ½ cup coconut milk

Day	Breakfast	Dinner
Day 3	1½ servings Turmeric Tea* 3¾ ounces canned sardines in tomato sauce ½ cup raw carrot slices ½ cup parsley ½ cup daikon radish 1 serving Beet and Red Cabbage Mixture* plus 2 tablespoons coconut oil ½ cup Kombucha Tea*	1 serving Basic Skillet Recipe* (Heart and Mustard Greens) 1 serving Brussels Sprouts, Bacon, and Cranberries* Salad: • 4 cups romaine lettuce • 2 cloves garlic • 1 tablespoon ginger root • dried oregano, to taste • 1 tablespoon extra virgin olive oil • balsamic vinegar to taste • 1 tablespoon sunflower seeds ¼ cup lacto-fermented okra pickles 1 cup cherries chamomile herbal tea ½ cup full-fat coconut milk
Day 4	1 serving Bone Broth–Carrot Soup* 1 serving Rosemary Chicken* 1 serving Beet Greens and Bacon* 1½ ounces raw almonds (soaked) ½ cup Beet Kvass* plus ½ cup water	1 serving Seafood Stew* (Paleo Plus version) 1 cup cooked butternut squash 1 tablespoon extra virgin olive oil Salad: • 4 cups bok choy • ¼ cup celery • 1 tablespoon sunflower seeds • 5 medium black olives • 1 tablespoon ginger root • dried oregano to taste • 1 tablespoon extra virgin olive oil • lime juice to taste 1 cup raspberries herbal tea ½ cup full-fat coconut milk

Day	Breakfast	Dinner
Day 5	1 serving Bone Broth–Pepper Soup* 1 serving Basic Skillet Recipe* (Collards and Ham) 1 serving Fruit Pudding* ½ cup Kombucha Tea*	1 serving Algerian Chicken with Asparagus* 1 cup Cauliflower Rice* 1 tablespoon extra virgin olive oil ¼ cup fermented sauerkraut Salad: • 4½ cups bok choy • ½ cup cilantro • ½ cup fresh orange sections • ¼ cup sliced cucumber with peel • 4 teaspoons extra virgin olive oil • lime juice to taste herbal tea ½ cup full-fat coconut milk
Day 6	1½ servings Bone Broth–Cauliflower-Turmeric Soup* Salad: • 3 cups kale • ½ cup radish • ½ cup sweet yellow peppers • ½ cup tomato • ¼ cup chopped onion • 1 tablespoon extra virgin olive oil • 1½ tablespoons chopped almonds (soaked) • balsamic vinegar to taste 3.5 ounce canned salmon ½ cup Beet Kvass* plus ½ cup water	1 serving Basic Skillet Recipe* (Pork Chops and Red Cabbage) ¼ cup kimchi 6 medium asparagus spears Salad: • 2 cups spinach • ½ cup sweet red peppers • ½ cup sliced cucumbers • ½ cup sliced mushrooms • 1 tablespoon extra virgin olive oil • lemon juice to taste 1 cup cantaloupe 1 serving Hot Cocoa*

Day	Breakfast	Dinner
Day 7	1 serving Bone Broth–Avocado Soup* ¾ serving Basic Skillet Recipe* (Steak and Mustard Greens) 1 serving Beet and Cranberry Mixture* 1 tablespoon extra virgin olive oil ½ cup Kombucha Tea*	1 serving Coconut Milk–Fish Soup* 1 tablespoon jalapeño pepper ¼ cup kimchi Salad: • 3½ cups romaine lettuce • dried basil to taste • ¼ cup sliced carrots • 1 teaspoon sesame seeds (raw, soaked) • 1 teaspoon extra virgin olive oil • lime juice to taste Mixed berries: • ¼ cup strawberries • ¼ cup blackberries • ¼ cup raspberries • ¼ cup full-fat coconut milk 1 cup chamomile tea 2.5 fluid ounces full-fat coconut milk (add to tea if desired)

Part Three

GOING BEYOND FOOD

Chapter 8

REDUCE TOXIC LOAD

Y OU'VE COME A long way. You've worked through the Wahls Diet, perhaps staying there, or you've progressed to Wahls Paleo, or perhaps
you've even moved on to Wahls Paleo Plus. If you are staying strong
with the dietary changes, you are almost certainly noticing some improvements, but you can do more. You can go further. In this next section of the
book, I will give you some non-food-related prescriptions that are all part of
the Wahls Protocol. First and foremost, let's talk about toxins.

We no longer live in the world inhabited by our grandparents. Since
World War II, we have relied on chemistry to lessen our work and enrich our
lives in many ways. Unfortunately, due to pollution of the air and water, pesticides and other chemicals used on agricultural products, chemical preservatives and colors used in drinks and processed foods, and food itself that has
been chemically manipulated (like hydrogenated oils and high-fructose corn
syrup), many of those chemicals end up inside us because we eat them, drink
them, inhale them, or touch them.

When substances that enter the body do not naturally occur there, they
are called xenobiotics, and these exotoxins can confuse the signaling that
goes on within and between our cells. A great and decades-long experiment

is being conducted, and we, the unsuspecting public, are the guinea pigs. Our living, working, and recreational environments are now loaded with toxins, more than ninety thousand of which are registered with the Environmental Protection Agency (EPA).

I've already talked about the chemical toxins in our food, both in plants and animals, in previous chapters; but food is not the only source of chemicals in our environment. Let's look beyond our dinner plates for a moment at the vast pollution and contamination in every aspect of our lives: arsenic-treated wood on play structures; off-gassing from the paint, carpets, and furniture in our own homes; residue from plastics; heavy metals in the water supply; and air pollution from factory emissions, vehicle emissions, power plant emissions, electromagnetic waves, microwaves, and Wi-Fi radiation (which can have biologic effects on our cells). We fill our mouths with mercury through our dental fillings; we wash our clothes and slather our skins with products that contain endocrine disrupters that can affect hormonal signaling in our bodies; and on top of that, we don't eat sufficient nutrients to help our bodies efficiently dispose of the toxins we ingest, breathe, absorb, and apply. It's a wonder our mitochondria work at all!

In her seminal environmental book *Silent Spring*, published in 1962, Rachel Carson wrote:

> *For the first time in the history of the world, every human being is now subjected to contact with dangerous chemicals, from the moment of conception until death. In the less than two decades of their use, the synthetic pesticides have been so thoroughly distributed throughout the animate and inanimate world that they occur virtually everywhere.*[1]

Many studies have linked various environmental chemicals with a wide variety of health issues, like neurodegeneration, mood disorders, diabetes, chronic heart disease, to cancer.[2] (You can see a chart from the Institute for Functional Medicine's Detoxification Course on my website, which provides more details.)

To confuse the matter further, in addition to all these environmental chemicals, toxins come from our own bodies. These are called endotoxins, because they are from our own chemical processes. They can be bacteria or

---

WAHLS DIARY ALERT

Answer any of these questions in your Wahls Diary:

- Do you worry about toxins?
- What toxins do you think you've been exposed to? Anything in particular beyond the average person living in the developed world? Do you have a job working with chemicals? Do you work on or live near a farm? Do you live near a factory?
- After you finish this chapter, list some of the ways you think you will be able to reduce your toxic exposure.

---

the waste products from chemical reactions. Normally, we can eliminate these efficiently, but if you are missing any of the nutritional elements necessary to keep the engine of detoxification running smoothly, you may have more trouble eliminating endotoxins as well as xenobiotics. Some people seem to handle the toxic load—both from within and from without—without much problem; but, depending on your genetic susceptibility, you may be particularly sensitive to the toxins inherent in our environment. The result is that the finely tuned symphony of life begins getting out of sync.

If you have MS or another autoimmune disease, chances are good that you *are* one of the particularly sensitive ones. The good news is that, while it is not possible to live a completely toxin-free existence, there are ways to drastically minimize your exposure to toxins. Most important, you must do two things:

1. Maximize your body's natural detoxification process
2. Minimize your toxic exposure

Promote Natural Toxin Elimination

Many of my patients test positive for heavy metals, and I was no exception. My lab tests showed I was toxic in numerous metals, so I detoxed naturally through my dietary protocol as well as gentle detoxing methods, like saunas, clay, algae, kelp, and targeted supplements (I'll talk about all these later in this chapter), until my body eliminated the toxic metals and my health was remarkably improved. Two years later, the follow-up labs showed that I had cleared out the excess heavy metals.

Many people have a name for the process of encouraging toxin elimination: cleansing. Trendy as cleansing may be, it's an ancient practice, and cleansing rituals are a part of many ancient traditions. Often, these cleansing rituals were associated with spiritual purification or healing: cold and hot springs, sweat lodges, mud baths, fasting; all are ways to help the body cleanse itself of impurities so it can work better.

Now we know more about the human body than our ancestors did. We know which organs specifically work to process and eliminate toxins. The main workers are:

- The liver
- The kidneys
- The sweat glands

Before we can understand how to promote the important work of the liver, kidneys, and sweat glands, it's important to understand how detoxification happens in the body.

Most toxins are fat-soluble, so they must be converted to water-soluble substances in order to be excreted in the bile (through the liver), the urine

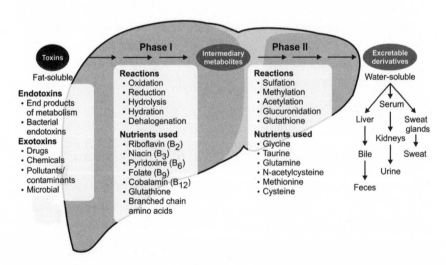

(through the kidneys), or the sweat (from the sweat glands). This process happens in two parts. In phase one, the toxins are converted to reactive metabolites using chemical processes like oxidation, reduction, hydrolysis, and dehalogenation. In other words, they are released from the fat and set free in the body. The toxin is then more active and actually more toxic to us because it is no longer trapped in the fat cells. But the body has a plan. In phase two, your cells attach a side chain to the newly active toxin. This could be another chemical structure, such as a sulfur group, a methyl group, or a specific amino acid. This makes the toxin water-soluble so it can be flushed out of the body. Every part of this process must work, however, in order to release the toxin from the body. If the toxin is converted to the reactive metabolite (phase one) but is not converted to a water-soluble state (phase two), it can actually be more damaging to the body. This is why people sometimes have negative experiences with detoxification. Once the toxins are ready to exit, we need to help them exit so they don't continue to circulate in the body freed from the fat, where they can do more damage.

There are important ways to do this, and fortunately they are not only easy but you are probably already doing them. The best way to do this is to eat your 9 cups of greens, color, and sulfur-rich vegetables, plus seaweed and organ meats, to facilitate this two-phase process and effectively eliminate the toxins. This will provide your body with all the substances it requires to effectively process the toxins to a state where they can be released. Specifically, be sure to get plenty of:

- Selenium and iodine (from seaweed)
- Zinc and coenzyme Q (from organ meat)
- Thiols (from sulfur-rich vegetables and greens)
- Flavonoids (from bright colors)
- Minerals (from iodized sea salt and seaweed)
- Complete amino acids (from animal protein or balanced vegetarian proteins combined to include all the necessary amino acids, as I talked about in chapter 6, "Wahls Paleo")

Adding spices with a favorable impact on detoxification can support your body's efforts even further by improving the efficiency of the detoxification enzymes in the liver, kidneys, and sweat glands (in part by impacting which genes in our DNA are turned on and turned off). The spices will help ensure the proper balance of the detoxification enzymes that are on hand to process and eliminate the toxins you encounter each day. Liberally add these herbs and spices to your food:

- Aloe
- Burdock
- Cayenne
- Dandelion root
- Dill
- Ginger

- Horseradish
- Parsley
- Peppermint
- Rosemary
- Saffron
- Turmeric

Other substances that can be valuable for detoxification include silymarin (from milk thistle seeds used for teas or supplements) and Pycnogenol (from maritime pine bark as a supplement; I'll talk more about supplements in the next chapter).

Nutrition is important, but there are some other great detox strategies I'd also like you to consider. Here are my favorites:

- **Sweat.** Many societies have sweating rituals as part of the purification process. The sweat glands are very effective at removing heavy metals, plastics, and solvents. The sauna causes the blood vessels to dilate for the cooling effect and increases the output of the heart. This is actually an alternative to aerobic exercise! (I discuss this further in the next chapter, "Exercise and Electricity.") Many with MS, however, are severely intolerant to elevations of body temperature. Do not use a sauna until you can tolerate it well. I needed to recover remarkably before I was able to tolerate taking a sauna and wasn't able to do this until six months into my recovery. When I was able to stand the heat, however, I went out and purchased an infrared sauna for my home. It sits next to the Endless Pool I swim in each day. I began taking a sauna four days a week as part of my detox protocol.
- **Mud/clay.** Clays have been used for thousands of years to rejuvenate skin and health. Clay baths for the body or face will extract heavy metals,

WAHLS WARNING

If people adopt my diet overnight, as the people who are entering our clinical trial do, it is common to experience "detox." Even a gradual introduction to the Wahls Diet at any level can result in a detox, especially if you have a particularly large burden of toxins, although it won't be as uncomfortable as a more sudden dietary change. Detox is a natural part of releasing toxins from the body. In most cases, the old adage applies: Better out than in! If you are prepared for the symptoms of detox, you will know what they are and not mistake them for a flare-up of your illness. They may include the following symptoms:

- Acne-like reactions in the skin (likely from bromine that is being excreted via skin)
- Headache
- Body aches
- Malaise
- Temporarily worsening fatigue
- Marked craving for sugar and carbs (by-products of dying sugar-loving yeasts and bacteria that are trying very hard to keep you eating a lot of carbs)

The good news is that these detox symptoms typically begin tapering within a couple of weeks for our clinical trial participants. In my clinical practice, I tell people to wind down the bad food as they wind up the good food over a week. When it is done that way, the detox symptoms are generally somewhat less bothersome. And remember what's happening when you feel them: The bad stuff is coming out!

solvents, and other toxins stored in the fatty tissues of the skin. Mud (clay) masks pull toxins from the skin even more actively than you can sweat them out. When I take my saunas, I put a mud mask on my face and body as I sweat and then I take a cold shower. You can purchase mud mask products in your local drugstore.

> ## WAHLS WARNING
>
> Note that clay, kelp, and algae will not only absorb toxins, they may also absorb medicines from your bloodstream or the medication you take by mouth. If you are on medication, let your doctor know if you plan to work to improve your detoxification, and follow your doctor's directions regarding the best way to do this so as not to interfere with your medication.

A wide variety of clays can be found in health food stores or through on-line stores. Mix these with algae (see the next bullet) and sea salt to make a paste, apply to your skin, and allow it to dry. Leave it on for thirty minutes, then rinse it off. Another way to use clay is to make a diluted clay bath in a bucket for soaking the feet. It's quite relaxing to mix this with magnesium salts. (Afterward, dump the muddy water in the yard so it doesn't clog your plumbing!) Or make a very diluted clay/water mixture and soak in the bathtub for thirty to sixty minutes. If you ever get the opportunity to go to a spa that offers mud baths, take advantage of this effective detoxifying therapy.

- **Algae.** Algae and kelp absorb released toxins so they cannot be reabsorbed back into the bloodstream. They are not only good for your diet but can be useful applied to the skin, with clay (as explained above) or in a seaweed mask.
- **Dry brushing.** This is a technique that increases detoxification through the skin. The technique is simple. Use a gentle brush or a clean, dry washcloth to stroke your skin, starting with your feet, in a gentle circular fashion up toward your heart. Do each leg, then your abdomen. Next, do each arm. This gently removes the old skin cells, rejuvenates the skin, and increases the ability of the skin to eliminate toxins. The whole process typically takes just five to ten minutes. You can do this daily if you wish.

Minimize Your Toxic Exposure

We encounter toxins in the environment all the time, but one of the most intense—and most easily controlled—is what touches your skin. The skin is your largest organ and it is important for toxin elimination, but what people don't always realize is that it also absorbs toxins from the environment. Think about all the soaps, lotions, sunscreens, and medicines you've applied to your skin. You soak those up and they enter your system. Read the labels: All of the chemicals named in the ingredient list will need to be processed and eliminated by your liver and kidney to keep you healthy. The term *organic* also applies to the products you put on your skin. Choose organic foods, and choose organic skin-care products as well—or products that are as natural as possible. Also consider how many products you really need to use. If you are bathing daily, washing your armpits and groin with soap, and eating a clean diet, you probably aren't going to need a lot of other personal-care products. You're going to look and smell great naturally. For instance, you may be able to skip an antiperspirant, which often contains aluminum, a heavy metal that has been implicated in dementia, Parkinson's disease, and neurodegeneration. If you do still want to use some sort of deodorant, look for a natural brand that doesn't contain aluminum. Or you can use a light dusting of baking soda instead.

WAHLS WARNING

The low-grade estrogen effect from the plastics, perfumes, solvents, and hormones in our foods and personal-care products has been implicated in early menstruation in girls as young as 7, falling sperm counts worldwide, increased problems with erectile dysfunction in men in their 20s (a common complaint in primary-care clinics), and infertility in women due to polycystic ovarian disease. They are also implicated as contributing to the development of obesity, metabolic syndrome, and diabetes. This is why they are called "endocrine disruptors." These compounds disrupt and confuse the hormone signals of our endocrine glands.

Your home is another potent source of toxins. The cleaning products and furnishings you use in your home can expose you to hundreds of synthetic compounds each day that interfere with your cells' chemical operations, often by gently nudging your hormonal system out of balance. If you clean up your indoor environment, you can minimize toxic exposure where you live, and that can make a big difference on your internal toxin load. Here are some strategies:

- Gradually replace synthetic carpets, curtains, and bedding with natural fabrics. These synthetic materials can release into the air chemicals that you breathe in for years. Good fabric choices for the home include wool, organic cotton, hemp, and bamboo fabric.
- Gradually replace all particleboard, plywood, fiberglass, fiberboard, and paneling in your furniture, cabinets, walls, and floors. These materials can off-gas toxic compounds into your indoor air. Replace them with natural hardwoods and bamboo.
- Paint only with low-VOC (volatile organic compounds) paint for indoor surfaces.
- Open your windows as much as possible to ventilate, and place a few green plants around the house; they will help detoxify your air. If you have allergies, consider a high-quality air cleaner for your bedroom, where you spend many hours of your life breathing deeply.
- Switch to natural or "green" household cleaners. Vinegar, baking soda, and hydrogen peroxide can take care of most jobs, or purchase natural cleaners. Clean your house at least every week to keep bacteria and mold in check.
- Replace all the plastic food storage containers in your home with glass ones. An economical way to do this is to save glass jars from foods like pickles and salsa, and use those to store leftovers.
- Replace Teflon-coated pans with stainless steel or enameled cast iron.
- Filter your water. There are many levels of filtering available; even a pitcher with a filter can reduce toxins in your tap water. A reverse-osmosis system is superior because it is the only way to remove the various drugs that have likely entered your water supply; it is what I have installed in our home.

WAHLS WARRIOR Q & A

Q: Will the Wahls Protocol help with PCOS (polycystic ovary syndrome), endometriosis, infertility, or other hormonal issues like PMS and hot flashes?
A: Once our endocrine glands begin to get out of sync, the chemistry of our cells begins to falter. These changes can make adult women hormonally much more like men, and adult men hormonally much more like women (think polycystic ovarian syndrome, infertility, erectile dysfunction, obesity, mood problems, and insulin resistance). The ovaries and testicles make the most potent sex hormones, which activate and develop the characteristics that make girls into women and boys into men beginning in adolescence. The adrenal glands also make sex hormones to a lesser extent, and fat makes sex hormones, too. In addition, there continues to be evidence that many synthetic compounds (e.g., plastics, solvents, fragrances, etc.) can fit into the sex hormone receptors and confuse our biology.[3]

Hormonal issues can feel like a huge problem, but in many cases the answer is relatively simple. Diet can make a huge difference for women suffering from PCOS and infertility as well as other hormonal issues like PMS and the symptoms of menopause. Also consider whether hormone disruption from plastics, solvents, fragrances, and pesticides could be contributing to hormone imbalance. Furthermore, unrecognized gluten sensitivity can be a factor in endometriosis, polycystic ovarian syndrome, and infertility problems. Many of these conditions are also related to insulin resistance. Stabilizing blood sugar and lowering insulin levels by decreasing carbohydrates and reducing the body's toxin load is the prescription. The more completely you can embrace Wahls Paleo or Wahls Paleo Plus, the more quickly insulin will normalize, and likely so will sex hormone ratios. Also, go meticulously organic and do what you can to improve the detoxification pathways and reduce hormone disruption.

And what about in your own mouth? If your mouth is full of silver fillings that contain mercury, a small amount of mercury vapor is released each day that you will absorb into your body. There is a relationship between the num-

WAHLS WARRIORS SPEAK

Knowing that I had numerous "silver" fillings and a "silver" cap that needed oral surgery to be removed, as well as a "mercury tattoo" [a tattoo with mercury in the ink], I took Dr. Wahls's advice and began the process of investigating my mercury levels. I had my urine, blood, and hair tested for mercury and, needless to say, I had high levels of it in my body. Because I'd experienced such marked improvements in my MS symptoms after following the Wahls Diet for a short period of time, I began the process of mercury detoxification immediately. I had all of the mercury removed from my mouth and I detoxify regularly in other ways. I continue to do dry body brushing; I take supplements, which include bentonite clay and additional B vitamins. I eat plenty of algae and cilantro; and, of course, I treat myself to a weekly clay (Aztec bentonite clay) footbath and facial. I loved learning about all the beneficial properties of herbs, spices, and teas from Dr. Wahls. Every day, I put a dash of cardamom in my tea, and I add turmeric to my bone broth.

—Debra K., Accord, New York

ber of mercury fillings in the mouth and the amount of mercury in the brain. Many people decide to have their mercury fillings removed, but I do not advise this without proper research and consideration. Removing mercury fillings can actually release more mercury into your body if it is done incorrectly. As the dentist removes the fillings, the drilling will vaporize some the mercury, which can then be inhaled and reabsorbed by your body. It is important to work with a dentist who has been specifically trained in the safe handling of mercury fillings to minimize the risk of increasing the mercury load that is released in the process. Look for someone who has been specifically trained by the International Academy of Oral Medicine and Toxicology (IAOMT).

Note that it has become increasingly popular for dentists to call themselves holistic, mercury-free, or biologic dentists because they no longer use

---

THE NEW TOOTHBRUSH

Ditch the fluoride-based toothpastes. In fact, ditch all commercial tooth-pastes. Instead try this: Put some cold-pressed coconut oil in the bath-room, draw the toothbrush across the coconut oil, and brush with that. Or you could use a few drops of olive oil, oregano oil, or tea tree oil, which will suppress the bacteria contributing to plaque development. The other thing you could do is to use baking soda. Although it is a bit abrasive for ongoing daily use, brushing a couple of times a week with baking soda will also help improve detoxification by increasing the alkalinity of your urine.

---

mercury/silver fillings. However, many of these dentists have not received advanced training in the safe removal of mercury. Do your research!

Another dental problem is the use of fluoride as a strategy to reduce dental decay and as an addition to city water. Fluoride is toxic to bone and brain cells and is associated with reductions in IQ of children.[4] Better to not use fluoride to prevent dental cavities; instead, eliminate white flour and sugar from the diet and stick with the Wahls Protocol, which will give you the intensive nutrition you need to fight dental decay.

All in all, detoxing isn't particularly hard, but it does require vigilance: pure food, a clean home, natural materials on and around you as much as possible, and a systematic nurturing of the body to help it eliminate toxins the way it is designed to do. It is the perfect complement to the Wahls food plan and an essential part of the Wahls Protocol.

Chapter 9

EXERCISE AND ELECTRICITY

I F YOU AREN'T mobile now and you change nothing about what you are doing, you're not going to become mobile in the future. This sounds obvious, but people don't often see it this way. They believe that rest will allow them to move more later, but as later gets further and further away, muscles begin to degenerate, and your whole physical system degrades. What happens when you don't start a car engine for years? At some point, it's going to seize up, and then it's going to take a lot more to start it than turning a key.

Because people with MS experience fatigue as the disease progresses, many physicians have been telling MS patients not to exercise. The belief was that this would reduce fatigue, leaving more energy for everyday life. Now we know how wrong this is. Numerous studies have shown that a wide variety of exercise programs, such as yoga,[1] strength training,[2] and aerobic training,[3] are very helpful for reducing fatigue and improving the quality of life for the person with MS.

I'm not going to tell you that you have to run a 5K or even walk around the block. Each person is different. You may be able to do things that someone else with MS can no longer do; yet another person with MS may be able to do things you can't do anymore. You can only do what is possible for you. What you must not do is neglect what is still possible for you. A downward spiral into immobility does not have to be your fate. Movement begets movement, and energy expenditure can, if done correctly, result in more energy, not less. Lack of mobility only leads to immobility.

You Were Designed to Move

Exercise has been essential for our species from the very beginning. For 2.5 million years, our ancestors traveled six to twelve miles a day on average, intermittently running as fast as we could to capture our food or, even more critically, to get away from predators or enemies. Our brains are hardwired to expect that level of activity.

Not only that, but brains depend on exercise for growth and maintenance. You might think that only your muscles, heart, and lungs benefit from exercise, but exercise directly impacts both your brain and spinal cord. Your brain literally depends on exercise for the growth factors it needs to thrive. Exercise stimulates the release of particular hormones in the brain that nourish brain cells (namely, nerve growth factor, or NGF), and brain-derived neurotrophic factor (BDNF) and other growth factors, which all stimulate the growth of brain cells and more synapses, or connections between brain cells.[4] If you don't exercise, your brain won't get this all-important growth-hormone "bath" and your body will react by pruning the unused neural connections and making fewer new connections. Your body also spends less time repairing those areas, and the result is atrophy and brain shrinkage. You are more and more likely to have early memory loss, declining social skills, and increased irritability and mood troubles.

The damage that results from a lack of exercise is cumulative. The amount of exercise that you do over your lifetime will impact your risk of developing Alzheimer's disease. Those with less exercise over a lifetime have a higher risk of dementia, and the theory is that the brain growth hormones you don't get when you don't exercise may actually contribute to the progression of Alzheimer's. And speaking of mood disorders, regular exercise, either aerobic or strength training, is as effective or even more effective than the Prozac family of medications for treating mood disorders like depression.[5] On a system-wide basis, exercise also lowers the excretion of cytokines that cause excessive inflammation.[6] In short, little or no physical activity is very bad for your well-being.

If you're not already on an exercise program, it is essential to start one, and this is an important part of the Wahls Protocol. Your exercise program should include stretching for shortened muscles, balance training, strengthening to

> ## WAHLS WARNING
>
> Before starting a new physical exercise program, particularly for those who are not doing any physical activity at all, it is important to speak with your physician and get clearance. This will give you a chance to ask for a physical therapy evaluation and to clarify what limitations you have based on your individual risk factors.

build muscles, and aerobic conditioning to improve endurance. Strength training generates the largest gains in nerve growth factors,[7] so do not neglect this important element! I urge you to begin a program of stretching and conditioning now, whatever your health status is. It will help protect your brain, improve your mood, and lessen the risk of heart disease, dementia, diabetes, obesity, and other chronic health problems.

> ## WAHLS DIARY ALERT
>
> In your Wahls Diary, track how often you exercise, for how long, and what you do. Also write down when you don't exercise and why. Your Wahls Diary can help hold you accountable—writing it down could increase your chances of getting up and doing it. Remember, no matter how small your movements or how short your exercise session, it still counts, and it's still better than nothing. The more you do, the easier it will become. Write it all down, and you'll also be able to track your progress as you get stronger in the months to come.

Getting Started

Most people do better with exercise when they are held accountable. There are many ways to do this. Although I've always been active, for years I kept an exercise calendar. I wrote down what I did every day—a quick summary of my workout in just a few lines in my weekly planner. You can use your Wahls Diary to do this. It's a way to be accountable to yourself. You might also consider exercising with a friend or reporting your exercise to a friend, who will ask you about it if you don't report back.

Or maybe you need something more. You may be more motivated to exercise if you make yourself accountable to a professional coach or a physical therapist. The advantage to working with a professional is that you have someone who can evaluate your progress and adjust your training program as you progress. If you have any impairment in your gait or balance, I urge you to see a physical therapist for a clinical evaluation. You can ask your physician for a referral. A physical therapist can evaluate precisely which muscles are strong and weak, how flexible you are, how good your balance is, how much endurance you have, and whether there are any corrections you can work on with your gait. If you don't have visible impairments, try an exercise therapist or athletic trainer for an assessment, personalized exercise program, and subsequent coaching. A good physical therapist and/or athletic trainer can design a specific exercise program for you and help you set and track specific goals. You will probably work with the therapist or trainer in the clinic or gym, and you will also likely get "homework"—exercises you can and should do on your own at home between sessions.

Even if you don't have access to a professional, you can design your own exercise program. There are many simple exercises you can do on your own that specifically target some of the issues that MS presents. These are primarily in four categories:

1. Stretching and lengthening
2. Balance
3. Strengthening
4. Cardiovascular fitness

I recommend doing a few exercises out of each category every day when possible. Or rotate through the days: stretching one day, balance the next day, strengthening the next day, cardio the following day. Do all four regularly at your own level for the most balanced program, to the extent that you are able. Let's look at each category separately.

Stretching

Dancers and martial artists are all focused on maintaining good flexibility. As a tae kwon do practitioner, I should have known to spend as much time on stretching as I did on strengthening, but I didn't do this as I became disabled. As a result, my calf muscles and hamstrings became shortened. I have spent years now working on stretching them back out.

Nearly everyone with MS develops shortened muscles, especially the calf muscles, hamstrings, and gluteal muscles. Muscle spasms and muscle stiffness are also common problems with MS patients, often because of decreasing activity. Doing regular stretching will help reduce the spasticity and stiffness greatly, but even if you aren't experiencing this problem, stretching and lengthening will benefit you. For anyone with MS, a regular stretching regimen can reduce spasms and muscle stiffness and help improve mobility. Stretching is also key for restoring or maintaining a normal range of motion, which is essential for mobility. It can also help reduce the trouble with leg cramps and spasms at night.

If your doctor has prescribed baclofen, which increases the neurotransmitter gamma-aminobutyric acid (GABA), it may be to help reduce MS-related spasticity and stiffness in your muscles. This can be helpful to many people but should be combined with a stretching program. With a good exercise program, medication may eventually become unnecessary. Research has shown that the combination of baclofen with a program of stretching is the most effective strategy to treat and prevent shortening of muscles, muscle spasms, and muscle stiffness.[8]

The following stretches are those I do and recommend. The images and summaries for the stretches that follow (and the neuromuscular reeducation exercises later in this chapter) are adapted from exercise education materials provided in the Toolkit from the Institute for Functional Medicine. Your therapist may have different or additional suggestions for you:

1. Soleus/Achilles Stretch

Stand about three feet from a wall with both feet flat on the ground. Place your hands against the wall. Step forward with your right foot, keeping both heels flat on the floor. Lean your hips toward the wall while keeping your left leg straight, to stretch your calf. Hold 10 seconds. Repeat with the other leg. Do a total of 10 times each leg.

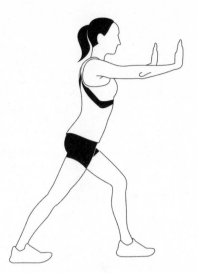

2. Hamstring Stretch

Sit with your legs straight out in front of you, feet against a wall. Hold your hands behind your back if you can. (If you cannot, rest your hands on the floor beside your hips.) Bend at the hips and lean your trunk forward until you feel a stretch in your hamstrings, along the backs of your thighs. Hold 10 seconds. Return upright. Do 10 stretches.

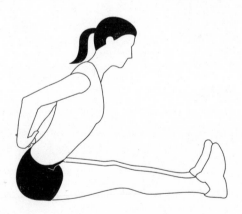

3. Gluteal Stretch

For your gluteal muscles (the muscles in your rear), lie on your back on the floor and pull your knees up across your chest. Do one leg at a time for a more intense stretch. Hold 10 seconds. Do 10 stretches on each side.

4. *Psoas Stretch*

Your psoas runs along the front of your hip and can get tight, especially if you sit frequently. Here's how to stretch it back out:

Place your right knee on a chair. Your left leg should be straight, with your foot flat on the floor next to the chair. Slowly bend your left knee until you feel a stretch along the front of your right hip. Do not arch your back. Hold for 10 seconds. Repeat on the other side. Do 10 stretches on each side.

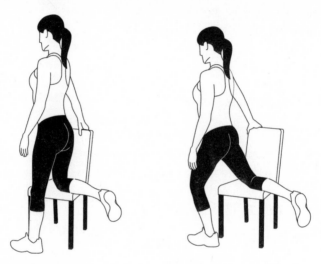

5. *Quadriceps Stretch*

Your quadriceps are four muscles on the front of your thigh. To stretch them, lie facedown on the floor. Bend your right knee. Reach your right arm back and grab your toe or ankle. Pull your foot into your backside until you feel the front of your thigh stretch. If you can't quite reach your foot, loop a scarf or towel around your foot and pull on that. Hold for 10 seconds. Repeat with the other leg. Do 10 stretches on each leg.

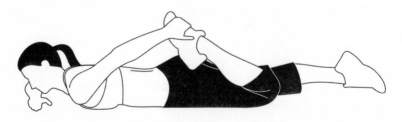

6. *Erector Spinae #1*

The next two stretches are for your erector
spinae muscles, which are the muscles in
your back around your spine. For this first
one, sit down in a chair and bend forward.
Reach down to grasp your calves with both
hands. Pull your body toward the floor.
Hold for 10 seconds. Relax. Repeat 10 times.

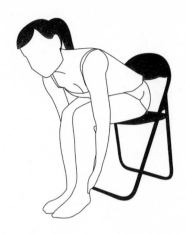

7. *Erector Spinae #2*

For this back-stretching exercise, get down on your hands and knees. If this is
painful, you may do this on a padded exercise mat or even on your bed. Place
your hands under your shoulders and knees under your hips. Slowly let your
back sag down and raise your head up. Don't push your back down; just let it
hang. Hold for 10 seconds. Then let your head hang down. Pull your stomach
in and arch your back up. Hold 10 seconds and return to a flat-backed position. Repeat 10 times.

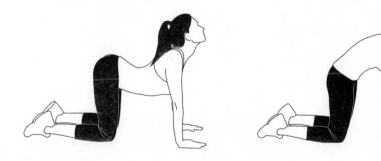

Balancing

Balance often becomes a problem for people with mobility issues. People with
MS and other autoimmune conditions may also have a loss of sensation in the
legs or feet, and/or issues with dizziness and impaired proprioception (not
having a good idea of where things are in space, like not realizing where your

foot is exactly). As we age, our ability to sense where we are in space diminishes, even in the best of circumstances. MS or any disease affecting the brain and muscles can speed the decline of this particular kind of awareness.

You can prevent or slow this loss by doing balance training. Your physical therapist can give you specific exercises, but an easy way to start is to simply stand on one foot for as long as you can. When I first started doing balance training, I did this in the hallway so I could easily touch the wall to regain my balance. I would lift one foot and start counting. My goal was to lengthen the amount of time I could stand on one leg. I can now do thirty seconds on either leg and have moved on to some Pilates and yoga poses.

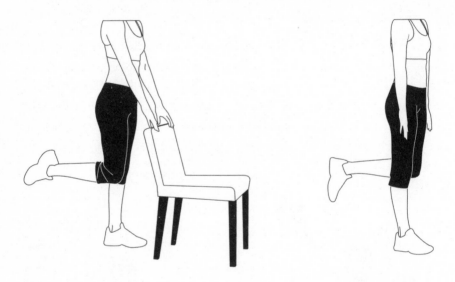

This is an excellent beginning exercise for anyone with balance issues. Start in the hallway or next to the kitchen counter so you can catch yourself when your balance falters. I suggest making it your goal to be able to stand straight up on one leg for thirty seconds or even one minute. Once you have achieved that goal, you can get more advanced by balancing on one foot while leaning forward with your arm reaching forward. You can also try this with your eyes closed, but be sure you have something to grab if you start to fall! Always stay safe when working on your balance.

Regular balance training can make a big difference in regaining your sense of where things are in space, and it can also help to prevent falls, which

---

WAHLS WARRIOR Q & A

Q: Why do MS feet turn purple, swell, and feel so disgusting, and what can I do about it?

A: The blood returns to the heart through the veins. The flow of blood from the legs and arms depends on the contraction of the muscles of the arms and legs. When the arms or legs become weak, there is less muscle pumping on the veins. The blood tends to back up, causing the swelling and the purplish discoloration. This is made worse by having more inflammation molecules in the blood. To help reduce the purple discoloration and swelling, two things are helpful: One, increase the contraction of muscles in the arms or legs. Doing more exercise and/or electrical stimulation of the calf muscles or arm muscles is helpful. Spending time with the arms or legs elevated above the heart would also help drain the extra blood back to the heart. Two, reduce the inflammation molecules and improve blood fluidity by eating more sulfur-rich vegetables. More bright colors and greens would also be helpful. I have observed these improvements in both our clinical trial and in my clinical practice.

---

can lead to serious injury. If you would like more guidance and structure in your balance training, consider a beginning yoga class or a yoga class for people with health issues, including "yoga in a chair." Yoga has many poses that are excellent balance training—at all levels.

Strengthening

Strength training is your next priority. Declining strength is a primary factor in falls and injuries, not to mention accelerated loss of mobility. Strength training combats this effect by utilizing the body's natural ability to adapt to whatever you do with it.

If you were already exercising regularly, you may also notice your strength decreasing slowly over time (although with the Wahls Protocol, you should be able to reverse this trend). I had been doing a daily workout for decades before

I was diagnosed. After the diagnosis, I knew that my strength training and swimming were going to keep me mobile, but despite my daily workout, my strength slowly declined. I had to change my ten-pound dumbbells for eight-pound dumbbells, and then eventually I had to drop to five pounds. Still I didn't let this stop me. I kept strength training to fight the decline.

Every patient is different, but there are a few strength issues that seem to plague MS patients. One particular strength issue we often see is weakness in the leg muscles that pick up the toes while walking. This was one of my first clear signs, when my wife, Jackie, noticed I was dragging my foot on a long walk. This often causes people to trip over their toes as they swing the leg forward and is a common cause of falls and injury. Strengthening the muscles that flex your ankle and toes upward can make a big difference in your stability. There are some easy ways to build this strength on your own:

1. Simply lift your toes and point your foot to the ceiling as high as possible. Count to ten. Repeat ten times. This is a simple place to start.
2. When that is easy, stand on your heels with your toes pointed up off the ground, your hand on the wall for balance. Hold for ten seconds. Repeat ten times, or do this throughout the day when you think about it.
3. When that is easier to do, then you can walk down the hallway on your heels with your toes in the air, again hanging on to the wall for balance.

You likely have other weak muscles that need training—most people do. Work on those, too. Having a therapist or trainer give you a specific strengthening program is important, because your program can be tailored to your individual needs. If you are still relatively mobile, I urge you to look for a group exercise class that would fit your interests and your schedule. Talk to the instructor, explain your health issues, and then discuss how he or she would approach having you in class. Tai chi, yoga, and Pilates are particularly good because of the strength and balance training involved.

If you never strength train, your body will think your muscle cells aren't important and won't devote resources to them. If you do strength train, then you are working the muscle cells to exhaustion, actually damaging them slightly. Your body, being adept at cellular repair, will repair the cells over the next twenty-four hours, rebuilding them to tolerate slightly more work, in response to your exercise. That is why you want to do strength training every other day: You need a day to recover and let your body make you stronger in response to your efforts.

Recovery time may not be necessary for your training at first. If you are very weak, your exercises in the beginning will likely be more aerobic than strengthening. If you don't work hard enough to damage the muscle cells, you won't need twenty-four hours for repair. However, as you get stronger, you can do more strength work. Your therapist or trainer will let you know when you are actually working your muscles hard enough that you need to do your strength training every other day.

There are also many strengthening exercises you can do at home, in addition to the ones I listed above to help keep your feet from dragging, such as those that involve weights or resistance bands. I strongly recommend you get guidance from a physical therapist or a qualified trainer, who can customize your program to exactly what you need.

Neuromuscular Reeducation

Before we move on to cardiovascular training, I want to tell you about a type of exercise that combines both balance training and strength training. It's called neuromuscular reeducation. Because these exercises help coordinate your brain and body, neuromuscular reeducation exercises are very useful for people with mobility issues as well as proprioception issues.

As you do these exercises your endurance will slowly improve, too, which will be good for your heart and can help you work up to a point where you are able to do cardiovascular exercise. They involve balancing on an exercise ball while smoothly and carefully doing certain movements. If you don't have an exercise ball, your local gym may have them available for gym use by members. They are also inexpensive to purchase at athletic stores or discount stores like Walmart, Kmart, and Target.

For every exercise on the following pages, keep a slight tilt in your pelvis to stabilize your lower back before doing any movement.

1. Flexion

Kneel behind the ball and grasp the ball with your arms, lacing your fingers together in front of the ball. Slowly roll your body forward on the ball and gently rock forward and backward. Work on maintaining your balance while smoothly performing this movement. (Stop if you feel any pain. Only go as far as you can comfortably while maintaining your balance.)

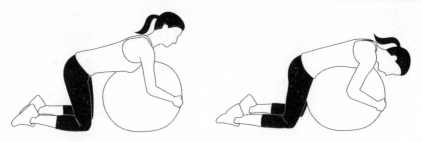

2. Extension

Squat with the ball behind you and place your back on the ball. Slowly roll your body backward on the ball. Reach above your head with your arms, gently rocking forward and backward. If you can, lean all the way back on the ball. (Stop if you feel any pain. Only go as far as you can comfortably while maintaining your balance.)

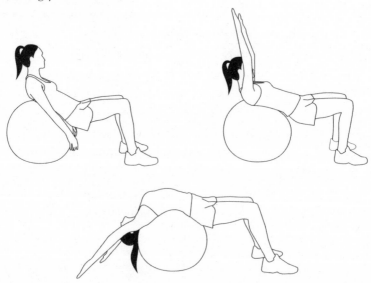

3. Lateral Flexion

Kneel with the ball on your right side and put your right arm on the ball for balance. Extend your left leg out to the left. Slowly roll your body on top of the ball. Reach above your head with your free arm. Repeat on the other side. (Stop if you feel any pain. Go only as far as you can comfortably while maintaining your balance.)

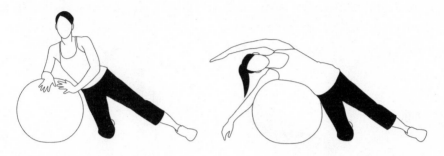

4. Seated Leg Lift

Sit on the ball with your knees bent at a right angle. Bounce up and down easily at first, then more energetically while maintaining your balance. Then lift one foot at a time, carefully maintaining your balance. When this becomes easy, lift one leg at a time and extend it parallel to the ground. Do not slouch!

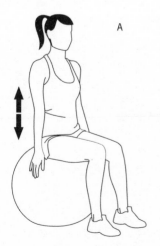

A

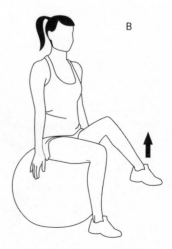

B

5. Downward-Facing Bridge

Kneel on the floor in front of the ball. Roll over the ball so it is under your stomach. Place your hands on the floor in front of the ball. Keep both sets of toes on the floor, feet about two feet apart. Extend one arm parallel to the floor, keeping the other hand on the floor. Lower the outstretched hand and then extend the other arm out parallel to the floor. Next, extend one leg out parallel to the floor, then return and extend the other leg out parallel to the floor. Once this becomes relatively easy, try extending one arm and the opposite leg parallel to the floor. Hold each position for a count of 10.

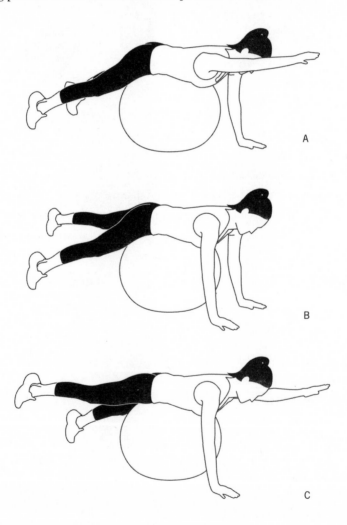

6. Upward-Facing Bridge

Sit on the ball. Walk out and roll down over the ball until the ball is between your shoulder blades, and your body is parallel to the floor. Lift one foot at a time, performing a small march. Then lift and extend overhead one arm at a time, parallel to the floor, while continuing to march. When this is easier, try extending one leg and the opposite arm and holding for a count of 10. Repeat on the other side.

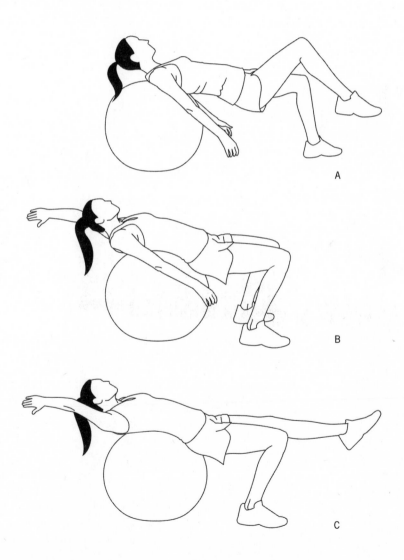

A

B

C

7. Curl-Ups

Solidify your core with this ab-strengthening version of sit-ups. Sit on a ball and roll forward so the back of your rib cage rests on the ball. Curl up and reach toward your knees with arms extended in front of you. If this is too difficult, place more of your back on the ball. When you can do this, try curling up with your arms folded across your chest. The most advanced level is to curl up with your arms behind your head, as pictured below. Be careful not to strain your neck during this exercise. Try to keep your neck relaxed so all the effort comes from your abdominal muscles. If you still feel a strain on your back, roll back so even more of your back is placed on the ball.

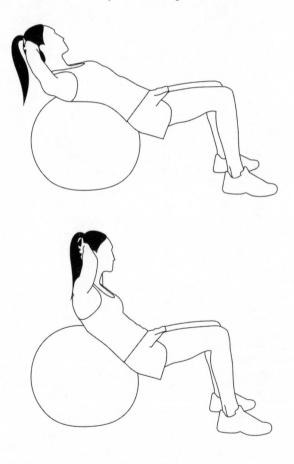

8. Superman

Place the soles of your feet against the wall and your knees on the ground (or on a mat). Rest your belly over the ball. Keep your chin tucked in. Slowly push off the wall and align your trunk and legs in a straight line. Hold for 10 seconds. Roll back. Try it again, reaching your arms out in front of your body like Superman, forming a straight line from feet to hands. Hold for 10 seconds and roll back. For the most advanced level, add a swimming motion, like you are doing the crawl stroke, alternating your arms as they reach overhead.

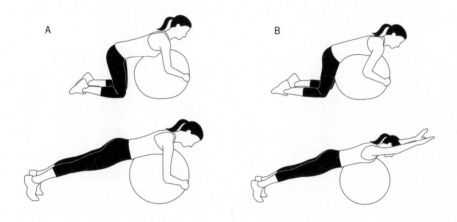

A   B

Cardiovascular Conditioning

When people think of exercise, they often think of cardio first. Cardio is important, but I want to emphasize that stretching, balance, and strengthening, as well as some targeted neuromuscular reeducation, are equally important for people with mobility issues.

Cardiovascular conditioning benefits the body in a different way from other exercises because it involves the heart and lungs. However, what constitutes a vigorous cardiovascular workout for one person might be effortless for another person, so it's hard to say exactly what you should be doing other than doing something that doesn't hurt but still gets your heart rate up, has you breathing more quickly than you do at rest, and maybe even gets you to break a sweat.

For me, aerobic workouts were always a part of life. I used to run until I had to slow down because of mysterious hip pain. I got into biking and then cross-country skiing. I picked up roller skis and started skiing on blacktops. I often took my children with me, pulling them behind me in a trailer either with wheels or skis. Jackie and I took them on easy biking trails through the woods and taught them to cross-country ski when they were old enough.

Soon, however, I found I wasn't able to cross-country ski using the faster skating technique. I was annoyed with myself, thinking I was getting old and out of shape, despite the fact that I had gotten up every day since college to work out before starting work. I hadn't missed a day in years. When I was finally diagnosed with MS, part of me felt relieved: I hadn't been a slug after all. There was a reason for my declining exercise ability.

However, I kept up because I knew daily exercise was important if I wanted to continue walking. For a while I walked uphill slowly on a treadmill for twenty minutes, but then that became impossible. That's when I discovered swimming.

Swimming is an excellent form of aerobic conditioning for people with MS and other mobility issues. I put an Endless Pool into my home in 2002, and I have to thank my mom for encouraging me to spend the money to do this. She reminded me that my health and stamina were incredibly important to maintain. If the pool helped me do that, it was worth getting. The Endless Pool is a pool with a current generator. It is a swimmer's treadmill. (For more information, see the Resources section at the back of this book.) I swam every day and did a weight routine with dumbbells. I have come to like swimming in cold water, particularly in the evening, so I do not heat my pool. I will swim in 65-degree water and ease myself into the water gradually, allowing my body to get used to the cold. (This isn't for everyone: Most people need warm water, or at least warmer than 65 degrees!) The cold water lowers my core body temperature, which—at least for me—seems to help me have a deeper, more restful sleep. I begin by doing the crawl stroke with my goggles and snorkel on so I don't have to worry about breathing technique or craning my neck. I'll swim for fifteen to thirty minutes in the evening and then spend time stretching.

You may not be able to put a pool into your house, but most communities have a recreation center with a pool, and many private gyms have pools. Even if you don't know how to swim, you can try walking in the water. The water provides resistance but also cushions joints for a potentially less injurious workout. I know many patients who "water walk" and get quite a good aerobic workout doing it.

Other options include water aerobics classes, which are generally easier on the body than regular aerobics classes. Or, if water really isn't your thing, do something different: Walk on a treadmill with bars to hold on to if you have balance issues, or try an elliptical trainer or a stationary bicycle. Rowing machines and reclining bikes are good options, too. Many of my patients do gentle yoga classes and Pilates classes, which can be adapted to different levels and abilities but provide stretching, strengthening, and an aerobic component, and use body weight and balance. Martial arts and CrossFit-type classes also improve strength, endurance, and balance but require a higher level of strength and endurance than many with MS will have.

Work with where you are right now. If you can only walk down the driveway and back, that's a starting point. If you can ride a stationary bicycle for five minutes, that's a starting point. Anything is better than nothing. If possible, again, I want to emphasize the importance of working with a physical therapist to evaluate your muscle strength, flexibility, balance, and gait and to create a personalized exercise program that covers all the exercise bases. However, you can get started today. You can start engaging your muscles again right now. Why waste any more time?

If you do some kind of cardiovascular conditioning on most days, or at least three days per week for as long as you can tolerate, you will be making good progress.

Vibration

Another workout I have come to enjoy that combines strengthening with balance and also has an aerobic component is whole-body vibration. I discovered whole-body vibration after reviewing another of Dr. Richard Shields's studies on the whole-body vibration machine.

The principle of whole-body vibration is that by standing on a vibrating platform your muscles make hundreds of tiny corrections each minute in re-

> ## WAHLS WARRIORS SPEAK
>
> *I've been in a wheelchair for seven years. I was diagnosed with RRMS in 1995, but that changed somewhere around 2002–2003 to secondary-progressive MS. Along with MS, I've had three surgeries for trigeminal neuralgia. I started the Wahls Diet about thirteen months ago but have been very strict on it for about six months.*
>
> *Since I've been on the diet, my right hand, which had been totally clenched into a fist since 2001, has started to relax and I've been able to cut down on my pain medications to less than half of what I used to take. Before the diet, I could stand up for only one minute while holding on to something and walk using a hemi-walker for about twenty feet. Now I can stand up for seven minutes and walk 160 feet. I used to do e-stim, but now use a full-body vibration machine twice per day, which is great for massage and my circulation. I continue to hope and pray that I will be able to walk and drive again someday, and I thank God every day that I was introduced to this diet.*
>
> *—Patricia O., Gainesville, Florida*

sponse to the changing position. Your body is also required to sense where you are in space, so it sends hundreds of messages each minute to your brain, which is great for your proprioception. All of the messages to and from your brain stimulate the release of hormones in the brain (the nerve-growth hormone family that stimulates repair and building connections, which I talked about at the beginning of this chapter). Your body is also stimulated to release hormones in the muscle, which in turn promotes muscular growth and repair in the muscles, tendons, and bones.

Dr. Shields is studying the impact of whole-body vibration for maintaining muscle and bone strength in paralyzed individuals. In the research literature, whole-body vibration has helped those who are deconditioned or have thinned bones to improve both bone and muscle strength.[9] It has also been used by Russian cosmonauts and American astronauts to stimulate more bone and muscle strength to increase the tolerance for space travel. Athletes have embraced whole-body vibration. Clinical studies have shown that whole-body vibration can have modest benefits for improving bone density and strength in those who have low bone-mineral density or who are deconditioned.[10]

When I heard about this, I was intrigued. I decided to give it a try. The model I picked up is the Vibra Pro 5500. I worked with my physical therapist to begin doing a strength-training program using whole-body vibration three days a week. I started with a low number of oscillations per second so that the gravitational forces that my body experienced would be minimal. Then very slowly and gradually I increased the length of time that I did each exercise and the number of oscillations per second. Ideally you will find a clinic or a gym that has a whole-body vibration machine so you can test this out for yourself and have your physical therapist or trainer assist you in designing a program specifically for whole-body vibration that matches what your body needs. I do not recommend doing this on your own, at least until you fully understand how to use the machine and you have a plan that has been designed specifically for you. These machines aren't cheap, either: Costs range from approximately $1,400 to $15,000 or more. See the Resources section for more information.

E-Stim

As you may remember from the introduction to this book, I discovered e-stim while reviewing a research protocol and was interested in how this therapy was being used on people who had lost mobility. I convinced my therapist to let me try a test session and found it to be of great benefit in restoring my strength and mobility. I have since incorporated it into the Wahls Protocol, and I believe it is a useful tool for reversing muscle atrophy and loss of mobility.

E-stim isn't the most comfortable experience in the world. Some people are more sensitive to it than others, and some people think that it is actually painful. It must be done *in addition* to exercise, not instead of exercise. Despite these inconveniences, however, you can grow more muscle with e-stim and exercise than you would by exercise alone.

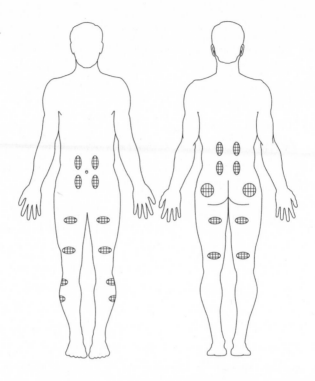

These are the motor points where I placed electrodes to stimulate the muscles that my therapist had identified as weak. Note that my physical therapist worked with me in placing the electrodes and testing which muscle was in fact being stimulated to confirm that the location was correct to stimulate the intended muscle group. Because we are all unique, each individual will often need adjustment of the location of the electrodes to get the desired muscle group.

Officially called neuromuscular electrical stimulation (NMES), e-stim is the application of tiny pulses of electrical current over the nerves that normally give your muscles the instructions to contract. In order to deliver this current, a therapist places electrodes over the skin in particular areas and hooks them to the machine with wires that deliver the electric pulses. A physical therapist has access to this equipment, although you can purchase e-stim machines online and use them at home to reduce pain. (Always work with a physical therapist or athletic trainer first to see where you need to apply the electrodes and to design a program that specifically addresses your unique needs. You may then be able to use your own machine on your own.)

E-stim was initially used by athletes to help them recover from injuries and surgeries more quickly. But electrical stimulation can be of great benefit, not just to MS patients, but to anyone who has experienced deconditioning for any health-related reason. E-stim has been studied and found to improve quality of life and function in people with advanced heart failure,[11] chronic lung disease,[12] osteoarthritis,[13] and rheumatoid arthritis.[14] It has been used more recently to help stroke victims recover function more quickly (even five years after the injury)[15] and has improved function in people with cerebral palsy, including improved use of affected legs, arms, and hands.[16] We are the first to publish results of using exercise augmented by neuromuscular electrical stimulation in the setting of multiple sclerosis.[17]

E-stim is useful for many aspects of MS. It can be used for overall fitness, but it is particularly useful to target specific areas of weakness. For example, e-stim devices such as the WalkAide and Bioness deliver an electrical current to the nerve going to the muscle that lifts the foot upward at the ankle, making it easier to walk without catching one's toes. Research has shown these devices to be helpful in improving walking speed and endurance.[18] Bioness also has devices to stimulate the thigh muscles and improve hand function.

Another usage for which e-stim has been approved is to treat problems

WAHLS TOOLS

E-stim electrodes are attached with sticky pads that are reusable and disposable. The reusable electrodes are self-adhesive and work for ten to thirty applications, depending on how thoroughly you clean your skin and how well you care for the electrodes. You can also use Carbonflex electrodes that do not have an adhesive gel but instead use elastic compression straps or compression shorts and socks to hold the electrodes in place. The Carbonflex electrodes can be reused for over a year. You need to moisten the Carbonflex electrodes with water to make them conduct electricity without excessive resistance (pain). I used the Carbonflex electrodes for years quite successfully. The larger the electrode, the more comfortable the current. I used three- and four-inch-diameter electrodes for the greater comfort larger electrodes provide. The supplies will range from $25 to $100 per month, depending on how many sessions are done per day.

with incontinence—that is, wetting and soiling accidents.[19] Poor control of the bladder and bowels can occur with MS as well as with many other auto-immune and neurological conditions, and even with simple aging. Doing Kegel exercises (practice squeezing the muscle to stop the flow of urine) can help, but it is now possible to use a vaginal or rectal probe to add electrical stimulation of the appropriate muscles. If you have problems with accidents, doing Kegels augmented by electricity may be quite helpful to you. The good news is that this treatment does have FDA approval and is covered by many insurance companies, unlike many other uses for e-stim. (See the "Getting E-Stim Treatment" box, below.) The Resources section at the end of the book contains more information on the devices that I have personally used. Your therapist may have other devices that she or he has more experience using.

GETTING E-STIM TREATMENT

Getting e-stim treatment may not be simple for you. Here's why: The FDA approval for the use of e-stim is not for specific disease states. That is because device makers would have to conduct clinical trials for every dis-ease state for which they wish to have an FDA-approved indication. That would cost millions for each disease state and be cost-prohibitive.

Instead, the medical device makers sought and obtained FDA approval for electrical stimulation of muscles for more general muscle-related issues like muscle spasms (see the list below and on the next page). The FDA has approved electrical therapy devices as either over-the-counter (OTC) or pre-scription-only devices. The OTC devices have less power and can be used only for muscle toning. The prescription devices can be used only under the supervision of an authorized practitioner, such as a physical therapist, and are approved for the following indications:

1. Muscle spasm
2. The prevention of disuse atrophy
3. Relaxation of muscle spasms

4. Muscle reeducation
5. Postsurgical stimulation of calf muscles to prevent blood clots
6. Improving range of motion

If your condition doesn't specifically sound like what e-stim is supposed to help, you may have trouble getting your doctor or physical therapist to refer you for this treatment. What many physicians and treating physical therapists don't realize is that there is a growing body of research that supports the use of e-stim to help people improve their strength and endurance.

Print out these two papers and take them with you to your appointment: *Neuromuscular electrical stimulation and dietary interventions to reduce oxidative stress in a secondary progressive multiple sclerosis patient leads to marked gains in function: a case report* and *Rehabilitation with neuromuscular electrical stimulation leads to functional gains in ambulation in patients with secondary progressive and primary progressive multiple sclerosis: a case series report.* It may be helpful to show peer-reviewed publications to your treating therapist to justify giving you a test session. You can get copies of relevant articles from my website, www.thewahlsprotocol.com, where they can be found under "Community Resources" (once you register for the e-mail newsletter). You can also remind your therapist that NMES is approved for muscle atrophy. If you are deconditioned and have muscle spasms and/or muscle pain, your muscles have likely atrophied. However, you will likely still have to pay out of pocket for NMES, as it likely won't be covered by your medical insurance.

Using E-Stim

If you want to investigate using electrical stimulation to assist your exercise training, here are some things to consider:

- **You still have to exercise.** E-stim is not a replacement for exercise. It is a way of supercharging the workout for your muscles so you have a chance of growing more muscle tissues. If you have the benefit of recovering good strength and balance, you will likely be advised to taper off the use of the e-stim and rely on the strength and endurance training alone. This is because that's the usual practice for athletes, and we are only now doing studies that focus on those with multiple sclerosis, so there are no published studies on long-term use of NMES or functional electic stimulation (FES). FES is an alternative way to use e-stim, in which the electrical current is timed to create a functional movement, such as how your muscles would react when riding a bicycle. You may, as some athletes do, however, choose to continue to train with the e-stim if you like what it does for you. Either approach is fine.

- **You need professional input.** You will need to have several training sessions at a clinic with a therapist to learn how to operate the device. There are many different companies and devices available. Your therapist or trainer may use Empi devices, such as the Continuum device I use (see the Resources section), or may have different devices in their clinic. You should be given a specific set of exercises to strengthen your muscles, and you can ask which exercises you should be doing while you are stimulating each particular muscle group. As you get stronger, the therapist will likely advance your exercises and may advance the duration and the intensity of the e-stim. This is all highly personalized to the individual. I urge you to have a therapist evaluate you and design a program specifically for you. Exercise and e-stim are individualized in our clinical trial for each participant. We do not use the same protocol for everyone because each person has a unique set of needs, and a professional can best help you determine what these are for you.
- **You may not tolerate the therapy.** Before you dive into e-stim therapy, you will likely have a test session, during which a therapist will determine whether you can tolerate the therapy. Not all people can tolerate the electrical sensations. In our clinical trial, we have had a couple of people find the electrical sensations to be too painful, but 80 percent or more can tolerate sufficient current to generate a strong contraction.

You can do it at home once your therapist is confident you can safely use the electrical therapy device, but stay in touch with your therapist. If e-stim

WAHLS TOOLS

E-stim has also been incorporated into exercise equipment. Restorative Therapies (www.restorative-therapies.com/ms) is a company that makes a functional electrical stimulation (FES) cycle. They use electrodes to stimulate the leg and/or arm muscles to push on pedals to maintain muscle strength and endurance. The original work on this was to determine how to use FES cycling to help paralyzed individuals maintain muscle, bone strength, and quality of life. The first patient population that the company targeted was people with spinal cord injuries. In a small pilot study of five patients with primary- or secondary-progressive MS, researchers found that patients tolerated the FES cycling and experienced faster walking time in the twenty-five-foot walk and higher quality-of-life scores. They report that they have 580 patients using one of their FES cycles. Now some doctors are using the FES cycles to help patients with multiple sclerosis.[20]

We are also conducting a small clinical trial using the FES cycles here at the University of Iowa and are submitting grants proposing a much larger study to the National Institutes of Health (NIH). In our study, we are comparing the effectiveness of different training protocols. Thus far, we are observing that the FES cycling is well tolerated and we're pleased with what we've observed. FES cycling is likely to be beneficial for improving strength and endurance, but the FES cycles are not FDA-approved as a treatment for MS. You can contact Restorative Therapies to see if there is a clinic near you that is using the FES cycle or inquire about having a trial period with a cycle to see if you might benefit. (Getting FDA approval is an expensive process, requiring two clinical trials that have at least two different study sites, with statistically significant results. That type of study costs millions of dollars to conduct.)

works for you, you may choose to buy your own device. The device should be portable and run on batteries. An e-stim device will typically have two to four channels, which translates into two to four muscles that can be stimulated at any given time. Devices that have sufficient power to help grow muscles as

WAHLS WARNING

Use caution if you could become pregnant: Never stimulate the abdomen or gluteal muscles if there is even a remote possibility that you could become pregnant, as the electrical current anywhere near the uterus could affect fetal development and lead to birth defects! Also, **no one should use an e-stim machine across the chest, brain, or neck.** Do not use an e-stim machine if you have an implantable electronic device, like a pacemaker, or a medication pump such as a baclofen pump for spasticity.

opposed to only toning muscles require a prescription to be purchased. Prices range from $100 to $1,300 or more.

Set goals, start small, and work your way up. If you get the opportunity to try this therapy, the general instruction is to stimulate the particular muscles that are weak for fifteen minutes a day if you want to prevent muscle atrophy, and forty-five to sixty minutes if you want to strengthen the muscle. That was why my personal goal was to add time gradually so I could stimulate each of my weak muscle groups sixty minutes a day. Note that for our extremely disabled study participants we needed to reduce the e-stim time to five minutes per muscle and slowly advance according each person's tolerance.

The reason for you to move your body is so you can live your life and not be limited by your disease. It's disappointing and frustrating when you can't do what you used to do, especially when you can't do things with your family that they want to do. However, the people who love you just want to be with you. That's the important thing. Rather than withdrawing into yourself, get up and move as well as you can. Every little bit is good for your body and helps engage you in your life, and with the Wahls Protocol your progress should be steady.

Chapter 10

WHAT ABOUT DRUGS, SUPPLEMENTS, AND ALTERNATIVE MEDICINE?

B EYOND DIET AND EXERCISE, there are many other interesting therapies to consider while on the Wahls Protocol. Many of my patients are very interested in what supplements they should be taking, and I have plenty to say about that. Another is alternative medicine. Should you also be trying some alternative treatments, and if you do, what will your conventionally trained doctor have to say about it? I have plenty to say about that, too, but the very first thing I want to address in this chapter is *the medication you are already taking.* You may already be thinking about this. If the Wahls Protocol is going to make you better, then you should be able to stop taking all those drugs, right?

Not so fast.

About Your Medications

A lot of my patients get very excited about the Wahls Protocol, and that's excellent. Excitement feeds motivation and helps people stick with the diet, even when it feels challenging. Many of these people, however, also get very impatient about the drugs or medications they are currently taking. They want the Wahls Protocol to improve their health (which it will), but they jump the gun and sometimes stop taking their medications in the hope that the Wahls Protocol will "fix everything" in a few weeks. This is not how it works.

You may begin to feel better almost immediately on the Wahls Protocol, but if you are on prescription medications, you must not stop taking your current therapy! This is very important. Do not stop any medication or intervention you are doing right now because you started the Wahls Protocol. Doing so could be disastrous.

It takes several months for the Wahls Protocol to reset your biology and begin the rebuilding process, and then your body must begin healing the damage that has already been done. If you stop your treatment now, you could very likely have another relapse or worsen before you get better. You will be discouraged, disheartened, and more likely to give up. Your friends and family will say, "See? It doesn't work. It's a waste of time and effort and money. Go back to what you were doing before." I can't say this strongly enough, so I am going to put it in a box in boldface for you:

> **You must stay on your current medications for your medical and psychological conditions!**

In my clinical trials, we do not have the patients stop any treatments, and you must not stop, either. Do the Wahls Protocol *in addition to* whatever you are doing now, then take a deep breath and be patient.

Over the next three years, a new you will be built, molecule by correctly made molecule. Your energy and mood will improve. Likely your blood pressure, weight, cholesterol, and blood sugar (if you are diabetic) will also improve. When you can see and feel the evidence of improved health because you can walk farther, do more, and have more energy, it's time to discuss reducing or tapering off your medication gradually, with your physician's supervision. Some other reasons to discuss tapering off medication after you are solidly on the Wahls Protocol:

- You are on Provigil and you can't sleep at night because the drug is keeping you awake.

- You are on blood pressure medication and now your blood pressure is too low.
- You are on cholesterol-lowering medication and now your cholesterol is too low (less than 200).

If these things happen, don't take matters into your own hands but do work with the doctor who is prescribing the medication. For example, your primary-care doctor may be prescribing medication for your cholesterol and blood pressure, and as those numbers improve, those drugs can likely be slowly decreased and potentially eliminated. Talk to your neurologist for questions about taking Provigil for fatigue.

But what about immunosuppressive drugs? This question is more complex. Your neurologist may agree that your disease has stabilized. Your MRI may show no new lesions. (Likely the lesions already there may remain forever.) However, your doctor may attribute your success to the drugs, not the Wahls Protocol.

Here the question becomes what to do. Do you continue to take the immunosuppressive medication or wean and discontinue? Unfortunately, I do not have research to guide you on this one. This is a conversation you will have to have with your primary-care doctor and your neurologist. I can only share my experience. One of the drugs I was on for MS-related fatigue was Provigil. After just one month into my new way of eating, my fatigue was greatly reduced. At three months I was sleeping less than four hours a night: Provigil is a stimulant—which is why it is commonly prescribed for fatigue—and my brain had so improved that the stimulant effect was keeping me awake. I wasn't fatigued anymore, and I also wasn't sleeping. It was clearly time to stop this medication, and my neurologist agreed.

When I started biking at six months, I told my neurologist that I no longer wanted to take the disease-modifying medication I was on (CellCept) but would go back on if the MS symptoms worsened again. He had me take half the dose for a week, then half that smaller dose the following week, and two weeks later I stopped completely. I have continued to do well even though I have not taken a disease-modifying medication more than five years.

Many doctors are happy to work with you as you improve, but unfortunately not all of them are open to the power of lifestyle modification. If you are not getting the kind of support you really want or feel you need, I would suggest finding a functional medicine physician to help you decide how to address the immunosuppressive-drug question. A functional medicine doctor may be more open to attributing your improvements to the changes in your lifestyle. I have successfully been able to get patients in my clinical practice off the immunosuppressive drugs they were on for their autoimmune conditions, but this was under my direct supervision.

What I see in my internal medicine clinical practice is that as patients fully adopt the Wahls Diet, each time we see them back in the clinic, they are looking healthier and younger. Time and time again I see blood pressures fall, blood sugars fall, moods improve, memory improve, and more. As your cells become healthier, it is likely that your organs will become healthier. As your organs become healthier, it is likely that you, the whole person, will have more energy, more vitality, and more good days and good feelings in your life.

As you become well, it will be apparent to you when you can begin negotiating with your doctor about which medicines to try tapering, and most doctors will see the changes as well and may be more than willing to help you navigate your new, healthier life. I invite you to have an opinion about which medications you want to discontinue first. Consider starting with the drugs with the longest list of side effects and the least immediate benefits to you. The more you can taper off drugs with unpleasant side effects that no longer benefit you, the better your quality of life will be. Just remember, it takes years to repair damage that has taken a lifetime to accrue.

If you are taking disease-modifying drugs and want to taper off those, ask for the package insert (or find it online) and read all of the side effects, then talk to your doctors about how many of your current health issues could be the result of the prescription medications. Let that guide your conversations with your doctors about which medications you want to begin tapering (very gradually) to see if you can come off them when your improved health justifies it.

About Supplements

A huge part of the Wahls Protocol is the infusion of the body, the cells, and the mitochondria with the essential nutrients required for the best possible functioning. This is accomplished primarily through diet, with the 9 cups of fruits and vegetables; the organic, grass-fed, or wild-caught meat and fish; the seaweed and organ meat and fermented food and coconut oil and all the other things I recommend ending up in your blender, in your soup pot, in your salad bowl, and ultimately in *you*.

But wouldn't it be a heck of a lot easier to just take some vitamins?

Vitamins and minerals act together to facilitate the chemistry of cells and must be kept in balance, but it is far better (if not easier) to achieve this balance through food, as I discussed in previous chapters. (Look back to chapter 5, "Mastering the Wahls Diet," for my longer explanation on this.) That being said, I do believe that in cases of deficiency, supplementation *in addition to the 9 cups* and the other required foods on whichever level of the Wahls Diet you are practicing may be helpful for some people. If you decide to take supplements, always talk to your personal physician prior to starting them. There are certain conditions for which certain supplements may be contraindicated and certain medications with which some supplements could react. It won't necessarily state this on the supplement package or the medication.

Also, I strongly urge you to begin one supplement at a time. Keep a log of how you feel in your Wahls Diary, write down any changes in symptoms you observe, and particularly note any head or belly symptoms or skin rashes. If you start several things at once and have problems, you will not know which caused the problem or which was helpful. It is worth being patient and adding things one at a time. If you have no problems after a week, you can add another supplement if you wish. This is the time for you to be a sleuth and pay attention to how you react to the introduction of each supplement.

It is very important that you understand we are all unique, with a unique set of enzymes for running the chemistry of our lives. A supplement that works fine for someone else with MS might not work well for you, and vice versa. Our needs and tolerances are highly individualized. This is why it is impossible for me to give a supplement program (or a diet program or exercise program) that will work for every single person. There will always be those people who have difficulty processing certain foods as well as certain supplements, and others that may need a higher dose than average.

Considering all of this, in addition to your medication, there are some supplements that might be of great benefit to you. These include vitamin D, essential fatty acids (including gamma-linoleic acid), vitamin E, and the B vitamin family (methyl B_{12}, methyl folate, and B complex vitamins, including thiamine, riboflavin, niacin, pantethine, and pyridoxine). In addition to these, I encourage you to also consider kelp, algae, and dietary enzymes. I will go through each of these later in this chapter.

Always talk to your doctor about whether you should be taking any or all of these supplements. I suggest beginning with a vitamin D test. Some people take a multivitamin/multimineral supplement also; however, that is much more likely to cause problems with nausea and GI upset. I generally do not have my patients use them routinely for that reason.

But first let's talk about making sure your supplement use is working rather than causing more problems for you.

Annual Tests

If you are taking supplements, it's important to have a CBC (or complete blood count, a blood test), a liver test, and a kidney test once or twice a year to be sure you aren't experiencing any toxic reactions that are compromising your liver, kidneys, or bone marrow (blood factory) due to those supplements or contaminants in the supplements. I also recommend several other annual lab tests to monitor anyone with a personal or family history of brain, heart, or other complex health issues for troubling signs. The following tests are all things your primary-care doctor should feel comfortable ordering. I have provided the target ranges that I use and the interventions I typically recommend for my patients, although your personal physician may work with slightly different targets and interventions. You are unique and may require refinement of these recommendations based upon your personal health circumstances. To get these tests, just request them from your doctor before your appointment.

Labs	*Target Range for the Wahls Protocol*	*Intervention*
Complete blood count (CBC), calcium, creatinine, and alanine aminotransferase (ALT)	Normal values for the target range. (A target range is the value the testing laboratory has defined as normal based on the values that occur in 97 percent of the population.)	These are safety labs to be sure your system is handling the supplements and processing them properly. If the levels become abnormal, you will need to discontinue any noncritical medications and reevaluate promptly to ensure things are normalizing again.
25-hydroxy Vitamin D (vitamin D25-OH)	50–100 ng/ml (nanogram/ milliliter) *or* 150–250 nmol/L (nanomoles/ liter) (British)	Adjust vitamin D dose up or down according to level. If vitamin D is above target range, then check calcium level to be sure the calcium level has not become elevated. If calcium is elevated, you will likely be directed to receive urgent if not immediate attention.
Folate and vitamin B_{12}	In top quartile of the reference range for that lab	Interpret with homocysteine (see Homocysteine, below).
Homocysteine	4 to 6.5 micromole/L	If low, eat more protein. If high, switch to the methyl forms of folate (methylfolate) and methyl forms of B_{12} (methyl B_{12}). (Note that less expensive forms of folate and B_{12} do not have the methyl group added.) Also a vitamin B complex like B-100. If still high once folate and B_{12} are optimized, see a functional medicine practitioner for guidance.
Highly sensitive C-reactive protein (hs-CRP)	Less than 1.0 mg/L (milligram/ liter) = low risk (ideal) 1 to 3 mg/L = intermediate risk Greater than 3 mg/L = high risk	If high, eat more vegetables and berries. If still high after consuming 9 to 12 cups/day, see a functional-medicine-practitioner for further guidance.
Fasting lipids	Triglyceride/HDL cholesterol ratio less than 3	A ratio greater than 3 indicates probable insulin resistance. Decrease carbohydrate intake and advance to Wahls Paleo or Wahls Paleo Plus diet. This may indicate need for more fish oil.
HDL cholesterol (good cholesterol)	HDL cholesterol greater than 60 mg/dL (milligram/deciliter)	If HDL is less than 60, decrease carbohydrates, increase vegetables and berries, increase fish oil, and increase exercise.

Labs	Target Range for the Wahls Protocol	Intervention
Total cholesterol	More than 160 mg/dL (milligram/deciliter) (preferably more than 200 for optimal brain function, although we do not know the optimal upper range for ideal brain function: 300 may or may not be too high). Note: If a person has coronary heart disease or cerebrovascular disease, the treating physicians will usually try to keep cholesterol below 200.	If cholesterol is 200 or less, lower or stop cholesterol-lowering medication. If no cholesterol-lowering medication, increase cholesterol intake, e.g., with ghee.
Thyroid-stimulating hormone (TSH) and free thyroxine (free T4)	TSH 0.30–5.00 micro international units per milliliter (IU/ml); free T4 in normal range according to reference lab	TSH is typically checked for those suffering with fatigue. There is some controversy over whether the upper limit of TSH should be 3.0, not 5.0. If the TSH is outside the target range, check free T4; if that is outside the target range, treatment for over or underactive thyroid is indicated.
Hemoglobin A1C	Less than 5.2 percent	Hemoglobin A1C is typically checked for diabetes. This correlates very well with the level of sugar oxidation of your LDL cholesterol. If hemoglobin A1C is greater than 5.2 percent, lower the carbohydrate content of your diet.

Vitamin D

A low vitamin D level is associated with higher rates of relapse and more severe disability, and higher levels are associated with higher levels of function.[1] Furthermore, low vitamin D levels are associated with higher rates of autoimmune disease, mental health problems, cardiovascular disease, and cancer.[2] For that reason I strongly urge you to monitor your vitamin D level and make getting it to an optimal range a priority.

The most natural and effective way to get vitamin D is simply to put your skin in the sun. Vitamin D is an interesting vitamin that actually acts somewhat like a hormone. We make vitamin D from cholesterol as a result of the ultraviolet radiation in sunlight hitting our skin. When this happens, the liver and kidneys transform the vitamin D into a more active form, and this allows our cells to read DNA instructions more effectively.

Unfortunately, instead of a continuous exposure to the sun the way our ancestors had, allowing a gradual increase in sunlight exposure over a season and a gradual increase in vitamin D levels and skin pigmentation throughout the summer, we spend hours inside. Think about how our Paleolithic ancestors lived and thrived. They spent most of their time outside. Although they usually slept in sheltered places, during the day they were out and about under the sun millennia before sunblock was ever invented.

We live much differently. We spend most of our time indoors. During summer, the heat and humidity in the outdoor world feels uncomfortable to us because we're not used to it and air-conditioning feels good. Even during nice weather, digital entertainment has replaced outdoor play for most people in developed societies. When we do go outdoors, our physicians—especially our dermatologists—warn us to apply sunscreen first. Of course you do not want to burn your skin, but one of the problems with sunscreen coupled with all this indoor time is that many children and most adults are still vitamin D deficient at the end of summer when our levels should be high enough to store vitamin D for the long winter.

Sunscreen blocks the frequency of light that our skin needs to make vitamin D, which is in the ultraviolet B range. The result is chronically low vitamin D levels, which increase the risk of infections, lung cancer, breast cancer, colon cancer, prostate cancer, heart disease, autoimmune problems, preterm labor, toxemia of pregnancy, schizophrenia, learning disabilities, and other mental health problems.

The lab vitamin D target range (meaning your vitamin D level as indicated by a lab test you can get from your doctor) is typically 20 nanograms per milliliter (ng/ml) to 70 ng/ml. Sometimes, it is stated as 30 ng/ml to 70 ng/ml. Because of this target range, many physicians will consider 31 ng/ml to be adequate, but with levels that low, the person is still at four times the risk for autoimmune problems and cancers as someone with a higher level. The

---

TEST YOUR OWN VITAMIN D

You can ask your physician to check a total vitamin D level and be sure you get the actual number, not just a note that it is "normal." Alternatively, you can get a home test kit and more information about the health impacts of vitamin D from the Vitamin D Council at www.vitamindcouncil.org. You can order kit(s) that have what you need to prick your finger, along with a card to collect the blood specimen in six circles. You let it dry and then send the card back to the lab. The lab is fully accredited, and you will receive a letter with the results and general advice about the target level.

---

hunter-gatherer societies and those who live in the sun 24/7 have values that range between 80 and 120 ng/ml. It is likely that this is the level most consistent with optimal health.

In my clinic, we base our target range on what a breast-feeding mother needs to have enough vitamin D for her baby in her breast milk: 55 ng/ml or greater. Our target range is 50 ng/ml to 100 ng/ml total 25-hydroxy vitamin D. I tell my patients that 80 ng/ml is an ideal target. In my clinical practice, however, I find that the vast majority (more than 90 percent) are below 30 ng/ml unless they are taking vitamin D supplements, working in an outdoor job with all-day sun exposure with the arms and legs (or torso) exposed, or using a tanning bed regularly. People with pigmented skin living farther from the equator than their ancestors (i.e., African Americans, Pacific Islanders, and Hispanics) are likely to have more severe deficiencies.

So what should you do about this? There are risks and advantages to increasing vitamin D through sun or tanning bed use (your skin) or through supplements (your gut), but my first recommendation is to follow nature's guidance and use your skin to make more vitamin D.

Vitamin D from the Sun

Exposing your skin to the sun is the natural way our ancestors got enough vitamin D, and it can work for you. Unlike taking vitamin D supplements, which can cause you to overdose on vitamin D (I'll talk about that next), your skin will not make too much. There are no reports of vitamin intoxication (excessive levels) from sun exposure, and there are studies that show achieving vitamin D levels of greater than 50 ng/ml through the skin leads to a superior immune function than can be achieved using supplements. With the sun, you will make vitamin D in the most appropriate amount and with the most benefit.

This means, however, that you will have to spend some devoted time exposing your skin to the sun and/or a tanning bed. More controversy! Yes, I am an advocate of using light to make vitamin D, even when it comes from a tanning bed. The key point is to gradually increase the time so that you do not get sunburns along the way. When you have enough sun exposure to get a slight pinking without getting a sunburn on your face, arms, and legs, your skin will have made 20,000 international units of vitamin D. There is also evidence that sun on the skin has positive immune effects independent of vitamin D levels.[3]

I tan once a week in a tanning bed during the winter for this reason using ultraviolet B light (UVB) in the 280 to 313 nanometer wavelength range, which is the light frequency involved in the initial steps of making vitamin D. I know what you are thinking: Tanning beds are associated with a higher rate of skin cancer and melanoma. Squamous cell and basal cell skin cancers very rarely metastasize or spread to distant sites. They are generally easily treated by cutting out the skin cancer. Melanoma, which is a cancer of the melanin (pigment-producing) cell, can metastasize and is much more aggressive and dangerous, even fatal, but it occurs most often in the non-sun-exposed parts of our bodies. Consider this, however: Hunter-gatherer societies, with their 24/7/365 exposure to sunlight, do not have a particularly high incidence of skin cancers or melanomas. The constant exposure, lack of sunburns, and a nutrient-dense diet may be a factor in why their risk of cancers appears to be much lower than ours.

Of course, you will have to weigh all these factors, and if you have a family

> ## WAHLS WARRIOR Q & A
>
> **Q: Are there specific benefits of the Wahls Protocol for osteoporosis, osteo-penia, and osteoarthritis?**
>
> A: Yes. Osteoporosis and osteopenia are strongly related to a lifetime of vitamin D deficiency and a high-glycemic diet, which tends to draw calcium from the bone. Add to that an increasingly sedentary life and there is very little drive to put calcium back in the bones. Reducing the high-glycemic foods, eating more bone broth, optimizing vitamin D levels to between 50 and 100 ng/ml, and, most important, getting more weight-bearing exercise will all help restore calcium back into your bones. Arthritis can also be helped by consuming a cup or two of bone broth every day so that your cells have the building blocks for maintaining and repairing the cartilage and ligaments around the joints. Eating three cups of sulfur-containing vegetables each day will also shore up joints, as will regular exercise. The Wahls Diet will also help to reduce the inflammation that is damaging the joints and provide the nutrients you need to begin repairs.

history of skin cancer or melanoma, you may be better off taking supplements. But if you like the idea of getting your vitamin D more naturally, I highly recommend more sun exposure, as long as you do not let yourself get a sunburn.

Vitamin D Supplements

Low vitamin D levels are associated with higher risk of worsening MS symptoms and higher rate of relapse.[4] For that reason I suggest that you get your level checked annually and work with your physician to optimize your level. Taking vitamin D supplements in place of or in addition to sun exposure has its pros and cons as well. If you take supplements, there is a risk that your vitamin D level could become dangerously high (greater than 150 ng/ml), leading to excessively high calcium in your bloodstream, kidney damage, even psychosis. This is because vitamin D is a fat-soluble vitamin. Fat-soluble vitamins have more potential for harm from excessive dosing than water-soluble vitamins. That is because the water-soluble vitamins (B and C vitamins) are excreted by the kidneys, whereas the fat-soluble vitamins are stored in fat, where they can accumulate and reach excessively high levels.

A vitamin D overdose is rare but possible. That is why it is so important to get a vitamin D level test and follow your vitamin D level regularly to know that you are in the ideal range and not becoming excessively high. If you are taking more than 2,000 international units (IU) of vitamin D, I urge you to have a vitamin D level test every three months until you have gotten your vitamin D level to the target level and then check it once or twice a year to confirm that you are keeping it in the target range.

Although your supplement needs depend on the latitude where you live, the pigmentation level in your skin, and the amount of time you spend outdoors without sunscreen, many people who live and work indoors need between 4,000 and 8,000 international units (IU) during the winter months when they cannot make vitamin D, and between 2,000 and 4,000 IU per day during the summer when they can get outside and get enough sunshine to have a dark tan, which will make enough vitamin D to maintain healthy levels.

Note that this is a wide dosing range, so the risk of toxicity from overdosing on vitamin D is real. Another problem is that as we increase vitamin D intake through supplement use, we can create a relative insufficiency of vitamins A, K, and E in the cells if those vitamins are not also increased. Eating liver, greens, nuts, and fermented cod-liver oil can be very beneficial for getting these fat-soluble vitamins.

Also, the amount of vitamin D that you need to take orally will depend in part on the efficiency of the enzymes that handle the production and use of vitamin D in your cells. These are called the single nucleotide polymorphisms, or SNPs ("snips"), that manage vitamin D. If you have several SNPs related to vitamin D, you may not be able to utilize vitamin D as efficiently and you will likely need a higher dose than those who do not have this issue. It is another reason that it is important to monitor your blood level so that you know you have achieved the target vitamin D level. Whatever your individual case, you need to follow blood levels for accurate dosing guidance. Personally, I not only tan my skin but I take additional vitamin D_3 in the form

> # HELPING VITAMIN D WORK BETTER
>
> For vitamin D supplements to work effectively, you also need vitamin K_2, especially vitamin K_2MK7. Your gut bacteria make vitamin MK7 from the vitamin K_1 in greens. It is also present in organ meat, fermented cod-liver oil, and high-vitamin butter oil from grass-fed cows. (Look for the casein-free version of these oils.) Be sure to eat plenty of these foods if you are taking vitamin D supplements. If you are already following the Wahls Diet, that should be no problem for you.

of vitamin D supplements and fermented skate-liver oil, and regularly check my levels.

Calcium

Because there is a lower intake of calcium in Wahls Paleo (approximately 950 mg) and Wahls Paleo Plus (750 mg) than in the Wahls Diet (1,450 mg), I suggest that you consider taking 250 mg calcium citrate once or twice a day depending on your gender, age, and which diet you are following. The RDA for calcium for men and for women under the age of 50 is 1,000 mg of elemental calcium. For women over the age of 50, and men over the age of 71, the RDA is 1,200 mg. It is important to intentionally and consistently eat calcium-rich foods—like eating the bones in canned salmon, as well as almonds, bok choy, and collard greens—but supplementation is an insurance policy.

The two main forms of calcium in supplements are carbonate and citrate. I prefer calcium citrate because you can take it with or without food and there is less risk of bloating, gas, or constipation than there is when using calcium carbonate. Calcium carbonate is less expensive but requires a good amount of stomach acid to be absorbed (and stomach acid declines after age 50). Also, it is important to note that vitamin D is required to absorb calcium efficiently from the gut, so it is important to monitor your vitamin D level as discussed previously. The percentage of calcium you absorb will depend on the total amount of elemental calcium consumed at one time; as the amount increases, the percentage of absorption decreases. Absorption is highest in doses of 500 mg or less, and doses of more than 500 mg have been associated with more adverse events.

Magnesium

Magnesium can be very helpful with reducing spasticity in muscles, improving restless legs syndrome, and improving sleep. (I'll explain more about this in the next chapter, "Stress Management.") Green leaves are a terrific source of magnesium. If you decide to take additional magnesium, you can take 350 to 400 mg of elemental magnesium by mouth every day as long as you have normal kidney function, but don't take more than that without working with your physician to be sure you are not overdoing the magnesium. Magnesium oxide is the least expensive form, but magnesium glycinate is the most easily absorbed into your cells.

Essential Fatty Acids (Omega-3 Fatty Acids and Gamma-Linoleic Acid)

The next supplement to consider adding to your routine is omega-3 fatty acid. I've already talked about this essential fatty acid when I talked about grass-fed meat and wild-caught fish (and also when I talked about problems with vegetarianism), but although you may be eating these foods, you still may not be getting enough.

There are two omega-3 fatty acids that are very important: DHA and EPA. Your brain needs docosahexaenoic acid (DHA) to make myelin. Eicosapentaenoic acid (EPA) is very helpful in lowering inflammation. You can see why anyone with MS or another autoimmune condition would benefit greatly from these compounds!

In our study, we have subjects take molecularly refined fish oil to increase both the EPA and DHA intake. This is an easy way to standardize intake for a clinical trial. Studies have shown, however, that eating foods high in DHA/EPA is more effective at raising the blood DHA/EPA levels than taking fish oil supplements. Eating wild-caught cold-water fish is best, but if you can't get enough, a supplement may be in order.

WAHLS WARNING

Fish oils can prolong bleeding time. As a result, we exclude from our study anyone who takes a medicine to thin the blood, such as Coumadin, Plavix, or aspirin. If you are on any medication to thin the blood, it is critical that you work with your physician regarding how much and what kind of omega-3 fatty acids you can safely take. If you are taking fish oil, do not take additional flax or hempseed oil without checking with your physician first to be sure you are not increasing the risk of bruising and bleeding. (Note that ground flax- or chia seeds you take for fiber if constipated should not cause a problem.) In my clinic, if a patient is on a blood thinner, I work with the doctor who is prescribing the blood thinner to see if he or she would be willing to replace the blood thinner with high-dose fish oil, since it does the same job. Sometimes that is appropriate and sometimes it is not.

There is also an interesting way to get the benefits of both, using a method of supplementation that traditional societies in the far north used for hundreds of generations: They fermented fish liver oils, which makes these oils even richer in nutrients and the fat-soluble vitamins A, D, and, to a lesser extent, K and E. This product preserves the essential oils in fish even better than if it were frozen or canned. Several traditional fermented cod- and skate-liver oil preparations are available from the company Green Pasture (www.greenpasture.org).

However, if you cannot or do not wish to take fermented fish liver oil, purified fish oil supplements can still be useful. Because of concern for mercury contamination, I suggest you look for highly concentrated, molecularly distilled fish oils such as Nordic Naturals Ultimate Omega or Solgar omega-3 EPA and DHA: They both have approximately 950 mg of combined DHA and EPA per capsule. If you go this route and take the molecularly distilled fish oil (as opposed to fermented cod-liver oil), you should also take vitamin E in the form of mixed tocopherols or tocotrienols at 200 to 400 mg per day.

(Note that 1 mg equals approximately 1.5 IU per day; some supplements are labeled with IUs instead of milligrams.) Without the additional vitamin E, you will increase the likelihood that the omega-3 fats will be rapidly oxidized in your bloodstream, which greatly reduces the benefits.

Ideally, ask your doctor to do a lipid panel that includes an essential fatty acid analysis to know what your bloodstream's omega-6-to-omega-3 fatty acid ratio is. This looks at the ratio of AA to EPA (arachidonic acid to eicosapentaenoic acid). Your goal is to get that ratio between 1.5 and 3. If you can't get an AA-to-EPA level, don't feel bad. I can't get the AA-to-EPA level at my hospital, either. I use a fasting lipid profile and work to optimize the HDL level as an indirect measure of the AA-to-EPA level. You will also want a hemoglobin A1C value to know how highly oxidized your LDL cholesterol is and a highly sensitive CRP to measure the inflammation level. The goal is to get the HDL over 60 with a CRP level of less than 1 and a hemoglobin A1C of less than 5.2 percent.

These are the numbers I look for in my clinic and what they mean:

- When triglycerides are above a 100 or there is a triglycerides-to-HDL ratio greater than 3, the insulin level is too high. I stress the need to further reduce the carbs/sugars and increase the omega-3 fatty acid intake. I encourage the person to move to or be stricter about Wahls Paleo or move to Wahls Paleo Plus. Note: This ratio is less reliable for people of African descent. In that case, it is better to measure insulin and glucose levels to simultaneously assess insulin sensitivity.
- If my patients have HDLs that are less than 60, I take that as another indication to increase the fish oil supplementation.
- If the hemoglobin A1C is greater than 5.2 percent, I urge the person to reduce his or her carbohydrate intake and increase the intake of healthy fats instead, and consider moving to Wahls Paleo or Wahls Paleo Plus.
- If a patient reports nosebleeds or excessive bruising, this is usually due to the blood-thinning effect. I hold the fish oil for a week and then resume at half the dose.
- You will want the CRP level under 1.0.

B Vitamins

Many people take vitamin B supplements because the B vitamins—including vitamin B_1 (thiamine), B_2 (riboflavin), B_3 (niacin), B_5 (pantothenic acid), B_6 (pyridoxine), B_7 (biotin), B_9 (folic acid), and B_{12} (cobalamin)—play so many important roles in the proper functioning of the cells. In our clinical trials, we want more specific information. I always check blood levels for folate, vitamin B_{12}, and homocysteine at entry into the study. I also do this routinely in

WAHLS WARRIORS SPEAK

I was diagnosed with MS in 2008 and a hair mineral analysis found that I had high lead levels. Blood tests around that time showed an exposure to tuberculosis, low blood protein levels, and elevated cytokine levels. Between my gluten and dairy intolerances, genetic predispositions, and stress triggers, my body couldn't detoxify and heal itself.

I found Dr. Wahls, started following her diet, and, after ten years of vegetarianism, I am slowly introducing meats and taking a coenzyme Q supplement and vitamin D daily. On the days that I don't eat fish or flaxseed oil, I take 15 millliters of high-dose EPA/DHA fish oil. I supplement my banana/kiwifruit/blueberry smoothies with lecithin, acai powder, hemp protein powder, mesquite powder, green tea powder, cacao powder/nibs, spirulina, chlorella, bee pollen, and flaxseed oil. The Wahls Diet satisfies my cravings for good fats and greens in a way that other diets didn't. It gives me direction and incentive because I know I'm eating to improve my myelin sheath, balance my GABA levels, and restore my mitochondria. I've had no relapses for one year and no drug treatment. I've felt improvements in energy levels [and] cognition, lessening brain fog, better balance, reduced weight, clearer vision, fewer migraines, better digestion, clearer skin, and shinier hair and nails. I can run again! My neurologist reported recently that I have no signs of disability. I am ecstatic to be able to keep myself healthy. It is intensive but it is a massive act of self-loving.

—Nissa P., Tasmania, Australia

> ## WAHLS WARNING
>
> Note that any vitamins or supplements that you take should be from a manufacturer that uses good manufacturing processes and has used a third party to test the product and confirm that the product is not contaminated with lead or some other heavy metal and in fact is what it says it is. ConsumerLab.com conducts independent testing of vitamins and supplements and ranks products according to their purity tests. A modest annual membership fee gets you access to their testing information. I think it is money well spent to know which products are the most safe and reliable.

my traumatic brain injury clinic and in my primary-care clinics for patients who have a personal or family history of a bad brain (neurological or psychological issues) or a bad heart (coronary heart disease, a valve problem, or a rhythm problem). I want to see the folate and vitamin B_{12} levels in particular in the top quartile (near the top) of the suggested reference range.

But what should you do? Ask for folate, B_{12}, and homocysteine levels. Your goal is to have your folate and vitamin B_{12} levels near the top of the normal range. You want your homocysteine level between 4 and 6.5 micromoles per liter. If your homocysteine is low, you probably need to increase your protein intake. If your homocysteine is elevated, increase your B complex, methyl B_{12}, and methyl folate. If it is still high after you have optimized your folate and B_{12} levels, you need to see a functional-medicine-trained physician who can do further evaluation and guidance to get the homocysteine optimized.

Coenzyme Q

Coenzyme Q is important for mitochondrial efficiency. It is part of the electron transport chain in the mitochondria that generates the ATP. (See chapter 1, "The Science of Life, Disease, and You.") As we mature, and particularly over the age of 50 years, it becomes more difficult for us to make enough coenzyme Q, and medications often compromise our ability to manufacture coenzyme Q. It has been used at doses ranging from 100 mg twice a day to 200 mg twice a day for heart failure[5] and at doses of 300 mg twice a day to 600 mg twice a day for Parkinson's disease.[6] I do not have studies using coenzyme Q for MS patients. Because the heart failure and Parkinson's studies were using only one intervention, it is likely that a smaller dose as part of an entire program of nutritional support (like the Wahls Protocol) would be effective. That is why in our clinical trial we used just 200 mg of coenzyme Q total per day. Eating heart (the richest source of coenzyme Q) and liver (also a good source) three times a week will also give you more coenzyme Q, creatine, lipoic acid, and other critical mitochondrial nutrition. Also, talk to your doctor about supplementing with coenzyme Q if you take statin drugs.

Algae

I already talked about seaweed in chapter 6, "Wahls Paleo," because these are actually functional foods rather than supplements. A similar food, algae, is more like a supplement, however, so I will mention it here.

Like seaweed, the cell walls of algae will also bind heavy metals, plastics, solvents, and other toxins, shuttling them out with the stool. Unlike seaweed, which grows in salt water, algae grows in freshwater ponds (chlorella or spirulina) or wild in the Pacific Northwest (Klamath blue green). All three types of algae are potent sources of vitamins, minerals, and protein, and all have been used by traditional societies as food sources for thousands of years.

You can take algae as capsules or in powder form. I have used all three types of algae, and I think there is benefit to rotating between the three forms. I look for organic algae from Maine, Canada, or Norway. (I avoid algae from Japan because of the radiation concerns.)

Algae tastes very green. Chlorella and spirulina are both somewhat better tasting than blue-green algae. Of course, if you take capsules, you won't notice the taste. Definitely take the algae in the morning, as many people are activated for several hours after taking algae. If you take it in the afternoon, you are more likely to have problems sleeping. When supplementing your diet with algae, pay attention to how you feel. Some people crave algae and do very well with it, while others find that it causes nausea or loose stools. If it disagrees with you, do not use it. Also, I periodically take a holiday from algae and omit it for one week each month. I do this in part because I get a pound

> ## WAHLS ON THE ROAD
>
> When I travel, it can be difficult to get as many greens and sulfur-rich vegetables as I prefer to have in my diet. If I am not getting my usual amount of vegetables, I will often take an additional dose of algae that day. When I take my algae, I put the spirulina, chlorella, or Klamath blue-green in a small glass of water to make what I affectionately call my "green whiskey." I drink it as a shot, very quickly. Other travel tips:
>
> - I often take liver jerky with me when I am traveling to make sure the nutrient density of my diet does not fall off while traveling.
> - I order vegetables, grilled meats, and salads with a wedge of lemon or balsamic vinegar, and berries when they are available.
> - I avoid sauces, dressings, and soups, as they often have hidden gluten and dairy.

of a single type of algae and use that until it is finished. If I were taking just a couple of capsules each day, or if I rotated which algae I was taking every day, there would be no need for the holiday. This is the same reason I want you to rotate your greens: They're great for us, but all greens have some toxins. If you rotate your greens, you have more benefit and less risk. So either rotate your algae or take intermittent holidays from it. I take one teaspoon of spirulina or chlorella or ½ teaspoon of blue-green, because it is more potent. During the summer when I am eating more fresh greens and a wide variety of greens, I stop the algae and resume in the fall when my garden greens are done.

Digestive Enzymes

Our modern bodies carry a heavy load: Not only must we digest cooked food that has had its enzymes destroyed by heat, but we also tend to eat diets high in sugar and carbohydrates that increase the demands on our digestive enzymes. Years of doing this exhausts the pancreas so that it is no longer able to produce the optimal amount of digestive enzymes for the food we consume.

While I recommend adding fermented foods to your diet in chapter 6, "Wahls Paleo," supplements of digestive enzymes can help your body do a better job of digesting cooked food.

There are several ways to take digestive enzyme supplements. You can either take one or two capsules with your meals to replace some of the enzymes destroyed by cooking, or you can take one to three capsules on an empty stomach thirty to sixty minutes before you eat. This is the preferable method, because your empty stomach will absorb the enzymes and receive even more benefits.

I take two enzyme capsules (the brand I take is World Nutrition Vitälzȳm; I have been very happy with them and recommend them highly) first thing in the morning and again at bedtime on an empty stomach, but I worked up to this. I recommend starting with one capsule and gradually working your way up, noting how well you do. When purchasing digestive enzymes, look to see if the product includes protease, bromelain, amylase, and lipase at a minimum. Digestive enzymes can increase the effect of blood-thinning medication and need to be used cautiously if you are taking any medication, especially blood thinners of any type, including fish oil. That is another reason for making changes in the dose very slowly.

Additional Dietary Fiber

If you develop problems with constipation, I suggest you take in more fiber. You could use freshly ground flaxseed or chia seed to make more fruit puddings and titrate your dose to the desired effect. That in my opinion is preferable to taking fiber capsules. However, if this isn't doing the trick for you, you might need more fiber. The intent is to take in enough fiber to poop two to three times a day without having an accident in your pants! Look for soluble fiber products made from psyllium husks, inulin, chia seed, or ground flaxseed.

Supplement Summary

This chart shows typical dosages for the supplements I generally recommend, but always check with your physician/health care practitioner prior to starting new vitamins or supplements.

Supplement	Maximum Daily Dose (unless otherwise directed by physician based upon personal evaluation)
Vitamin D	Variable: Follow blood levels and take the amount recommended by your doctor.
Calcium citrate	250 mg elemental calcium once or twice a day if on Wahls Paleo or Wahls Paleo Plus diet
Magnesium	350 to 400 mg of magnesium glycinate daily
Docosahexaenoic acid (DHA)/ eicosapentaenoic acid (EPA), fish oil, or fermented cod-liver oil	2 grams DHA/EPA *or* 2 grams fish oil *or* 2 grams fermented cod-liver oil
Mixed vitamin E tocotrienols or mixed tocopherols	400 mg, if taking fish oil or DHA/EPA
B complex multivitamin, preferably B-100 (higher potency)	1 caplet
Methyl B_{12} (this form is preferable than a cheaper form of B_{12}, cyanocobalmin)	1,000 mcg (Let it dissolve slowly under your tongue and it will be absorbed into your bloodstream more efficiently than if you swallow it.)
L-methylfolate (levomefolic acid)	1,000 mcg
Coenzyme Q	200 mg
Algae (capsules or powder)	2 to 8 capsules or up to 1 teaspoon of powder (½ tsp if Klamath blue-green)
Dietary enzymes: protease, bromelain, amylase, and lipase	4 or more capsules on an empty stomach; may interact with blood thinners
Fiber (freshly ground flaxseed or chia seeds; best to soak 24 hours, then grind and blend)	As needed to have 2 soft bowel movements daily

Optional Supplements

There are some additional supplements that are often promoted for people with brain problems like autism, MS, neuropathy, Parkinson's, memory loss, and mood disorders. You may have heard about them or considered taking them, so I will weigh in. Note that many of these same compounds are promoted for people with heart failure and diabetes. These supplements are not part of the Wahls Protocol but you may consider them, especially if you are not making progress after six months with excellent adherence to the protocol. (Always work with your personal physician if you begin taking any supplement, whether part of the Wahls Protocol or not.)

- **Zinc, iron, and copper.** It is important for your zinc, iron, and copper to stay within optimal range—neither too low nor too high. Excessive copper and iron as well as zinc deficiency either in combination or individually have been associated with increased risk of neurodegenerative disorders such as Parkinson's and Alzheimer's dementia.[7] The increase in copper can occur in part from the copper used in water supply lines or the use of supplements that include copper. The excess iron can occur as a result of supplement use or cooking with cast-iron cookware. Because the uptake of copper is coupled to zinc, avoiding copper supplements (often present in multivitamin-multimineral supplements) and taking zinc (at low levels such as 30 mg daily or three times a week) may reduce the risk of excess copper or zinc deficiency. A baseline zinc level is also a consideration if you plan to take zinc on a regular basis, so make sure you do not overshoot and create a copper deficiency. Because iron is a necessary cofactor for many enzymes in the brain, it is necessary to have an optimal iron level. For that reason, any iron supplementation must be monitored with iron levels to be sure that your iron level does not become too high. Eating organ meats three times a week (rich in minerals) is better than taking supplements, because you are more likely to avoid creating excess or deficiency problems. This is another reason that I believe eating nutrient-dense food is safer than supplementation done without monitoring the levels of the specific vitamin or minerals levels.

- **Other brain and heart supplements.** Supplements other than the ones I've recommended earlier in the chapter often used in functional medicine practices to help support brain cell process include lipoic acid, carnitine, and creatine. Any or all of these may or may not be helpful to you. At a dosage of 300 to 600 mg/day, lipoic acid has been shown to be helpful in treating painful diabetic nerve damage.[8] Lipoic acid (600 mg) combined with carnitine (1,000 mg) and varying levels of coenzyme Q (100 mg to 600 mg twice a day; see previous section) are used for Parkinson's.[9] The combination of lipoic acid, B vitamins, and coenzyme Q has also been shown to be protective in a variety of animal models with brain troubles related to mitochondria that fail[10] and heart failure.[11] Note that two organ meats, liver and heart, are excellent sources of very bioavailable B vitamins, lipoic acid, and carnitine, as well as coenzyme Q. They are also all found in sardines, oysters, mussels, clams, and kidneys in forms that are more readily absorbed and utilized by the body than the synthetic versions in commercial supplements. You will also have less concern about whether the supplement may be contaminated with heavy metals or solvents from being grown in contaminated soils or during the manufacturing process. I'd rather you spend your money on buying and growing food.

- **Fasting boost.** When fasting, even for the twelve to sixteen hours suggested in Wahls Paleo Plus, your efforts will be boosted by a resveratrol supplement. This will further stimulate positive changes to your mitochondria.[12] You can get resveratrol naturally from black-colored berries such as aronia and blackberries, purple grape juice, and red wine, or you can take it in supplement form at a dosage of 250 mg once a day.

- **NAC (N-acetylcystine).** Take 500 mg to 1 gram daily. NAC is approved at much higher dosing for use in acute poisoning and Tylenol overdose and to reduce the risk of damage to kidneys with the use of intravenous contrast for X-ray studies. When I am concerned about detoxification for a particular patient, I may recommend 500 mg to 1 gram of NAC daily for additional detoxification support.

- **Turmeric.** This orange cooking spice helps rebalance the phase 1 and phase 2 detoxification enzymes in your liver and kidneys. I often take turmeric (½ to 1 teaspoon a day, in water like a shot or with coconut milk as a tea) and have patients who need additional detoxification support take turmeric tea regularly.

- **Organic sulfur compounds.** These are sometimes given as supplements to support detoxification enzymes, reduce cancer risk, and reduce excessive inflammation: sulforaphane, indole-3-carbinol (I3C), and diindolylmethane (DIM).[13] They are all present in the cabbage family of vegetables, which is why the Wahls Diet includes 3 cups of sulfur-rich vegetables.

- **Antioxidant supplements.** This series of supplements is often used to boost detoxification, reduce inflammation, optimize homocysteine levels, and/or improve the cholesterol profile. Many functional providers will suggest adding some of these when additional interventions are needed, based upon the person's evaluation. I have listed the supplement and put in parentheses the food source for that compound so you can see how the Wahls Diet was designed to maximize these important nutrients: resveratrol (skins of vegetables and dark berries), ellagic acid (berries), quercetin (green tea, onions, and berries), epigallocatechin gallate (EGCG; green tea and yerba maté), aged garlic extract (garlic family vegetables), hydroxy-tyrosol (olive oil that is not heated), and anthocyanins (purple and black vegetables and berries).

- **Aged garlic extract.** This has been shown to reduce oxidative stress, improve endothelial function, and improve blood flow[14] through the sulfur components within the garlic family of vegetables. Of course, you could just eat more garlic.
- **Zeolite and clay toxin binders.** Some integrative health providers push a number of toxin-binding compounds such as bentonite clay and/or zeolite. These compounds act like sticky flypaper to absorb the toxins that the liver transformed from fat soluble to water soluble and excreted into the

WAHLS WARRIOR Q & A

Q: Why did you simplify the supplement list since your first book, *Minding My Mitochondria: How I Overcame Secondary Progressive Multiple Sclerosis (MS) and Got out of My Wheelchair*?

A: I have learned a lot since I wrote *MMM* and have had a lot of additional research come in. One thing that has become very clear: It is best to individualize the protocol. In patients taking a long list of supplements, I have seen more problems with nausea, abdominal pain, and loose stools. For that reason, in my clinic I start with the short list I have provided in this chapter, check labs, take a careful history, do an examination, and then personalize the recommendations. Additions after this point will be more likely to have a positive effect, and the risk of side effects is lower. Requiring fewer supplements is also more cost-effective. I urge all Wahls Warriors to discuss the supplements you want to take with your health care practitioner to decide if they are worth considering for your circumstances, and monitor your reactions to each new supplement carefully. Add them one at a time and make dose changes slowly. Meanwhile, try to get as much of your nutrition from food as humanly possible!

bile. The toxins will stick to the clay and/or zeolite, you will not be able to reabsorb the toxin back into the bloodstream, and you will excrete the toxin. They also absorb nutrient metals like zinc and magnesium. Therefore, if you are going to take these internally, do so only under the direction of a physician.

- **Joint supplements.** These are often used for joint support for those suffering with degenerative joint disease or rheumatoid arthritis and include glucosamine, chondroitin, and methylsulfonylmethane (MSM). The best food source for these compounds is bone broth made with knucklebones, chicken feet, and sulfur-rich vegetables.

Finally, remember that targeted use of supplements may be very beneficial, particularly if the homocysteine remains elevated, but keep in mind that the Wahls Diet is designed to increase your intake of these nutrients naturally.

Complementary and Alternative Treatments

I am a conventionally trained internal medicine physician practicing at an academic center, so it's probably not surprising that, prior to my diagnosis, I was skeptical of alternative and complementary medicine. I believed people were wasting a great deal of money on these alternative, unproven therapies—that is, until I became a patient with a progressive disease for which there is no cure.

In my research, I found numerous studies showing that MS and other autoimmune patients use complementary and alternative medicine treatments, usually as adjuncts to their conventional medicine treatments. How could I not consider this option when I had so few choices left?

That is when I began looking at alternative medicine. Yet, I did this with the eye of a conventionally trained doctor: In everything I read, I looked for some common sense, and sometimes I found it. Not always, but sometimes. When I found evidence, I kept an open mind. There are many alternative medicine modalities that are not science-based. This is where you have to be careful. When I looked at alternative therapies, I asked myself whether the treatment balances potential benefit with potential harm in a responsible

WAHLS DIARY ALERT

If you decide to try any new therapy, keep detailed notes in your Wahls Diary about how you feel before the treatment begins, what you hope will improve, and how long you are going to try the new treatment before deciding if it is helpful or not—say, three months. Put a note in your Wahls Diary on the day you are going to reevaluate how you are doing, and put a note on your calendar, too. Then make notes once a week about how you are feeling. When the date comes for you to reevaluate how you are feeling, you will have a little more information to decide if the new treatment is helping you or not. Sometimes it takes stopping the new intervention to realize how much it is benefiting you.

way, even if the treatment isn't FDA-approved. Is there any research backing it? Does it make scientific sense? I urge you to ask yourself these questions before trying something new:

1. What are the risks? They should be minimal. For example, going gluten-free for two weeks to see how your body reacts has very little, if any, risk.
2. How much will it benefit the specific disease I am suffering from? Is there any proof that it will, or that it has done so in others with my specific disease? Are there published studies in peer-reviewed scientific journals? Pubmed.gov is where I search.
3. How much will it benefit (or potentially worsen) my overall health? Is there proof that it has done so in others?
4. How much will it cost to do this, how often, and what kind of monitoring, if any, is needed if I try this? Is there a way to test whether it is working?
5. Does it make sense in terms of potential mechanism of action? Would a doctor or scientist say it is impossible, just improbable, or actually quite possible?
6. Can I do it easily on my own or with my family's support?

7. How will I decide if it is improving the quality of my life or my family members' lives enough to continue?

Even if the therapy you want to try doesn't pass every test, you may still want to try it. We all have our own level of risk tolerance. Some people prefer to wait for clinical trials that garner FDA approval for a drug or surgical treatment. If that is what makes you comfortable, then that is the appropriate choice for you. (You may, however, want to read the package insert of potential side effects for those prescription drugs!) Others do not want to wait and are more comfortable seeking new things to try to improve the quality of their lives, even if they aren't proven just yet. However, I do recommend that you evaluate new treatments with this rubric and create a plan that will help you decide if the intervention is helping you. I suggest doing this for every new treatment (FDA-approved or not) that you begin. Keep a record of your progress and don't hide what you are doing from your personal physician.

The list of potential alternative therapies is a long one, but there are some that I find particularly low-risk and potentially useful for MS, autoimmune problems, and other chronic diseases, as well as for other brain issues. There are other alternative therapies that I did not include on the list because of space limitations.

Low-Risk Alternative Therapies

- **Reiki /Healing Touch/Therapeutic Touch.** This is a form of therapy that supposedly manipulates energy so it moves better through the body, promoting balance and healing. The use of Reiki, Healing Touch, or Therapeutic Touch therapy uses light or proximity-only touch to interact with the biofield energy of the body. *Biofield* is the term used to describe the field of weak electromagnetic energy surrounding the human body. With the development of quantum mechanics, the tools to build monitors that can measure these fields now exists, and it is the same quantum mechanics that allow for magnetic resonance imaging (MRI) scanners that have become critical to imaging the brain. Reiki and Healing Touch/ Therapeutic Touch techniques interact with the person's biologic energy, using the energy of the person who is giving the therapy to provide support to the person receiving the treatment. Biofield therapies are being added to cancer treatment centers and have been shown to be clinically helpful in reducing pain and improving quality of life, and are now being shown to improve immune cell function.[15]

- **Movement therapies.** This group includes practices like yoga, Pilates, and tai chi. These three styles of movement all include stretching, balance, strength training, and awareness of your position in space. As such, they are all excellent for improving the connections between your brain and your body. I do both yoga and Pilates as part of my morning workout. I have also attended tai chi classes. If you can find a good, experienced instructor, I recommend any of these therapies highly. Another option is to obtain a DVD and begin doing them at home. The advantage of an instructor is that she or he can be very helpful in learning how to do the moves correctly, adapting them to where your body is presently, and helping you advance what you are doing as your strength and balance improve. (For more on these and all types of exercise, review chapter 9, "Exercise and Electricity.")

- **Bodywork.** This includes body manipulation by someone else, as you would experience in massage and reflexology. Our skin is filled with skin receptors that send information back to our brains. The touch that we feel can help down-regulate the number of inflammation molecules and restore a more optimal balance to the hypothalamic-pituitary-adrenal function.[16] In other words, massage can reset your stress hormone levels back to idle. For years I could not tolerate massage therapy, as even the lightest massage felt painful to me. Now, however, I find that massage, even the most vigorous deep-tissue massage, is very helpful. It is relaxing and provides a deep sense of calm and contentment following the massage. If you can have massage therapy on a regular basis, by all means, do so. If all you can do is simply massage and stroke your own skin—or have a family member or friend do this for you—you will still enjoy plenty of benefits. Even if you do get massages, I also recommend that you spend some time stroking your face, ears, hands, and feet daily.

- **Reflexology.** This is the art of applying pressure to specific locations in the feet to reduce symptoms and improve function. Studies of reflexology and multiple sclerosis have shown benefits in reducing pain and fatigue.[17]

This next list of therapies come with a slightly higher risk, but you might want to consider them.

Moderate-Risk but Potentially Beneficial Alternative Therapies

- **Chiropractic care.** Many people with multiple sclerosis have lesions in the cervical (neck) spinal cord. If the cervical bones are not in proper alignment, they can put pressure on the spinal cord. Chiropractic manipulation, if done properly, can lessen malalignments and decrease the pressure. In a study of chiropractic care to the neck using forty-four multiple sclerosis patients and thirty-seven Parkinson's disease patients published in the *Journal of Vertebral Subluxation Research* (a chiropractic journal), 91 percent of the MS and 92 percent of the Parkinson's patients improved.[18] If you have cervical lesions, an evaluation by a chiropractor may be beneficial to you, but choose someone with a good reputation who has experience treating patients with your disease.

- **Acupuncture.** Acupuncture is a therapy involving the insertion of tiny needles into predetermined points on the body. Practitioners study where these energy centers are and which ones can be stimulated to resolve particular issues. Acupuncture can be done using needles or electrical stimulation of particular points in the body to improve the flow of energy, or *chi*, through the body to reduce symptoms and improve function. In two studies of the use of acupuncture to treat fatigue in the setting of multiple sclerosis, benefit was shown. In one study, twenty subjects who had fatigue that was not helped by drug therapy underwent twelve sessions of acupuncture. Fifteen of the twenty had clinically significant reductions in fatigue.[19] In another study of thirty-one patients with relapsing-remitting MS who were given immune modulator drugs and acupuncture therapy or sham therapy (a placebo), the active acupuncture group had greater reductions in pain and depression than the placebo group.[20]

- **Pulsed electromagnetic therapy.** Magnetic forces may have biologic effects on our cells, in part due to the documented improvement of the flow of electrons through the electron transport chain in mitochondria in an electromagnetic field. There have been several uncontrolled small studies that have shown the benefits of using pulsed electromagnetic fields (PEMF) in the setting of MS. There has now been a randomized, double-blind (meaning neither the patient nor the investigator knew who had active treatment), placebo-controlled study that used two study sites to examine the effect of PEMF in multiple sclerosis. In this study, subjects received four weeks of therapy, then a two-week washout period, and then two weeks of the other therapy. One hundred seventeen subjects completed the study. There was significant improvement found for fatigue and overall quality of life for the active device (the device that actually delivered PEMF, as opposed to the sham device or "placebo device" used in the study). No benefit was seen for bladder control.[21] In another study using PEMF, using Bio-Electromagnetic-Energy-Regulation (BEMER) therapy, thirty-seven subjects were randomized for a double-blind twelve-week treatment of active therapy versus placebo and were then followed three years after the initial randomized crossover controlled trial. Again the PEMF was associated with reduction in fatigue and improved quality of life in the short-term and longer follow-up studies.[22]

- **Detoxification/colonics/cleanses/chelation.** There are many practitioners whose goal is improving detoxification pathways of the kidneys, liver, and sweat glands. Some of the practitioners use intravenous drugs to pull out the toxins. The potential harm of intravenous detoxification is that more toxins will be pulled from the body than the liver, kidneys, and sweat glands can process, which will lead to the transfer of the toxins back to the storage sites in the lipids (fats) in the body, including the brain. For that reason I would be very cautious about any intravenous detoxification strategies. Other detoxification strategies (beyond those I talked about in chapter 8, "Reduce Toxic Load") include colonics or colon hydrotherapy, which is the use of water or other fluids to wash out the colon. Although the FDA regulates the devices used to introduce the fluid into the colon, it does not regulate the practice. Conventional medicine does not consider colonics to have any scientific merit. I cannot find any studies of colon irrigations in PubMed.gov, nor do I have any experience with colonic lavage, personally or in my patients. Therefore I cannot give you an opinion on its benefits and/or potential harm. Intravenous chelation therapy is costly and potentially hazardous if not done correctly. Work with a physician who has been trained and certified so that you are not harmed by removing the toxins more quickly than your liver and kidneys can metabolize the toxins. When that happens the toxins are transferred from your belly fat to the fat in your brain—not a good thing to do!

Finally, there are a few approaches I do not recommend.

Alternative Therapies I Do Not Recommend

- **Color therapy, crystal therapy, and aromatherapy.** There isn't really anything wrong with these harmless therapies. If you are using these as part of your meditative practices to lower your stress level or improve your sleep, please continue to use them. They are certainly not dangerous. However, I cannot find any published peer-reviewed literature offering proof of their effectiveness or supporting their use specifically for autoimmune conditions (though I admit those studies may exist and I simply have not found them).
- **Bee venom, scorpion venom, and other biologic toxin therapies.** These have been reported to be remarkably useful for some individuals in uncontrolled studies of MS and other autoimmune conditions, but randomized controlled studies have been mixed at best.[23] I chose not to pursue those therapies because the risk for adverse reaction is significant.
- **Stem cell therapy.** This is a medical treatment with significant risk and costs involved. There are limited published papers supporting its benefits. However, I expect that if the underlying environmental factors (diet, toxins, food sensitivity, hormonal imbalance, etc.) are not addressed, the benefits will not be permanent.
- **Liberation therapy (angioplasty for blocked vessels) for chronic cerebrospinal venous insufficiency (CCSVI).** I discussed this earlier when I reviewed Dr. Paolo Zamboni's work studying patients who have clogs in the veins that drain the brain.[24] Liberation therapy is a costly surgical

procedure with significant risks, and I expect that if the underlying environmental factors (diet, toxins, food sensitivity, hormonal imbalance, etc.) are not addressed, the benefits achieved will likely not be permanent. (I do understand, however, why those with severe disabilities consider this intervention.)

Navigating a disease can be difficult and frustrating, especially when you don't feel like you are making progress. However, unproven, risky treatments are not the answer. Stick with sound, sensible approaches that feed your cells and promote repair and healing. Stay on your drugs and work with your personal physician to individualize these concepts for you. As you provide your cells the building blocks they need to do the chemistry of life properly and remove the toxins that interfere with doing the chemistry of life properly, your cells will begin repairing themselves.

Chapter 11

STRESS MANAGEMENT

S TRESS, BOTH PHYSICAL and emotional, is necessary for life. Growing up on a farm gave me excellent bone density because of all the stress on my bones from manual labor. When humans enter a weightless environment, with no gravity pulling on bones and muscles, our bodies begin to lose strength and shrink. Likewise, our brains need the stress of learning and adapting to change in order to produce the hormones (nerve growth factors) that nurture brain cells and direct them to make new connections. Without the stress of learning, our brains make less nerve growth factor and begin the process of atrophying (shrinking).

This is an adaption from our Paleolithic days. We needed that spurt of energy from our adrenals to get away from predators or catch prey for dinner. That spurt of adrenaline and surge of cortisol that come from physical or emotional stress sharpens our vision and hearing and improves muscle strength and endurance. We are more likely to get away and survive.

This applies to our lives now, too. A quick burst of energy, pressure, activity, learning, and then relaxation is the healthiest way to benefit from stress. This can help you jump out of the way of a speeding car, have a good workout, learn a new language or how to play a musical instrument, or remember what you have to do tomorrow—then relax with a "Phew! I'm glad that's over!"

Stress, however, is meant to be acute, not chronic. Chronic high stress without that important recovery period is maladaptive, damaging the body and the brain. After stress, our bodies are supposed to rapidly metabolize (process and eliminate) the stress hormones circulating through the system so we are back to a safe state of "idle." When our adrenals are constantly putting out stress hormones, however, we can't get back to that important safe state. Our chemical processes (metabolism) become deranged as a result, leading to excess inflammation in the body and in the brain. We are more likely to become obese and/or diabetic, have clogged arteries (atherosclerosis), have mental health problems, develop autoimmune problems, and even create ideal conditions for the growth of cancer cells. Chronic stress wears down the body and uses all your internal resources, distracting them from building and healing. Just the fact that you have a chronic disease puts you into a state of chronic stress.

Your Autonomic Nervous System

The stress response is complex, but one way to look at it is through the lens of the autonomic nervous system. This is the set of nerves that connect brain to body and that help us identify whether we feel safe or unsafe at any given moment. This is very important for your health because the autonomic nervous system also governs all the things that happen in your body automatically, like digestion, breathing, and the beating of your heart.

The part of the autonomic system that reports when you are safe and all is well is called the parasympathetic system. When that system is in charge, your cells know they are safe and can focus on doing the work of living. That means digesting food, making hormones, removing toxins, and building proteins to create new cells, support your immune cells, repair damage, and grow.

There is another part of the autonomic nervous system that kicks in when your brain signals that you are not safe and are indeed acutely threatened. This is called the sympathetic nervous system. When the sympathetic nervous system takes over, everything changes. The work of living, including digestion, normal hormone production, detoxing, and protein building, comes to a screeching halt. Your cells switch gears, priming the body for only two things: either to run away or to fight an attacker.

In order to do this, two glands—the adrenals and the thyroid—change tactics. You can think of them as the tortoise and the hare. The adrenal glands are the hare. They respond rapidly to a threat, immediately revving up the metabolism and secreting stress hormones like adrenaline, noradrenaline, and cortisol. These make your heart speed up, enable your eyes to see more acutely, and divert blood from your bowels to your muscles so you can run faster and longer. They also make your blood sugar and insulin levels increase so you have more energy with which to run. That's all very effective—for a short time. Once the threat has passed, our bodies quickly metabolize or break down the stress hormones and we go back to a safe state, digesting our food and conducting the chemistry of life normally.

Meanwhile, the thyroid has a longer view. It adjusts the metabolism according to what the adrenals are doing. If there are a lot of threats, the metabolism may stay idling at a higher speed, just to make sure the engine is ready to go whenever necessary. However, if the adrenals are always pouring out stress hormones and don't get to calm down because the brain never signals that the threat has passed, and the thyroid thinks the motor has to be racing all the time, we don't get that all-important recovery period. Over time, this exhausts the adrenal glands, and they lose their reserve. At that point the person begins to develop adrenal fatigue, which just feels like plain old bone-tired chronic fatigue. The adrenals may look "normal" from a conventional medicine perspective, but the adrenal reserve is compromised. Your body will do the best it can to keep your metabolism running. When the adrenals can't keep you energized, your thyroid will pick up the baton to keep your energy and metabolism up; but when your thyroid can't keep up with your continual stress, it, too, will begin to fail. By that time you are likely experiencing deep fatigue.

Now your hormones are out of whack, and this can cause widespread trouble in your body and brain. In addition, chronic stress can also damage the lining of the blood vessels throughout the body, including the ones in your brain and in your heart, and the lining of your gut, causing leaky vessels, a leaky brain, and a leaky gut, which puts you at greater risk for developing

WAHLS WARRIORS SPEAK

I have a traumatic brain injury that occurred during a bicycle accident in 2008. Secondary to that, I've dealt with epilepsy, aphasia, cognitive problems, memory loss, major depression, vertigo, and the inability to go back to my previous position as a pediatric nurse practitioner. A few years after my accident, I was craving a diet high in dark green vegetables, fruits, and salmon, and my doctor recommended that I meet Dr. Wahls. Among the many improvements I've noticed since starting the diet three years ago, I've been able to cut my antidepressant medication in half because my depression has improved a great deal, as has my mental clarity. I truly love and need exercise, so I do cardio or strength-training exercises nearly every day. I meditate and nap daily, get a massage once a month, and use deep breathing whenever I'm stressed out. Being out in nature and having some quiet time alone are so necessary for me. I also utilize my medical knowledge to share my story of survival with others. I believe all of these have helped me, and giving talks when I'm able has been a wonderful experience.

—Bridgid R., Coralville, Iowa

or worsening your autoimmune problems. Our cells simply aren't built to work that way over the long term, continually bathed in high levels of stress hormones.

The Stress/Insulin Resistance Connection

In addition to the damage to your blood vessels and hormone levels, stress can also lead to system-wide inflammation by causing an increasingly common and dangerous condition called insulin resistance. Here's how it works. As I mentioned earlier, stress hormones acutely increase our blood pressure, heart rate, blood sugar, and insulin levels. But when there is a constant elevation of stress hormones in the body, that leads to a chronic overelevation of blood sugar, which then produces chronic high levels of insulin to keep that blood sugar under control.

One of insulin's main jobs is to shuttle sugar out of the blood to keep the level in a safe range. It drives blood sugar into muscle cells and more importantly into fat cells, especially the ones around your middle, also known as visceral fat. The problem is that visceral fat is hormonally very active, making lots of cytokines (little protein molecules that act like hormones) that markedly increase inflammation in the bloodstream and in the brain. The more sugar in the bloodstream from either eating a high-carbohydrate diet or chronic elevation of cortisol (or likely both), the more likely the stressed, sugar-eating person is to develop insulin resistance.

Once that happens, the pancreas responds by making more and more insulin, which also leads to more and more visceral fat, which will make more inflammation cytokines and hormones that are responsible for revving up the inflammation in your bloodstream. To make matters even worse, these changes also increase a person's appetite for carbohydrates, further driving this entire cycle. It's a downward spiral. Continuing to eat a high-carbohydrate diet when you are fighting inflammation is like dripping gasoline on a fire while the firefighter (your doctor) is trying to put out the fire with water from the hydrant (conventional medicine). You are making it much harder to put out the inflammation fires as long as you keep your insulin levels high. Go to the root cause and lower the stress hormones through the stress management techniques we will talk about in this chapter *and* lower carbohydrate intake. (Wahls Paleo is ideal for this.)

If the "doors" in the muscle and organ cells become resistant to letting the glucose in, so that it remains in the bloodstream, despite insulin's efforts to push it out, the doors will get more and more "stuck" over time. The high sugars are dangerous, so the body goes into alert mode and the pancreas pumps out even more insulin. An insulin-resistant person needs much more circulating insulin than a healthy person to keep the blood sugar in the normal range. If this is happening to you, you may be diagnosed with metabolic syndrome, which is considered a precursor or warning sign that diabetes is in your future. If you continue the way you are going, your pancreas will eventually lose the ability to keep your blood sugar in the safe range. Diabetes is the

TEST YOUR INSULIN SENSITIVITY

A simple test for insulin sensitivity is the fasting triglyceride/HDL cholesterol (good cholesterol) level in the bloodstream. A ratio of greater than 3 suggests insulin resistance and that the insulin level is way too high. Keep in mind that this ratio is less predictive in people of African descent. If that group includes you, ask your physician to check your blood glucose along with an insulin level to check insulin resistance or sensitivity. The best way to improve insulin levels is to reduce the demand for insulin production by eating a diet high in protein and healthy fat and very low in carbohydrates. Wahls Paleo and Wahls Paleo Plus fit the bill perfectly: They are both intentionally lower in carbohydrates, greatly reducing or eliminating starchy vegetables and starchier, sweeter fruits.

result. You will begin spilling sugar into your urine, and the damage to your blood vessels and brain cells dramatically increases. People often have diabetes for many years before it is diagnosed, inflicting damage on the nerves and brain cells all the while.

In addition to the very real risk of diabetes, insulin resistance is also associated with higher rates of brain problems like apoptosis (brain cell death), more damage to nerves (like painful diabetic neuropathy), and more amyloid protein tangles typical of Alzheimer's dementia. That is because insulin interferes with the enzyme that normally clears these harmful protein tangles.[1] The visceral fat produces cytokines, which drive up the inflammation in the bloodstream and brain, making autoimmune problems worse. Insulin resistance is also a major contributing factor in the development of atherosclerosis, polycystic ovarian syndrome (a leading cause of infertility), hirsutism (facial hair on women), erectile dysfunction, and low testosterone in men. Insulin resistance wrecks your hormones and metabolism in many profound ways.[2]

In short, insulin resistance is increasingly recognized to be associated with increased risk of harm to the brain and nerves, damage to your blood vessels, the development of early dementia, and the screwing up of your sex hormone balance. You don't want to go there!

Stress Management the Wahls Way

You know stress is bad for you. The question is: How do you get your stress hormones back to the resting state or idling, so your body can recover and your chemistry can normalize again between bouts of healthy stress?

Fortunately, stress management is an important part of the Wahls Protocol, and it's not difficult. In fact, it feels fantastic. All you have to do is switch the autonomic nervous system control from the sympathetic back to the parasympathetic to signal that you are safe. This reduces the demand for stress hormones and gives your poor adrenal glands a break.

How do you do this?

There are many ways of reducing stress, so choose the activities you enjoy the most. I recommend doing something stress-relieving several times each day, such as one thing in the morning and one thing in the afternoon or evening. Every single one of these activities is something you could not and would not do if you were in an emergency situation. If you were in danger, would you be meditating with your eyes closed? Would you be strolling through a park or working in the garden or writing in your journal? Of course not. Activities like these will trigger the brain to signal the adrenals that they can relax again. You are meditating, so all must be well. This helps the whole cascade of stress response actions in the body go in reverse and you eventually, with some practice, get back to your normal state.

Here are some ideas, and remember my prescription: Two per day!

- **Spending time in nature.** Walking or jogging outside in the fresh air and sunlight is incredibly rejuvenating and a good way to de-stress, especially if you spend a lot of time indoors feeling tense.
- **Gardening.** Gardening has multiple benefits: It is light exercise; you are outside in the sunlight, producing more vitamin D; and you are in nature. You are also doing something productive, like beautifying your yard or growing your own food. It also has a distinct calming effect on people.
- **Exercise.** Any kind of exercise (aerobic, strength training, stretching) can work for stress relief. See chapter 9, "Exercise and Electricity."
- **Meditation and/or prayer.** I'll talk in more detail about meditation and

prayer later in this chapter, but meditation can be done just a few minutes several times a day.

- **Journaling.** Write in your Wahls Diary about the problems you are facing or have faced in the past. Spend at least forty-five minutes over the week writing about your deepest concerns or struggles. No one else has to see the journal. You don't have to read the journal entries again, and you should write in pen and not correct yourself. This is called free writing, and it helps you develop new insights into your experiences. This actually helps the brain send less energy down the sympathetic nervous system to the adrenals. That translates into less adrenaline and cortisol in your system, resulting in better immune cell function and better health. Continue to journal a few minutes each day or fifteen minutes three times a week.

- **Regular contact with a supportive group of people.** When people have a supportive group of peers, they are more successful at adopting behaviors that promote health. Dr. Mark Hyman completed a project with the Saddleback Church in Lake Forest, California, where he coached the church through the adoption of health behaviors to combat obesity and diabetes, with tremendous success.[3] Dr. Hyman taught the church community about functional medicine and diet, but the small support groups the church formed to help their members along seemed to have the greatest impact. I suggest you do something similar for yourself. Find a support group of like-minded people and you will feel your stress drop.

- **Contemplate your higher purpose.** Finding that higher purpose beyond the self can provide inner calm, direction, and guidance that is reassuring and healing. (See chapter 3, "Getting Focused.")

- **Forgive.** Carrying a grudge for prior injustices and wrongs burdens the person who continues to hold the grudge.

- **Yoga.** With its focus on breathing and postures, yoga also reduces stress hormones. There are many different types, from strenuous to meditative. Almost anyone can find a variety that they enjoy.

- **Massage.** Our skin expects to be touched, massaged. While receiving a deep-tissue massage has many measurable health benefits,[4] getting a daily professional massage is impractical. In our clinical trial we teach people to give themselves a simple self-massage as part of their daily routine. They

WAHLS WARRIORS SPEAK

In addition to daily exercise and deep breathing, I spend time in nature every day and, occasionally, I meditate for about ten minutes. Learning many new cooking techniques has also been good for my brain. One improvement since starting the Wahls Diet and retiring is that I have resumed piano lessons. Playing piano is therapeutic for my weak left hand, which has begun to function better, a wonderful development because I am left-handed. Playing piano is also good for my cognition, and I have developed a deeper appreciation of music. That's good for my brain, too!

Like Dr. Wahls, I am a Unitarian Universalist. I am surrounded by a terrific community of friends! They are quite a reassuring comfort and source of strength, security, and love. I'm not just feeling sorry for myself and thinking about my health concerns. While my activism is limited now due to my low energy levels, I remain connected to the larger issues in our world and maintain a global perspective. I just make sure to bring my own meals to the frequent potlucks endemic to my UU social life.

—Toni C., Cave Creek, Arizona

can use an essential oil (such as grapefruit, lavender, or sandalwood), or an omega-3-rich oil (like walnut oil), or no oil at all. I ask them to begin by massaging the sole of the right foot and all of the toes. The fingers should press as firmly as desired into the ball of the foot and the arch then massage the toes. Repeat with the left foot. Then, using both hands, gently massage the calf and leg muscles, pulling toward the heart. This will improve the return of lymph fluid to the heart. Move to the right hand and massage the palm of the hand and the fingers. Massage the left hand. Next massage the arm, stroking toward the heart. Massage both earlobes between the fingers, then move around the entire earlobe and ear. Then massage the forehead, cheekbones, and chin. Massage the scalp. Do the massage yourself as part of your evening routine, just before bed or upon arising.

- **Take an Epsom salt bath.** Chronic elevations of stress hormones lead to depletion of minerals, especially magnesium. That is why Epsom salt (magnesium sulfate) baths can be so soothing. They help reduce the stress hormones and begin to replenish the magnesium.

The Importance of
Sleep for Stress Management

Sleep is incredibly important for stress management, especially for people with autoimmune conditions. Many people who are stressed have trouble sleeping even as they suffer from fatigue. The relationship between sleep quality and duration and health has been well established across multiple studies,[5] and because sleep problems are more frequent in those with MS than the general population, and restless legs are a common problem for MS patients,[6] this is worth dealing with right now.

Sleep is an important part of maintaining the health of all mammals. We need to sleep. It's a requirement for life. Without sleep, our brains will become disorganized. We will hallucinate and become psychotic and nonfunctional. For our bodies, sleep is equally critical. During the eight or nine hours of sleep that our biology requires, the body doesn't consume as much energy because it doesn't have to move, digest, or engage in rational thought. That leaves more available energy for toxin removal, hormone manufacture, and infection fighting. When we fail to get enough, our bodies may not complete those important tasks, increasing the chance of developing problems due to excess toxins, inflammation, and hormone imbalances.

Even with my MS fatigue, I never slept a lot. I liked thinking I needed only five to six hours of sleep to function normally. This was back in the days when I was reading scientific literature at night after my family was in bed. Once a week, I'd crash and sleep a lot—sometimes ten hours—then I'd be back to not needing much sleep.

When I learned how critical sleep is to normal biology, I began to rethink my strategy and address my sleep behaviors so that I could get a regular seven to nine hours of sleep. Even if you think you thrive on less than seven hours of sleep a night, your body is paying a heavy price. You will be at a much higher risk of heart attack, obesity, diabetes, early memory decline, and autoimmune problems. Your cells need you to sleep if you want to have optimal health. That is why I pay attention to sleep now.

Sleep is such a natural activity that it may seem strange so many people have trouble with it. However, if you look at how we live, it isn't such a surprise. We do many things that interfere with getting a good night's sleep. Here are some of the most common and what you can do about them to improve your sleep:

- **Caffeine.** People often drink caffeinated beverages throughout the day to compensate for not having enough energy (often because their diets are so poor), and that caffeine can stay in the system for hours, increasing wakefulness even when it's time to sleep. Some people are much more sensitive to the effects of caffeine than others. For best sleep, stop drinking caffeinated beverages after 11 a.m. and switch to drinking a chamomile tea or an herbal blend with chamomile in it in the evening.
- **Alcohol.** People often drink alcohol in the evenings "to relax." However, alcohol can interfere with sleep quality throughout the night. On the Wahls Protocol, I prefer to limit alcohol use to "occasionally" (three or fewer drinks per week). Consuming it more often may compromise the health of brain cells. Also, consuming alcohol increases the probability of awakening in the middle of the night with difficulty resuming sleep. For this reason, do not consume alcohol for two to three hours prior to going to bed.
- **Sleeping pills.** People often use a variety of medications to induce sleep (sleeping pills like Ambien or other preparations intended for different uses, like Benadryl or NyQuil). These also interfere with the normal sleep cycle and should not be used for more than three days in a row. In numerous studies, individuals who used benzodiazepines or antihistamines—the classes of medicines most often used as sleeping pills—had a higher risk of falls and hip fractures.[7] Definitely not worth the risk.
- **Irregular sleep hours.** Many people stay up too late or go to bed at different times every night. People also use electronic devices late into the night, sitting on the computer or watching television. Because we want to finish what we're doing or watching, we tend to prioritize that over sleep.

EPSOM SALTS

Epsom salts are an excellent remedy for relaxation. Make an Epsom salt bath (with warm or cool water) part of your regular evening routine. Taking a bath for twenty to thirty minutes just before bed will relax you, and Epsom salts can also help support your body's detoxification processes, as well as providing supplemental magnesium and sulfur.

This confuses our bodies. If you set up and strictly follow a bedtime routine—such as always having a cup of chamomile tea, listening to relaxing music, having a warm bath, and then meditating, praying, reading, or journaling before bed—your body will get in the habit of relaxing and will naturally induce sleepiness.

- **Exercising at night.** Aerobic exercise during the day can actually improve sleep later, but exercise right before bed can make sleep more difficult for some because it is stimulating.
- **Stress.** Most of us have chronic elevations of stress hormones that keep us alert, making it more difficult to initiate and maintain sleep. Manage your stress!

A few more sleep-inducing tips:

- Taurine is a sulfur-containing amino acid found in fish that boosts the production of gamma-aminobutyric acid (GABA). Taurine supplements (500 mg) and a few cups of chamomile tea may also help to induce natural sleep. Meditate, pray, or write in a journal right before sleeping.
- Write a note to yourself about the issues that you want to address in the coming days, or make a to-do list for the next day. This can prevent your waking up to fret about what you have to do or what you don't want to forget during the night. Once it's down on paper, you can release it from your mind.
- Give your face, ears, hands, and feet a massage with lavender oil as soon as you get into bed.

- Try to sleep between eight and nine hours every night. You won't believe how much better you'll feel if you can get in this habit!

About Melatonin

Much of our ability to get a good night's sleep has to do with the brain's ability to manufacture melatonin, the hormone made by the pineal gland that is key to the wake-sleep cycle. Your brain secretes melatonin (making it out of serotonin) in response to the world becoming dark, and increases in melatonin are associated with shorter times to falling asleep. You get to sleep a lot faster if you have a melatonin spike in your brain in the evening with the onset of darkness.

The problem is that our current lifestyles conflict with the melatonin cycle. For instance, we use artificial lights, which confuse the brain. Is it the sun? Is it daytime? Your brain doesn't know. Also, melatonin is a potent antioxidant and anti-inflammation molecule. You want to have your brain making plenty of it! Here are some things you can do to help regulate your melatonin cycle:

- Have some daylight exposure in the morning or noon hour and spend at least thirty minutes looking into the blue sky or clouds to get your dose of natural blue light to your retina, which will help your brain to trigger your melatonin cycle.
- Go to bed just after sunset, ideally between 8 and 10 p.m.
- At dusk, put on yellow glasses to block the blue light spectrum. I tell my patients with sleep problems to use glasses that block the blue light spectrum when the sun goes down. You can wear these up to two hours before going to bed. This corrects the natural light exposure to your eyes and therefore your brain, increasing the production of melatonin, because the blue portion of the light is what suppresses the melatonin surge. I often use low-blue-light glasses when I am awake past sundown, working in my home. Depending on the time of year, that could mean I wear the glasses for just a few minutes or for several hours before going to bed.
- Wear a sleep mask at night so your eyes see only darkness when you are in bed. Because many with MS have balance issues, you will want to leave

some kind of yellow light on to avoid nighttime falling if you do have to get up. When you do, don those yellow glasses so that you don't stimulate your retina with the blue light spectrum.

- Although fixing light exposure is the most effective way to boost your melatonin, you can also take melatonin by mouth. Take 1 mg of melatonin one to three hours before you wish to sleep. Check with your physician regarding the top dose for you. Melatonin is best kept for intermittent short-term use. Fixing your light exposure is the real solution for correcting your melatonin levels.

IF YOU HAVE RESTLESS LEGS SYNDROME

Restless legs syndrome (RLS) is a disorder in which people have an uncontrollable urge to move their legs, usually in the evening when relaxing or at night when trying to sleep. RLS can involve feelings of pain, cramping, spasms, electrical sensations, tickling, itching, or a "crawling" feeling in the legs. It can also be characterized by an intense need to move the legs without any particular feeling in the legs. It can occasionally affect other limbs, but the legs are most common.

Although primary RLS is idiopathic, meaning there is no known cause, it has been observed at higher rates than in the normal population in people with autoimmune diseases as well as with neurological disorders like Parkinson's disease and peripheral neuropathy, and with other conditions like diabetes, thyroid disease, fibromyalgia, and attention deficit hyperactivity disorder (ADHD). The underlying mechanism for restless legs has to do with a drop in the dopamine neurotransmitter level in the brain. Dopamine levels fall in the evening, allowing us to sleep, but that drop in dopamine may also trigger RLS symptoms.

The biggest problem with RLS, other than being an annoyance and sometimes painful, is that it can severely interfere with sleep. The frequency of restless legs increases with age, but even young people in their teens can develop restless legs. The treatment from conventional medicine is to prescribe medications that boost available dopamine to counteract the effect and/or to prescribe benzodiazepines at night to make the person sleep more deeply. (This will increase the risk of falling and also the risk of dependence and addiction to benzodiazepines.) I prefer to use alternative and complementary approaches, including getting sufficient iron, B vitamins, omega-3 fatty acids, magnesium, calcium, and trace minerals. You should get all these things in sufficient amounts on the Wahls Diet, Wahls Paleo, or Wahls Paleo Plus.

You might also try using menthol or camphor ointment applied to the legs at bedtime. Ointments like Vicks VapoRub, Tiger Balm, and Bio-freeze provide a mild topical anesthesia to the leg and help calm the restlessness. Reapply as needed.

Finally, boosting your brain's ability to make gamma-aminobutyric acid (GABA) may be helpful, both for restless legs syndrome and for helping the brain calm down, making it easier to fall asleep. In addition to taurine supplements (mentioned earlier in this chapter), compounds that boost your brain's ability to make GABA include N-acetylcysteine (NAC, 500 mg to 2 grams) and lipoic acid (600 mg). Prescription medications that boost GABA, including baclofen and gabapentin, can also be helpful in extreme cases. Many people with MS are on one or both of these compounds any-way because of muscle stiffness or spasticity (baclofen) or pain (gabapen-tin). Somewhat higher doses may resolve the restless legs for you. Talk to your doctor about seeing if a higher dose is an option for you.

It's rather amazing that stress and sleep deprivation can have such a profound effect on the body, but they do. Manage that stress proactively and take these important steps to getting a full, sound eight to nine hours of sleep per night, and you will be taking a huge leap forward in your healing because your body will have the biochemical environment and the time it needs to perform the many subtle and pervasive cellular repairs, corrections, and manufacturing you require.

Chapter 12

RECOVERY

You've come a long way. You've worked through the Wahls Diet, perhaps staying there, or you've progressed to Wahls Paleo, or perhaps you've even tried out Wahls Paleo Plus. You've instituted changes in your routine. You may be exercising more, practicing stress management, and sleeping better. Now it's time to step back and take a look at how far you've come. This is your chance to assess your progress. Are your improvements greater than you expected? Are you right on track? Or are you not seeing the results you hoped to see?

If you are seeing dramatic results, I am overjoyed for you! If you are seeing mildly positive results, know that you are headed in the right direction. If you are not seeing results yet, I will help you determine what to do next in this chapter. People are impatient. People with chronic illness are even more impatient—they want to be well! At least, they want to be well right up until they give up on ever feeling better.

Do not give up! Recovery is a highly individual process, but I've watched it happen time and time again, in my traumatic brain injury clinics, in my primary-care clinics, even in my own family. People are standing up to witness about their own recoveries in my public lectures. And me? I'm walking.

Riding my bicycle. Working. Enjoying my family. Writing a book. I can't believe how far I've come.

Great Expectations

Many of my patients have very high hopes for the Wahls Diet, and many of them see their hopes fulfilled. For others, however, when progress is slow, it can be incredibly frustrating. They see what happened to me and they want those same results, but my road was an incredibly long one. Do not give up hope.

There is always hope. We constantly replace our cells and the molecules within cells. The lining of your gut is replaced every week to two weeks. It takes about a year to replace your skin. It takes approximately one to three years to replace the cells in your liver and kidney. Blood vessel cells (endothelial cells) are continually repairing themselves. It takes seven to ten years to replace the myelin insulation around the nerves in your brain, in your spinal cord, and out to your body. It takes fifteen years to replace the muscle cells in your heart. It takes twenty years to replace the minerals in your bones and teeth.[1] It is happening right now, inside you. Every day your cells are replacing molecules, replacing mitochondria, growing more mitochondria, and rebuilding themselves. It may happen quickly or slowly, but it is happening.

However, we all have a unique combination of genetic vulnerability because of the mix of efficient and inefficient enzymes that we have, courtesy of our DNA from our parents. If you have more inefficient enzymes, it will take fewer insults to make disease happen to you, and it will take more work to reverse the process. Depending on who you are and how you are made, there will be variations in the rate of healing.

This may be a good time to repeat the Medical Symptoms Questionnaire you filled out in your Wahls Diary when you began the protocol. You may have progressed more than you realize. When you begin to feel better, it's easy to forget how bad you used to feel. You are unique, so I can't give you an exact timeline of what your progression should look like, but I can give you some averages based upon what I have seen in my clinics, in my followers, and in the practices of other functional medicine health care practitioner colleagues:

WAHLS WARRIORS SPEAK

I was diagnosed with RRMS in 1985 and SPMS in 2004, and I started the Wahls Diet in June 2012 after hearing about it from my mother. I feel as if the disease has halted as opposed to progressed. I used to walk with two sticks, but now I just use one. In addition to improved balance, I've noticed much more strength and energy and an increase in my walking speed. I practice water exercise and stretching daily, and I use e-stim and Reiki as well. With the diet, I love eating organic fruits and vegetables, and I have fun looking up new recipes that fit in the Wahls Protocol. These are early days in my recovery, but I know there will be great things in the future.

—Debra F., Napa, California

- **More energy.** Fatigue is usually the first thing to improve. Many will see energy begin to improve within a few weeks, but nearly always within the first three months. This is often accompanied by improved mood and motivation.
- **Better mobility.** Mobility usually takes longer and is less predictable. Many will see mobility improvement, however slight, within six months, but it could take a year or more to begin seeing improvements in your ability to walk. For others, the most that may happen is halting the steady decline—its own victory. The reasons for poor walking ability are varied. It could be a problem with the balance-sensing part of the brain, problems with the muscles of the legs or torso, poor coordination, generalized and diffuse weakness, or problems with pain. In addition, much depends on how severe the damage is, how severely disabled you are now, how much of the Wahls Protocol you adopt, and what your burden is of broken biochemistry, toxins, hormone imbalance, and genetic vulnerability. I had one patient take up jogging and another began lifting weights at the gym after just six months on the Wahls Protocol. Others have had their energy, memory, and mood improve, but walking hasn't changed much, even after a year. One patient told me that even though she is still not walking, and in fact has lost some functions in the last year, the losses are occurring at

a much slower rate and she is much better than she was in many other ways, including energy, thinking, and mood. For her, this is a huge success.

- **Improvements in diabetes.** People with diabetes—often those who are overweight—who start with Wahls Paleo come back reporting that they are losing weight without being hungry and have more energy than they have enjoyed in years. In many cases, we see blood sugar going down into the normal ranges within two weeks, leading to steady reductions in the medications needed to control blood sugar. Because your blood sugar rapidly improves as you adopt the Wahls Protocol—sometimes within days, certainly within two or three weeks of fully adopting the protocol— it is critical to work with your diabetes doctors and monitor your sugars closely to adjust your medications as you improve. The more completely the patients adopt the diet and the protocol, the more rapidly the sugars normalize.

- **Improvement in blood pressure.** High blood pressure develops because the proteins designed to provide elastic support to blood vessels become oxidized and stiff from the high levels of inflammation, blood sugar, and insulin in the bloodstream. As you adopt the diet and protocol, those incorrectly made, oxidized, and stiff protein molecules are replaced with correctly made, flexible molecules. We see blood pressure steadily improve over the next three years, with the medications needed steadily declining, often down to none.

- **Improvements in heart disease symptoms.** Patients with heart disease— who are usually overweight, and many of whom are diabetic—report weight loss, more energy, and better lipid levels. Again, the root cause of clogged arteries is the high level of inflammation in the bloodstream, the cholesterol that has been oxidized by the high sugar in the diet, and the high levels of inflammation and stress from poorly working mitochondria. The Wahls Protocol improves all of those things. People who have heart failure are often on medications that interfere with the body's ability to manufacture ubiquinone (coenzyme Q), a crucial element for the heart muscle. Helping the person improve his coenzyme Q, B vitamin, and mineral status is key. The improved blood pressure, better blood sugar, lower insulin levels, lower inflammation, and more effective mitochondria do wonderful things for people suffering with heart disease. People typically feel noticeably more energetic within three to six months, sometimes within weeks.

- **Fewer abdominal complaints.** Those with autoimmune problems like rheumatoid arthritis or inflammatory bowel disease report fewer abdominal complaints and more energy, again typically within three months. It is common for those with chronic abdominal complaints, ranging from irritable bowel to severe inflammatory bowel disease, to find that once they go gluten- and dairy-free, their abdominal discomfort dramatically improves. Some can tell things are improving within two weeks when experiencing dramatic improvement, but some improve slowly over three to six months. The vast majority report that the diarrhea and belly pain are markedly lessened and usually completely gone within two weeks

- **Weight loss.** I have consistently observed that people who are overweight steadily lose weight with minimal hunger when they adopt any of the Wahls diets. The weight loss begins with the first week of full implementation of any of the three diet plans and is usually sustained until the person is back to a normal body mass index (healthy weight), often the weight they had in their early twenties.

- **Improvement in headache severity and frequency.** Chronic, often daily headaches are a common, disabling problem in our society. Again, many of my patients and followers with chronic headaches discover that unrecognized gluten and/or casein sensitivity is the root of their daily headaches. In my clinic, I suggest a two-week or month-long experiment on a gluten- and dairy-free diet to see if the headache frequency reduces. At the end of the trial period I have them try a test meal with gluten. The following week I have them do a test meal with dairy. In nearly every case, headache frequency and severity steadily diminish and often disappear on Wahls Paleo, and the gluten meal triggers a recurrence. The dairy meal will trigger a recurrence in about 80 percent. This convinces patients to eliminate gluten and usually dairy permanently. It's also an opportunity to test other foods they have given up, to see if they also cause reactions. I also have patients keep a food symptom diary in which they write down the ingredients of what they are eating each day and whether they develop a headache in the next seventy-two hours, then look for patterns. Many find multiple sources of sensitivity or allergy.

- **Less irritability.** Irritability is another common problem with anyone who has had any kind of psychological or neurological problem, including concussions, post-traumatic stress disorder, depression, and autoimmune disorders involving the brain. We each have 10 billion brain cells with 10 trillion connections between those cells. If we have had a concussion, severe psychological stress, or chronic inflammation in the brain due to MS or some other autoimmune problem, some of the connections between brain cells are strained and/or broken. As a result, brain cells have less cross-talk between them. People can have brain cells ready to engage in mortal combat over nothing at all, just to protect the person, and without that cross-talk, those brain cells aren't "supervised" and don't have much feedback about whether a situation is a big deal or whether they are prompting an overreaction. (Frankly, the reason we aren't all in jail for fighting everyone we meet is that our brains have cross-talk going on that restrain us.) When people who are suffering from irritability start the Wahls Protocol, typically within ninety days of adopting the lifestyle changes, they tell me that things are beginning to improve: The kids are not as annoying, it is often easier to get along at work, and they are not fighting as much with their spouses. These are huge improvements in quality of life.

Troubleshooting the Wahls Protocol

If you haven't improved as much as you would like, it's time to assess what you are doing. One potential reason for an upward tick or a lack of progress is new exposure to potential food allergens, molds, stress, toxins, or infection. If your Medical Symptoms Questionnaire (MSQ) score is greater than 40, toxin overload is likely a factor contributing to your health challenges. Go back to the detox chapter and think about what you might have been exposed to. People with high MSQ scores often have problems with toxins or toxin elimination; this is unfortunately quite common in people with any type of brain disorder, obesity, and/or diabetes. Another potential cause is excessive stress hormones due to unresolved conflicts and other stressors. Remember, those high cortisol levels derail the healing environment.

The most common problem I see in my patients when they aren't improving, or are improving too slowly, however, is certainly compliance. What sometimes happens is that patients are excited and perfectly compliant at first. Over time, however, following the diet strictly may become difficult, especially if you are doing well and think that this gives you license to take it easier. You will be tempted to cheat as you feel better. You might also be tempted to cheat if you aren't feeling better and it seems like too much work for no payoff. In either case, the old familiar comfort foods that you eliminated when you started the diet may creep back in because you don't realize that the very reason you are doing so well is because you have been following the rules so carefully—or that the very reason you aren't doing well is because you have never really strictly followed the rules!

Sometimes people slide back into bad habits so gradually that they don't realize it. A little exception here, a little splurge there, and suddenly you're having a relapse. In the clinic, if the MSQ is slowly improving or under 20, we consider that a satisfactory score. But I should also tell you that the longer

WAHLS DIARY ALERT

Keeping motivated is tough when temptation is all around you. To help you keep track of what you are actually doing, especially if you are not progressing as quickly as you would like, it is critical to record what you do every day, including what you are eating and whether you are meeting the goals for the Wahls Diet, Wahls Paleo, or Wahls Paleo Plus.

Writing down your dietary plan as well as your symptoms in your Wahls Diary will also help you keep it all organized as you keep track of the guidelines for the level of the diet you are currently on and how well you are meeting those requirements. It can also be a great source of inspiration. See how far you've come when you're having a bad day by looking back at your initial Medical Symptoms Questionnaire or reading what you wrote about what you were eating, how you felt, and how much you were moving and doing on a day in the past. Your Wahls Diary is your support system here, so make the most out of it. If you aren't writing it all down, you are missing a tremendous opportunity.

the person is on my program, the more likely he or she is to get the score all the way down to near zero! If the MSQ begins to rise or gets stuck and stops falling, we explore with the patient or study subject how well they are complying with the study diet. Nearly always, our people with rising scores admit that they have been slacking off and allowing prohibited foods back into their diet. One woman thought that by eating twelve servings of vegetables each day, she could have pizza and ice cream with her friends on the weekly girls' night out. It would be wonderful if this trade-off worked, of course, but in her case these little indulgences were sabotaging her progress. When she stopped the pizza and ice cream and went back to 100 percent compliance— gluten-free and dairy-free in this case—her energy improved.

If you find it hard not to "cheat" on your food plan, to slack off on your exercise, or to think you don't really need stress management, just remember, it's not about getting away with something. The Wahls Protocol exists to help you, not to restrict you. It is your ticket to a better life. Keeping that in mind, think about the last two weeks, and check any boxes that apply:

☐ Have any gluten grains crept back into your diet? Have you had gluten even once in the last two weeks? This can cause a major reaction in gluten-sensitive people.

☐ Have you been eating sugar? Even natural sugars like raw sugar, honey, and real maple syrup will feed the bad bacteria and yeasts in your gut.

☐ Are you eating dairy? A little cheese here and there?

☐ Have you been eating eggs, since they are on "regular Paleo," and you thought they would be okay even though you might be sensitive to them?

☐ Are you really eating your 9 full cups of vegetables and fruits? If you are on Wahls Paleo Plus, are you getting at least 6 full cups of vegetables and fruits?

☐ Are your vegetables and fruits evenly distributed between leafy greens, sulfur-rich vegetables, and deeply colored vegetables and fruits, or are you eating a lot more colorful fruit than anything else?

☐ Are you getting enough animal protein? Remember, you need at least 6 ounces per day, and preferably closer to 12 ounces. On Wahls Paleo, you need 9 to 21 ounces.

☐ Are you eating mostly organic produce and organic, wild-caught fish and/

or grass-fed meat? (Chemicals and other impurities in your food could be interfering with your recovery, even though you are getting sufficient nutrients.)

☐ Are you following all the rules for the dietary level you've chosen?

☐ Are you limiting cooking oils to only coconut oil and animal fat as prescribed?

☐ Are you eating enough fat? If you are on Wahls Paleo Plus, are you eating enough coconut oil and/or coconut milk every day?

☐ Did you go off your medication prematurely? (You may be able to do this eventually, but you must not stop before you and your doctor determine you are ready.)

☐ Did you have an emotional setback and lapse into other bad habits because you were upset?

☐ Do you have unresolved stress with family, friends, or coworkers?

Nobody is perfect. We make mistakes and bad decisions. Sometimes we go off our diets or stop taking our medicines because we are hopeful that we are better and don't need to try so hard anymore. This kind of regular evaluation is incredibly useful and informative as you track your own progress and continue to take charge of your own health because you will have a record of when things aren't working. I encourage you to complete the MSQ once a month for a year and use the scores to monitor your progress. Whenever you see an upward tick in the score, you will know it's time to reexamine how well you are implementing the whole protocol.

If you began to see progress but then your progress stalled, it may be time to move up to the next dietary level. If you are on the Wahls Diet, consider advancing to Wahls Paleo. If that's not quite giving you the rapid results you want, it may be time to move up to Wahls Paleo Plus.

What a Functional Medicine Doctor Can Do for You

If you are following the Wahls Protocol carefully and you still aren't seeing the results you want to see, it may be time to consult a functional medicine doctor who can evaluate you in a highly individual way that a book could never do. A functional medicine doctor will approach your health from the broadest possible standpoint. As part of the initial evaluation, a functional medicine health care provider will likely have you complete several detailed questionnaires about your life's story, from the time you were in your mother's uterus. You will answer questions about the various infections, vaccinations, toxin exposures, and health issues that led to this point in your life.

After reviewing those forms, your doctor will ask more questions and then do a physical examination. The next step is to look at the various health problems that you have experienced and how those problems fit into the big picture of how your body works. There are seven big-picture physiologies a functional medicine doctor will consider:

1. Energy production (how well your mitochondria work)
2. Assimilation (how well you digest and absorb nutrients)
3. Defense and repair (how well and appropriately your immune cells are working and the health of your "old friends" living in your bowels, your nose, and your skin)
4. Biotransformation and elimination (how well you process and eliminate the harmful compounds that your cells encounter, including both the trash the cells make as they do the work of living and the toxic stuff we absorb through our skin, our lungs, and our gut)
5. Communication (how effectively your cells can communicate with one another through hormones, neurotransmitters, and other signaling molecules)
6. Structural integrity (the structural integrity of the tiny things like cell membranes as well as big things like muscles, ligaments, and bones)
7. Transport of fluids through the body (blood and lymph)

Your functional medicine doctor will also want to understand your personal health behaviors, which are the bedrock of health (or disease). These are the very things that you have been tuning up and optimizing as you implement the Wahls Protocol: (1) Sleep and relaxation, (2) Exercise and movement, (3) Nutrition, (4) Stress and resilience, and (5) Relationships. When all of that is complete, the functional medicine health care provider will tell the story back to you of how your problems fit into the matrix, what the antecedent risk factors are (your genetic vulnerabilities), what your triggers are, and what is likely keeping your disease active. This will help your doctor explain where your various health problems fit in the seven physiologies and how your health behaviors are likely contributing positively or negatively to your current health.

Once the matrix has been completed, then you and your functional medicine doctor will develop a plan to move forward together. If you are following the Wahls Protocol, you will already be doing many of the things functional medicine recommends, but this careful individual assessment can tell you much more about how you as a unique being can benefit from additional targeted guidance.

As you progress, your functional medicine doctor will also be there for you, helping you to adjust your plan based on your individual reactions to the lifestyle, vitamin and supplement usage, and other changes and prescriptions. For those tough cases that don't respond sufficiently to the Wahls Diet, this is your best plan for making faster progress.

Functional Medicine Tests to Consider

One of the benefits of visiting a functional medicine provider is that you will have access to certain kinds of tests that conventional medicine doesn't normally use. The types of testing that a functional medicine health care professional[2] can request and evaluate include the following:

Genetic Tests

Genetic testing is usually an ethical quagmire when it is used to predict if you might have a specific disease such as Huntington's disease or cystic fibrosis or the gene increasing the risk of developing breast cancer. That is not the type of testing I am discussing. Instead, the type of testing I am discussing here is to look at how efficient some of your enzymes for running your cell chemistry are, particularly the ones involved in how you eliminate toxins and manufacture brain neurotransmitters. Once you understand which enzymes are not optimal, you can use dietary choices, vitamins, and/or supplements to bypass the less effective enzymes and lower the risk for a variety of health problems such as brain disorders, heart disorders, toxic overload, and even cancer.

I have used labs associated with Genova Diagnostics to do genetic assessments to understand my own genetic risks. Genetic testing doesn't tell you everything, however. For example, it can tell you which enzymes are mutated, but it won't necessarily tell you about function. You can, however, assume that mutated genes are probably less effective (often but not always the case), and this may be helpful in understanding which vitamins and supplements can make up for this.

Toxin Load Assessment

For someone with an autoimmune problem who continues to struggle, understanding the body burden of toxins may be very useful. Often this is done with a twenty-four-hour urine collection and a provocation agent to draw toxins out of fat storage. Depending on the clinical circumstance, the test may be for heavy metals, solvents, or pesticides. Often the person also has a genetic vulnerability in their detoxification enzymes that exacerbates the toxic effect. If the person is toxic, the next decision is whether to do a long, slow detoxification that is based on food or to effect a more rapid removal using chelation under the direct supervision of a physician trained and certified for managing chelation therapies.

Nutritional Testing

It is possible to have a comprehensive assessment of your nutritional status in terms of your levels of vitamins, minerals, essential fats, and antioxidants, and to look at how efficiently your mitochondria can generate energy, how well your brain cells can make neurotransmitter molecules, how well you produce myelin, and more nutritional details. These types of tests are helpful in showing how well your own personal chemical factories are functioning and where the blocks (inefficient enzymes) are located. A functional medicine physician can then guide you to the foods, vitamins, and nutraceuticals (herbs) that can help unblock the ineffective biochemistry. This may be a good alternative to using genetic testing to identify which enzymes are not working as effectively. See the Resources for a list of labs that offer nutritional testing.

Gut Health

You may need to have a comprehensive assessment of your gut function. The beginning assessment might be DNA analysis of your stool, which would outline bacteria, yeasts, and parasites living in your bowels. Many of the labs also do analyses for sensitivity to the common nutraceuticals and pharmaceutical agents in order to treat the troublemakers that may be contributing to your problems.

Other labs do cultures and microscopic examination to look for the yeasts, bacteria, and parasites. The key point is to find a lab that has extensive experience, as most conventional physicians do not routinely have access to labs that are experienced with the evaluation of dysbiosis (microbial imbalance). The comprehensive gut health assessment will also look at digestion enzymes and acid production in the stomach.

Food Allergies and Sensitivities

If you need a lab test to convince yourself or your family member to give up gluten, dairy, or other potential foods that are creating trouble, then food allergy/sensitivity testing is money well spent. Since I can't get these tests in the VA, I need to convince people to go gluten-/dairy-/egg-/soy-free for a month and assess how they do; but if you have access to food allergy tests and you want to go that route, ask your functional medicine doctor about the best ones for you. These tests are controversial. Many conventional physicians do not agree that they are accurate or that they relate to any clinical signs of allergy. A good reason to do the tests, however, is because many people have delayed reactions to foods. Although most reactions to food occur within seventy-two hours, occasionally the delayed reaction can be as long as seven to fourteen days. If you are still having trouble after adopting the Wahls Paleo or Wahls Paleo Plus diet, it can be helpful for you to get a food allergy assessment of some type and eliminate the foods to which you are sensitive. They may be foods you never suspected.

Getting evaluations for food allergies can be done in a variety of ways, and each has its drawbacks:

- **Elimination diet.** The gold standard for understanding whether you have a food sensitivity or allergy is completing an elimination diet, in which you essentially go on a supervised fast and then, starting with the food least likely to be troublesome, reintroduce foods one at a time every other day (or sometimes every third day). During this time, you keep a detailed food symptom diary and monitor your pulse rate before and after eating each new food. Any food that evokes a jump in heart rate or a problem symptom such as pain or fatigue is put on the suspect list and removed from the diet for six months and then retested. This is difficult to do on your own and is most effective under the supervision of a nutritionist or functional medicine doctor because you will be less likely to cheat, which would completely skew the results.
- **Modified elimination diet.** Another approach is to go on a diet that eliminates the most common allergenic or sensitizing foods: gluten, dairy, eggs, soy, corn, potatoes, tomatoes, eggplant, peppers, citrus, peanuts, shellfish,

ANOTHER TEST TO TRY

Another strategy to understanding sensitivity/allergy to foods and other inhaled proteins is the Pulse Test.[3] The Pulse Test was created by the allergist Dr. Arthur F. Coca. This is a physiologic test that monitors whether the pulse and/or heart rate increase after exposure to a food item or something in the environment. This involves monitoring the pulse every two hours for three days to see what the low and high pulse rates are and recording everything that you eat or that comes into contact with your skin. Using the Pulse Test can be a bit tedious, but if you are willing to do the work of recording and look for the patterns, it can be a very helpful tool.

and fish. You eat strictly organic foods to avoid genetically modified foods and toxins. After six months you test the ingredients one by one to look for reactions. The reactions can be headache, fatigue, abdominal complaints, rash, allergy symptoms, asthma, or acne. As you heal your gut and stop having a leaky gut, some sensitivities may diminish to the point where you could have the offending food once a week without problem (but if you return to daily consumption, you are likely to develop problems with that food again).

- **Blood test.** One blood test option is the ALCAT (Antigen Leukocyte Cellular Antibody Test) and is marketed by Cell Science Systems. It is capable of assessing delayed responses to 350 different foodstuffs for food sensitivities (as opposed to allergies, which is an immediate reaction mediated by the immunoglobulin IgE). Another option is to measure blood levels of immunoglobulin IgG and/or IgA in response to various foods. Because 2 percent of the population does not make a normal amount of IgA, if you have a negative test, you should also check your IgA levels to be certain that you can make a normal amount of IgA before trusting that negative test. See the Resources section.
- **Stool test.** You could get what I unceremoniously call the "poop test" for the most common food groups. This is more sensitive than the blood test because abnormal antibodies to foods are secreted in the stool sooner—

WAHLS WARNING

Many people ask me about gluten sensitivity testing and are surprised to learn that I do not recommend getting a blood test for gluten sensitivity through your primary care doctor's office. A negative test does not rule out gluten sensitivity, and even though your doctor will likely tell you that you can eat gluten, you actually should not. The test is not worth the money spent and could even slow down your healing. I have had many people with a negative blood test for gluten sensitivity experience remarkable improvements to their health after going gluten-free.

---

sometimes years sooner—than they are detectable in the bloodstream. However, this test detects fewer food items. You can get your own stool test from EnteroLab without a doctor's order, but insurance won't cover it. Another advantage of stool testing is that EnteroLab will do genetic testing to see if you have the genes that put you at risk for developing gluten sensitivity, and they can also test for sensitivity to dairy, *Saccharomyces cerevisiae* (baker's yeast), eggs, soy, and nightshade vegetables (potatoes, tomatoes, eggplant, and peppers). The stool test is also less likely to give a false negative.

Infections

We are used to thinking of an infection as an acute illness caused by a virus, bacteria, fungus, or parasite. Our immune cells begin attacking the infecting agent and a war ensues. If we win, our immune cells clear out the infection and we return to good health. If we lose the war completely, we die.

There is also, however, a middle ground. When our immune cells are unable to clear the infection completely, it may continue to smolder. For example, people who have irritated gums (when they brush their teeth vigorously, their gums bleed) have a low-level infection of their gum tissue that can increase inflammation and the probability of developing an autoimmune disease, heart disease, stroke, diabetes, and other chronic diseases.[4] As vitality declines, we are more likely to be infected with something else. If we don't have the proper nutrition for our immune cells or we have too many toxins impairing the immune cells, we have troublemakers living in our bowels, our hormone signals are confused, and our white blood cells are less capable. As a result of any of those factors, our immune cells are less effective at clearing the infection. Furthermore, once a person's immune system is weakened by having one of these chronic infections (or overgrowths in the bowels), they are more susceptible to having a coinfection with a second organism or more.[5]

If you are still struggling with fatigue and brain symptoms, it may be very helpful to have a comprehensive assessment to test for these types of chronic infections or coinfections, especially if the Wahls Protocol is not resolving issues like chronic fatigue—which could be due to a viral infection (such as Epstein-Barr, herpes 6 virus, and herpes simplex) or a bacterial infection (such as *Borrelia burgdorferi*—Lyme disease—chlamydia, and *Bartonella*).[6] A functional medicine doctor can evaluate you for the possibility of these indolent chronic infections. If you do have an infection or coinfection with several organisms, a functional medicine doctor may treat you with nutraceuticals, pharmaceuticals, or a combination of both, depending on the type of infection and your individual health situation. Some protocols require years of treatments to clear infections, particularly if there are multiple infecting agents, so finding someone who has considerable experience evaluating and treating chronic infections will be essential.

Hormonal Balance

Hormones are the molecules that our cells use to communicate and regulate how the other cells in the body will function. They instruct other cells to work harder and faster or when it's time to relax and slow down. When the hormones are finely tuned, your body works like a beautiful symphony; but when the hormones get out of balance, health declines.

Classic signs of hormonal imbalance include fatigue, foggy thinking, and irritability. Immune cells become less effective when hormones are imbalanced, and you may become more vulnerable to both infection and cancer. People with hormonal imbalance may also be much more likely to develop an autoimmune problem.

Everything you do impacts your hormones, and your hormones impact everything you do. Scientists continue to discover that our bodies have multiple layers of hormone communication that provides many layers of feedback to help keep the potassium, sodium, calcium, magnesium, and other minerals in the correct concentration in our bloodstreams and in our cells. Maintaining an optimal hormone balance means providing your hormone-secreting glands (pituitary, adrenal, thyroid, ovaries, and testes in particular) with support so that each gland has a healthy reserve.

The Wahls Protocol should accomplish this for most people, but if you are still having trouble, you may need a more comprehensive assessment of the interplay between your adrenals, thyroid, pituitary, and sex hormones to understand and correct persisting hormone imbalances. Consult a functional medicine doctor who has experience in hormonal balance for more advanced hormonal testing and a more natural but specifically targeted program of nutrients, supplements, and medications, if necessary, to address your issue. A functional medicine doctor will view your hormonal imbalance based on the big picture of your physiologies and personal health behaviors, so your treatment will be more comprehensive and individualized.

These are the primary tests that could be done in a functional medicine clinic. They are generally not covered by health care insurance, often because they are not yet FDA approved. The tests can cost many hundreds to many, many thousands of dollars if you investigate every potential imbalance, so your functional medicine doctor will likely recommend only the tests that are indicated based on your functional medicine matrix and then help you prioritize which ones to obtain first.

In my clinical practice, I rely on careful history and laboratory evaluations that I can obtain through my conventional pathology departments. We then focus on maximizing all the health-promoting behaviors of the Wahls Protocol. I refer those who want to pursue the comprehensive testing I discuss here to another functional medicine provider in the community to complete the testing. I see terrific results without advanced testing, but at times it may be very helpful when the person is not responding despite full implementation of the Wahls Protocol.

Finding a Functional Medicine Practitioner

Many functional medicine practitioners come from the ranks of conventionally trained medical professionals: medical doctors (M.D.s), osteopathic doctors (D.O.s), advanced registered nurse practitioners (A.R.N.P.s), physician's assistants (P.A.s) and nutritionists and registered dietitians (R.D.s), and more. To find a functional medicine practitioner near you, go to the Institute for Functional Medicine website at www.functionalmedicine.org and click on "Functional Medicine Resources." Then click on "Find a Functional Medicine Practitioner." You will then be able to enter your address and how far you are willing to travel. You will be presented a list of individuals who have completed the training course called "Applying Functional Medicine in Clinical Practice." The Institute for Functional Medicine is creating a certificate program for those individuals who have completed additional training and have successfully passed an examination. The individuals who pass the certification process will be an Institute for Functional Medicine Certified Practitioner, or IFMCP. This is a relatively new qualification and the earliest that practitioners will be able to complete certification is 2014, so this list will probably grow over time.

Once you have some names, visit a few (if you have more than one option). Ask some questions so you can get to know the practitioner and whether you will feel comfortable working with her or him. Some questions to ask:

1. Where and when did you get your training in functional medicine?
2. What percentage of your practice is functional medicine?
3. Do you assess and treat problems related to high body burden of toxins, food allergies, gut microbiome problems (the ecosystem of bacteria, yeasts, and parasites that is living in your bowels), or problems with troublemaking bacteria, yeasts, and parasites.
4. Do you take medical insurance? (Note: Most of the providers do not take medical insurance because it would not cover all of the time involved. The assessments and evaluations are expensive and time-consuming, and some providers, like myself, may choose not to do much testing, pre-

ferring to focus on a careful history, physical examination, and lifestyle intervention.)

If you cannot find someone close to you who is in the Institute for Functional Medicine database, you can still look for health care providers with an integrative medicine background or interest. Talk to the provider about the issues of toxic load, food allergy and sensitivity, the microbiome (who is living in your bowels), digestion and assimilation issues, and hormone issues to see if the practitioner is trained and has a good knowledge base in those areas. Naturopathic doctors (N.D.s) and doctors of chiropractic (D.C.s) are often more focused on using nutrition than M.D.s or D.O.s. In fact, they receive more training in nutrition than most medical doctors and can do these types of comprehensive evaluations and treat with food and nutraceuticals. They are definitely health care providers to consider.

If you still can't find anyone, work with your primary-care physician as you adopt the Wahls Protocol. Many primary-care physicians are more open-minded to the power of diet and lifestyle interventions than the subspecialists and are willing to learn about different approaches to healing, especially for chronic issues like autoimmune disease that aren't responding to conventional treatment. The best doctors rely on a good history, a thorough physical exam, and basic lab tests. You can help lead your primary-care doctor to do just that.

This is the Wahls Protocol, in all its simplicity and complexity. Now it's your turn to make it what you want it to be. You can simply adopt the Wahls Diet. You can go all the way to Wahls Paleo Plus. You can integrate an exercise program, cleansing techniques, supplements, alternative medicine, stress management, and of course the Wahls Diary. You may or may not take on the services of an official functional medicine practitioner, but the bottom line is this: *You* are now in charge of your own health. Your future, your progress—even your happiness—is up to you. Your destiny is in your hands, and that is a wonderful and powerful thing to know. I hope you will make the most of it. Your future can be filled with health, hope, vitality, and connection. I've given you the tools. Now it's up to you to use them.

EPILOGUE

The End of My Story,
The Beginning of Yours

YOU KNOW MY story of decline. You know I got out of my wheelchair. Now I'd like to finish that story.

When my body began to heal, I didn't fully understand what was happening at first. In spite of the changes occurring with amazing speed, I still did not consider that I might recover. I had accepted for years that people with secondary progressive MS did not improve. It did not occur to me that the improvements I was experiencing could continue. It was not until nearly six months after my symptoms began to reverse that I first dared to wonder if recovery might be possible.

I began to dream of biking again. On Mother's Day weekend in 2008, I was feeling so much better and my mobility had improved to such a great degree that I decided to try riding a bike. I went to the garage, picked up a helmet, and walked to my bike. Five years earlier, when I got the wheelchair, I'd given my bike to my son, Zach. Now I wondered if I was ready to take it back. I adjusted the seat downward, clicked on my helmet, and began rolling the bike out.

My kids heard me in the garage and came to investigate. Zach grabbed the bike from me and called out for Jackie to stop me. We all looked at one another. I told Jackie that if she thought I wasn't ready, I wouldn't attempt it. She responded by getting out her bike helmet and bike and told Zach and Zebby to jog alongside me.

We all got into position. Jackie gave the all-clear that there was no traffic. I pushed off. The bike wobbled, but I did not fall. My kids cheered as they ran behind me. Tears streamed down my cheeks as Jackie and I pedaled around the block. When I stopped, Zach, Zebby, Jackie, and I all stood together, holding one another and crying. I had a new future ahead. I had proof: I had ridden my bicycle. My steady decline was not the rule, not anymore. I was rewriting my future and who knew what it might become! I still have tears in my eyes when I tell that story. It is and always will be miraculous to me.

Doctors and scientists don't often believe in miracles. My getting up from that chair wasn't really a miracle from a scientific perspective, even though it felt like one to me at the time. My getting out of the chair and onto a bicycle was just the facts related to my body's ability to regain strength and health. We may not fully understand all the facts, but it's science that my team is working hard to reveal. This is the basis of the clinical trials we've undertaken in order to understand the mechanisms of why the Wahls Protocol is effective and who can best be helped by it.

Our first paper is now published, describing the preliminary data on the first ten subjects with secondary progressive MS who experienced a statistically (and more importantly, clinically) significant reduction in fatigue. We have had all of our subjects complete twelve months of the protocol, and we are now writing up the findings in four more papers, describing the changes in fatigue, walking ability, balance, cognition, mood, nutritional status, blood biomarkers, and MRI findings. We have additional studies underway testing the Wahls Diet vs. the Wahls Paleo Plus vs. usual care. That study will be finished in December. We have another study testing the effect of exercise and electrical stimulation alone, so that we can determine how much of the benefit is due to diet, and how much is due to exercise and electrical stimulation.

New ideas always meet both skepticism and enthusiasm from scientific colleagues. Our work will be no different. We will have champions and detractors. But we will keep doing our work, submitting our papers, applying for grants, and raising money through the Wahls Foundation to continue and expand our work. If you'd like to become a member of the team and donate to the Wahls Research Fund, please see the Appendix for more details on how to support our research team.

Money is incredibly hard to get for research, with less than 2 percent of applications being funded now. Researchers must show preliminary data with grant applications to have any hope of getting their grants funded. I can tell you that the Direct-MS charity, which has seen our preliminary data in our two most recent grant applications, has been excited by our work and has given my lab additional funding to expand our research! We have several more groundbreaking trials planned to test the Wahls Protocol's ability to intervene in other chronic health conditions. We are also testing a new protocol, focused on diet alone, and we have another one that is testing the effect of just exercise and electrical stimulation of muscles to see how much benefit is due to the diet versus the exercise and electrical stimulation versus the diet plus all of the other interventions. Preliminary results are thrilling—stay tuned for that news as it develops!

I also remain committed to public education. I have created a website and newsletters, recorded my lectures, and given lectures around the country. I do webinars, interviews, radio shows, and talk shows. I cannot wait for my colleagues to catch up. Yes, I will continue to do the research to deepen my understanding and publish those findings in peer-reviewed scientific journals, but I will also continue to teach people directly, because nobody should have to wait for information like this. Scientific inquiry is a long and complex process, often taking twenty to thirty years for proven successful treatments to become accepted clinical practice or the standard of care. Why wait for accepted clinical practice to catch up when you want to begin turning your health around *today* using the commonsense things under your control, like the food you eat and what you choose to do every day? Let the public choose whether to take back their own health by learning how to adopt the many wonderful health behaviors embedded within the Wahls Protocol. Let the public decide whether the Wahls Protocol works for them and their loved ones. I don't want you to have to wait for study results to try the commonsense, low-risk interventions that the Wahls Protocol represents.

I acknowledge that not everyone is helped in my clinics or in my trials. Not everybody will be able to adopt all of the Wahls Protocol, and not everyone will be able to get up from the chair. But what if you could? What if you will? The Wahls Protocol has already worked to reverse debilitating health symptoms in hundreds of people. Why shouldn't you be one of them?

Everybody can maximize their own functioning. One person's best may be quite different from another person's best, but you can be *your* best. It may be that you have a condition that is associated with steady progressive decline such as Huntington's disease or Lou Gehrig's disease (ALS). The Wahls Protocol may not be able to make you fully well, but by following it you can have the best function that is possible for you. We're learning new things every day about the body and disease, but what I do know is this: When you align yourself with what nature intends for you, remove impediments to your biochemical functioning, and restore what your mitochondria and cells are missing, you can maximize your biochemical health at the cellular level to optimize your life, whatever your health challenge. The Wahls Protocol gave me my life back. Give it the chance to restore yours.

WAHLS RECIPES

Adopting any of the Wahls Diet plans is a challenge. Reducing and/or eliminating grain and dairy means we have to reimagine our breakfasts without the cereals, pancakes, breads, and eggs typical of the standard American breakfast. I recommend that you start the day with a smoothie that provides some of the 9 cups of vegetables and fruit and high-quality protein. The following section provides guidance on the creation of smoothies for your household. Experiment with flavors.

Basic Smoothie

YOU CAN USE anything that qualifies for your 9 cups in a smoothie, especially greens. To begin with, most of us need the sweetness of fruit to mask the bitterness of greens. Soy, almond, or coconut milk will also mellow the flavor nicely. Boxed milks often have extra calcium added, which is helpful, since by decreasing dairy you are lowering your intake of that essential nutrient. Always check the nutrition label to verify.

The ratio I recommend starting with is:

- 1 part greens
- 2 parts fruit or juice or 2 cups organic soy milk (Wahls Diet only), coconut milk, or other nut milk, preferably unsweetened
- Add water and ice and combine in a high-speed blender until desired consistency.

There are endless smoothie combinations: combine kale, collard greens, romaine lettuce, beet greens, or cilantro with blueberries, strawberries, grapes, peeled orange segments, pineapple, and mango as well as other vegetables like broccoli or cucumber. Beets yield a brilliant magenta smoothie. As you get more used to the taste of green smoothies, you can gradually shift your ratio until you get greens and fruits in an approximately 1:1 ratio or switch to greens only and an approved nondairy milk. You can also add greater proportions of coconut milk. Having fat with your greens reduces bitterness and also lowers the glycemic index of the fruit in your smoothie. I personally always use full-fat coconut milk in a can to make smoothies and soups and to add to my teas.

You can also add a few unexpected nutrient boosts to your smoothies. Spices such as cinnamon, cardamom, ginger, or nutmeg can also cut the bitterness and add more nutritional benefits. I like to add 1 to 2 tablespoons of nutritional yeast, because it is a powerhouse of B vitamins, minerals, and RNA. Great stuff! Use nutritional yeast whenever you can in your smoothies or sprinkled on top of your vegetables. You'll get a lot of wonderful nutrition. The yeast in nutritional yeast is *Saccharomyces cerevisiae* that has been killed. Still, the inactive *Saccharomyces cerevisiae* is believed to suppress the harmful *Candida albicans* that can overgrow with a high-carb diet. Occasionally, some people have headaches with the nutritional yeast. If it bothers you in any way, omit it.

My breakfast protein sources are usually leftover meat from the previous night's dinner, liver pâté, or pickled herring. That way my breakfasts are fast and easy. When I was still eating three meals a day, my lunch was essentially a repeat of breakfast. I took a thermos with some of my morning smoothie in it and leftovers from the night before. Again, quick and simple.

SKILLET MEALS

IN THE EVENING, after both Jackie and I have worked all day, we usually have a skillet meal for dinner. I'm typically the chef in our house, and when I get home I prefer to be able to eat within twenty minutes of starting to cook. If it takes more than twenty minutes to make something, it is much less likely that I'll have that dish often. Skillet meals fit the bill: simple dishes with animal protein, lots of vegetables, and savory spices. These meals are prepared in a skillet on the stove and are generally ready in less time than it takes to cook a frozen pizza. Using my family's big skillet, I add coconut oil and some wine or vinegar, then I sauté onions or mushrooms and add meat. Since I tend to like my meat rarer than the rest of my family, I put my piece in three to four minutes after the others. Two minutes before all the meat is finished cooking, I add other vegetables, and that's it. I can usually have the meal done within fifteen minutes from the time I start, and I serve the meal from the skillet. Because the meals are prepared and served in a single skillet, there are fewer dishes in the cleanup.

Before I give you the basic directions, here are a few general things to keep in mind:

- Grass-raised and grass-finished means an animal was fed grass until slaughter. This should be your first choice. Grass-raised, grain-finished means the animal was fed grain during the last six weeks of its life, which skews the omega-6-to-omega-3 fatty acid ratio unfavorably but is still preferable to conventionally raised meat.
- Farm-raised fish means grain-fed fish, which leads to a much higher omega-6 fatty acid level than found in wild fish. Look for wild-caught fish.
- Garlic and other members of the onion and cabbage families all contain sulfur. This sulfur stabilizes in the crushing and cutting of the vegetable. Therefore, if you are cooking with these vegetables, crush, mince, and/or chop them and then allow them to sit for five to fifteen minutes prior to cooking. You'll lose less of the sulfur-rich antioxidants as you cook the food.
- Seaweed: Remember that ¼ teaspoon powdered kelp equals 1 teaspoon dulse flakes. You can use them interchangeably in the recipes, and I encourage using a variety of seaweeds for maximal health benefits. Alternating between kelp and dulse is superior to using the same seaweed each day. *Remember that it is important to introduce seaweed and algae into your diet gradually.* If you eat too much of these too suddenly, it can cause problems with your thyroid. Follow your tastes and gradually increase the amount. When you are accustomed to it, have up to 1 serving per day. The amounts listed are optional and you can always leave seaweed out of any recipe if you choose, but do try to have it at least a few times per week, as recommended at the Wahls Paleo level. I recommend adding seaweed because collards—and all cabbage family vegetables—compete slightly with the

iodine uptake in your immune cells and all of your endocrine glands, including the thyroid.

- Vinegars: I like balsamic vinegar. It does have more sugar, but it also has more antioxidants and flavonoids than other vinegars. Other vinegars I particularly like are unpasteurized, unfiltered apple cider vinegar with the "mother" or "SCOBY." (SCOBY stands for symbiotic colony of bacteria and yeast—these are terms referring to the bacterial colony that transforms fermented alcohol into acetic acid to make vinegar.) Also try wine vinegar, rice vinegar, and coconut vinegar. Feel free to experiment with other vinegars. You can also substitute citrus juice for vinegar in any recipe.
- Sea salt has trace minerals but does not contain iodine. Be sure you are cooking with plenty of seaweed if you use sea salt. I use iodized sea salt for the iodine boost.
- Black pepper and other spices support cellular health; use spices and experiment with new ones.
- Cook at lower temperature for more nutrition. Mix water, vinegar, or wine with cooking fat to keep the temperature lower as you cook on the stove.

Do feel comfortable modifying these recipes by adjusting seasonings to taste and using the meats and vegetables that are available in your community and beloved in your culture. It is far better to use your local greens than kale or mustard greens that have been shipped in. Rotate through the varieties available to you and try new combinations. The magic is in eating fresh, in season, and local. As my mother said, recipes are only suggestions. These are my suggestions for easy meals.

Basic Meat and Greens Skillet Recipe

SERVES 4

THE BASIC PRINCIPLE of this versatile recipe is to cook meat in a skillet with coconut oil, vinegar, and spices, then to add greens in the last 2 minutes of cooking. I chop chard, mustard greens, spinach, and most other varieties of greens but usually add kale whole because kale leaves are delightful to slice with your steak knife as you go. Experiment with the types of animal protein, cuts of meat, and seasonings you use, and remember to rotate through different greens to maximize the health benefits. If you feel the greens are bitter, add up to 2 tablespoons of vinegar, lime juice, or lemon juice. The bitterness is the alkalinity of the food, so a bit of acidic liquid will often mellow that out.

Any variety of meat and greens will work well together using this recipe. Zebby is particularly fond of salmon and cooked greens, while Zach really likes steak and has come to enjoy his nearly as rare as I eat mine. Jackie and I consider heart to be like a very fine filet mignon. It's a terrific source of ubiquinone, or coenzyme Q. (Eating brain is another more potent source, but few are doing this now.) We get bison hearts from our local butcher and they are marvelous. Ideally, we have heart once a week. My great-grandmother knew that heart, liver, and kidneys were a vital part of family nutrition. I like to make enough meat to have leftovers for a quick and easy breakfast.

Here are the basic proportions:

1 tablespoon coconut oil

Your favorite seasonings to taste (experiment!): garlic (add with greens), ginger, fresh or dried herbs (basil, rosemary, thyme, etc.), dried spices (cumin, curry powder, chili powder, turmeric, paprika, even cinnamon)

1–2 tablespoons vinegar and/or citrus juice: apple cider vinegar, balsamic vinegar, lemon juice, lime juice, red wine vinegar

1 teaspoon organic kelp powder, like Starwest Botanicals organic kelp powder (optional)

1 teaspoon iodized sea salt

1–2 pounds meat or fish: nitrate-free bacon (cooked before the main protein source, with excess fat drained from pan), ham, steak, chicken, turkey, pork, salmon, lamb, heart, liver

6–7½ cups greens and other vegetables: broccoli, collard greens, kale, mustard greens, spinach, turnip greens, plus cabbage, carrots, eggplant, mushrooms, onions

❖ Add coconut oil to a large skillet with cover over medium heat. Add seasonings, vinegar, kelp powder, and salt. Add meat or fish, and simmer until it is cooked to your liking. Keep in mind that the more done the meat is, the more tough it is likely to be. I like my meat rare, so I cook it for about 5 minutes. Add greens, and steam for another 1 to 2 minutes. Before serving, I slice the meat into thin slices. If it is too raw for some at the table, put the slices back in the skillet for another minute to make them well-done.

Algerian Chicken/
Algerian Vegetarian

SERVES 4

MY DAUGHTER AND I enjoy an Algerian restaurant in Elkader, Iowa, and decided we needed to add Algerian flair to our repertoire. It does take a bit longer than basic skillet meals, but it is delicious! This is a flexible recipe that you can make vegetarian if you wish. It can be enjoyed at the Wahls Diet (served over quinoa with red pepper), Wahls Paleo (served over cauliflower rice, spaghetti squash, winter squash, yams, or sautéed cabbage), or Wahls Paleo Plus levels (replace the green beans with asparagus).

4 cloves garlic, minced

1½ pounds chicken, with skin on (You can use breasts, legs, or thighs. Omit for vegetarian version.)

1 14.5-ounce can chopped tomatoes

2 cups sliced leeks

1 cup Bone Broth (page 345; use vegetable broth or water if vegetarian)

1 medium-size banana pepper, sliced

1 medium-size carrot, sliced

1 tablespoon coconut oil

2 teaspoons ground turmeric

1 teaspoon ground cinnamon

1 teaspoon ground cumin

1 teaspoon organic kelp powder, such as Starwest Botanicals organic kelp (optional)

½ *teaspoon iodized sea salt*

4 cups green beans (Wahls Diet/Wahls Paleo) or 4 cups asparagus
    (Wahls Paleo Plus)

2 cups chopped cilantro, with stems separated from leaves

❖ Mince garlic and let sit for 15 minutes prior to use to allow sulfur to stabilize. Add garlic, chicken, tomatoes, leeks, Bone Broth, pepper, carrot, coconut
oil, spices, kelp powder, and salt to large skillet over medium heat. Simmer for
15 minutes. Add green beans or asparagus and chopped cilantro stems to the
skillet and simmer for another 5 minutes. Stir in chopped cilantro leaves just
prior to serving.

Rosemary Chicken

SERVES 8

ROSEMARY AND CHICKEN go together beautifully. Rosemary is an easy herb to
grow in your garden or container garden.

6 cloves garlic, minced

2 teaspoons chopped fresh rosemary

2 pounds cut-up chicken thighs, skin on (or any cut of chicken)

1 medium eggplant, sliced

1 pound mushrooms, sliced

2 large carrots, sliced

2 tablespoons distilled vinegar

1 tablespoon coconut oil

½ *teaspoon organic kelp powder, such as Starwest Botanicals*
    organic kelp (optional)

½ *teaspoon iodized sea salt*

❖ Mince garlic and let stand for 15 minutes. Put rosemary under the skin of
the chicken. Place garlic, chicken, eggplant, mushrooms, carrots, vinegar, coconut oil, kelp powder, and salt in a skillet. Simmer for 20 minutes. Serve.

Liver, Onions, and Mushrooms

SERVES 4

THIS RECIPE IS ADAPTED from my great-grandmother's cookbook *The 1890 Compendium of Cookery and Book of Knowledge*, which has a chapter devoted to the use of organ meats, liver, heart, brain, sweetbread (thymus), and kidney. Chicken liver is milder than the other livers, so it is a good place to start. You can also make this in the oven, baking at 250 degrees for 1 to 2 hours, which is my favorite way to prepare liver. In that recipe, one lays the bacon pieces between the liver slices, which rest on top of the onions and mushrooms. We intentionally make enough to use the leftovers to make liver pâté, which I have for breakfast.

> *½ pound bacon (nitrate-free)*
> *½ pound mushrooms, sliced*
> *1 teaspoon organic kelp powder, such as Starwest Botanical*
> *   organic kelp (optional)*
> *1 pound onions, chopped*
> *1⅔ pounds chicken livers*
> *1 tablespoon balsamic vinegar*
> *½ teaspoon iodized sea salt*

❖ In large skillet, fry bacon. Pour off all the fat. Add mushrooms, kelp, and onions, and cook for 3 to 5 minutes over medium-low heat. Add livers, vinegar, and salt. Cook over medium heat for 2 to 3 minutes. Make sure to leave the livers medium-rare because overcooking will make them tough.

Liver Pâté

2 SERVINGS

WHILE LIVER PÂTÉ is not a skillet meal in the traditional sense, I put it here, because each time I make liver and onions I intentionally make enough to make a batch of pâté. I use this liver pâté as my morning protein after having liver and onions. We particularly enjoy it with turnip, rutabaga, radish, or kohlrabi slices. Celery is also good.

> **Liver, onions, and mushrooms**
> ¼ *cup olive oil, coconut oil, or ghee*
> ¼ *cup balsamic vinegar (or Bragg apple cider vinegar)*

❖ Take your leftover liver, onions, and mushrooms—about half of the preceding recipe—and add it to a food processor with oil and vinegar. Process on high until smooth. If it seems too thick, add more water or vinegar to make a runny pudding consistency. Store in the refrigerator.

Wahls Pizza

SERVES 1

GIVING UP PIZZA was difficult for my family. While it is possible to find gluten-free pizzas, it is more challenging to find pizzas that are both gluten-free and dairy-free. Zebby and Jackie often have pizza while I stick to Wahls Paleo Plus. Here is an example of how you can use gluten-free tortillas as a crust to build your own pizza. Add a bunch of vegetables, your meat of choice, and a dairy-free cheese such as Daiya (www.daiyafoods.com), and you are set. Serve with a large salad and you have comfort food to make the transition a little easier for you and your family. Be sure to read the ingredient labels of the gluten-free products to know that they are gluten-, dairy-, and (ideally) egg-free, too.

Note: The amounts in this recipe are for two 6-inch corn tortillas, but if you decide to make your own version on a larger gluten-free pizza crust or gluten-free tortilla to share, add more ingredients according to your taste. It is important to use the optimum amounts of Daiya on pizza for the best performance. These are the amounts I have found work best: 10-inch gluten-free tortilla = 4 ounces; 12-inch = 5–6 ounces; 14-inch = 8 ounces; 16-inch = 10 ounces; 18-inch = 12 ounces. If you like the convenience of frozen pizza, Daiya also makes a frozen dairy-free, gluten-free pizza now.

2 6-inch corn tortillas (or gluten-free flour tortillas)

¼ cup pizza sauce (look for sauce without sugar or gluten)

¼ pound ground beef, browned

¼ cup chopped sweet red peppers

¼ cup chopped onions

¼ cup sliced black olives

¼ cup spinach

1 clove garlic, minced

6 ounces soy-based imitation cheese (you can find nondairy cheese
   substitutes in health food stores and regular grocery stores)

❖ Place the tortillas on a large cookie sheet. Place the pizza sauce and beef on the tortilla. Add the peppers, onion, olives, spinach, and garlic to each tortilla. Top with the gluten-free, dairy-free cheese alternative. Bake at 375 degrees, or until the cheese melts, about 5 to 10 minutes. Alternatively, you can broil the pizzas in a toaster oven or put the tortilla in a large covered skillet and cook on the stove over medium heat until the cheese melts, usually 2 to 3 minutes. Carefully slide the pizzas out of the oven, toaster oven, or skillet, and serve.

Rawmesan

MAKES 16 SERVINGS

THIS IS A VEGAN RECIPE that tastes much like Parmesan cheese. (Of course, you don't have to be vegan to enjoy it on your Wahls Pizza or cooked veggies.)

½ cup nutritional yeast

½ cup ground walnuts

½ teaspoon iodized sea salt

❖ Combine ingredients in a food processor and process in short pulses until the mixture resembles Parmesan cheese.

SOUPS

Bone Broth

MAKES VARYING AMOUNTS,
DEPENDING ON HOW MUCH WATER YOU USE

BONE BROTH WILL KEEP in the refrigerator for three days, in sealed airtight glass jars, or in the freezer for three months. The more bones you have in the pot, the longer you should let it steam and simmer to increase the collagen and minerals in the broth. Knucklebones and chicken feet add a lot of gelatin and collagen. My goal is to have 1 to 2 cups a day, especially during the winter.

Water (filtered or reverse-osmosis water), enough to fill the pot or
 Crock-Pot
1 onion, chopped
3–4 cloves garlic
2–4 tablespoons cider vinegar (1 tablespoon per quart of water
 added is a good place to start)
1 teaspoon kelp powder or 1 tablespoon dulse flakes (optional)
½ teaspoon black pepper
½ teaspoon iodized sea salt
Bones (knucklebones are particularly good)
4 chicken feet (optional but recommended)
Any vegetables in your fridge that are getting a little bit limp

❖ Heat the water to steaming or a light simmer and add the rest of the ingredients. Simmer anywhere from 4 hours to 2 days. If any foamy materials come to the top of the pot, skim them off and discard. After you turn off the heat, allow to cool. Strain out the vegetables and bones.

THE POWER OF BONE BROTH

People spend a lot of money on expensive joint supplements for arthritis. These include substances like glucosamine, chondroitin sulfate, and methylsulfonylmethane (or MSM, another sulfur-containing compound). People also spend a lot of money on hyaluronic acid joint injections. I prefer a more natural approach: Get all these joint-strengthening, bone-building substances and more by making your own bone broth and drinking it every day. Bones with cartilage and tendons attached have more glucosamine to help benefit bones and joints even more. Those with a lot of marrow have more DHA fat, which, as I mentioned earlier, is really good for you, too!

Bone Broth–Avocado Soup

MAKES ABOUT 2½ CUPS

THIS WILL MAKE a lovely thick creamy soup. If it is too thick, simply add more broth or water.

2 cups Bone Broth (page 345)
⅓ can full-fat coconut milk
1 avocado, pitted and peeled
2 cloves garlic, crushed
1 teaspoon grated fresh ginger

❖ Mix all the ingredients. Blend in a high-powered blender until smooth. You may wish to heat again, although this soup is equally wonderful cold.

Bone Broth–Carrot Soup

SERVES 1

1 cup Bone Broth (page 345)
⅓ can full-fat coconut milk
½ cup cooked or raw carrots
1 teaspoon minced fresh ginger
½ teaspoon ground turmeric

❖ Bring the Bone Broth to a simmer over medium heat. Stir in remaining ingredients. Puree in a Vitamix or other high-speed blender.

Bone Broth–Cauliflower-Turmeric Soup

SERVES 1

1 cup Bone Broth (page 345)
⅓ can full-fat coconut milk
½ cup cauliflower florets (cooked or raw)
1 clove garlic, minced
½ teaspoon ground turmeric

❖ Bring the Bone Broth to a simmer over medium heat. Stir in remaining ingredients. Puree in a Vitamix or other high-speed blender.

Bone Broth–Pepper Soup

SERVES 1

1 cup Bone Broth (page 345)
½ cup chopped red peppers
⅓ can (or more) full-fat coconut milk

❖ Bring the Bone Broth to a simmer over medium heat. Add remaining ingredients, and then blend in a Vitamix or other high-speed blender.

Coconut Milk–Fish Soup

SERVES 4

THIS IS A FAMILY FAVORITE. It's very easy to adjust this to any combination of seafood, or even poultry.

> 6 cups Bone Broth (page 345)
> 1 13.5-ounce can full-fat coconut milk
> 1 teaspoon organic kelp powder, such as Starwest Botanicals
>   organic kelp (optional)
> ½ teaspoon iodized sea salt
> 5 cups chopped bok choy
> 3 cups chopped broccoli
> 1 medium carrot, sliced
> ½ pound shiitake mushrooms, sliced
> 1 tablespoon thinly sliced ginger
> 1½ pounds Chinook salmon
> 2 tablespoons lime juice

❖ In large kettle, add broth, coconut milk, kelp powder, salt, vegetables, and ginger. Add additional water if you want more broth in the soup. Bring to a simmer. Add salmon and lime juice. Bring soup to a boil. Turn off heat. Let kettle sit for 10 minutes and serve.

Seafood-Tomato Soup

SERVES 4

THIS SOUP IS MARVELOUS and the saffron is a wonderful addition. We alternate between this and the Coconut Milk–Fish Soup. Both are very big hits with both Zach and Zebby. Neither takes long to make.

4 cups Bone Broth (page 345)

1 18-ounce bottle clam juice

1 14.5-ounce can chopped tomatoes

4 cloves garlic

1 cup chopped sweet red pepper

1 cup chopped sweet yellow pepper

1 leek, sliced

1 teaspoon organic kelp powder, such as Starwest Botanicals
*   organic kelp (optional)*

½ teaspoon iodized sea salt (or to taste)

⅛ teaspoon saffron

½ pound scallops

½ pound shrimp

❖ Place broth, clam juice, tomatoes, garlic vegetables, kelp powder, salt, and saffron in a large pot over medium heat. Simmer 5 minutes. Add scallops and shrimp to the pot. Bring to boil. Turn heat off, let sit 5 to 10 minutes, then serve.

Kale-Sausage Soup/ Vegetarian Kale Soup

SERVES 4

THIS RECIPE IS PARTICULARLY GOOD for winter meals. Zach enjoys it with kale and sausage, but any type of leafy green will work well. You can also use any variety of sausage you like or omit it entirely to make the recipe vegetarian.

8 cups Bone Broth (page 345; or vegetable broth, if vegetarian)

4 cups chopped kale

2 cups chopped sweet potato

1 cup chopped onion

1 medium banana pepper, sliced

1 teaspoon organic kelp powder, such as Starwest Botanicals
*   organic kelp (optional)*

½ teaspoon iodized sea salt

4 bratwursts (If vegetarian, omit or substitute 2 cups black-eyed peas, canned or cooked from dried, though soaked is best to decrease the lectins/phytates.)

1 13.5-ounce can full-fat coconut milk

❖ Add broth, vegetables, kelp powder, and salt to a Crock-Pot or soup pot. Add brats and simmer for at least 30 minutes, or add black-eyed peas, which will be tender in 30 minutes if they were soaked first. Fish out the sausages, slice them, and add them back to the soup. Add coconut milk, stir, and serve.

Red Chili with Beans

SERVES 4

You can use louisiana hot sauce or other pepper sauce on the table to make your chili as hot as you like. Jackie prefers a milder chili, but Zebby and I like it hot. Zebby probably has the hottest taste preference of us all. The heat from the hot sauce is capsaicin, which has been a traditional treatment for chronic nerve pain. If you soak the beans overnight and sprout them, the cooking time is shortened, plus you will have reduced the lectins and phytates.

8 cups Bone Broth (page 345)

1 pound ground bison meat

1 cup chopped onion

1 15-ounce can black beans, drained

2 6-ounce cans tomato paste

1 medium carrot, sliced

1 jalapeño pepper, minced

1 teaspoon chili powder

1 teaspoon organic kelp powder, such as Starwest Botanicals organic kelp (optional)

½ teaspoon iodized sea salt

❖ Put all ingredients in kettle. Simmer 30 minutes.

Seafood Stew

SERVES 4

THIS STEW IS great with oysters or scallops, and it can be varied to fit the Wahls Protocol level you've selected. For the Wahls Paleo version, double the amount of seafood and keep the rest of the recipe the same. For Wahls Paleo Plus, use 1 pound of seafood but omit the butternut squash.

1 13.5-ounce can full-fat coconut milk

2 cups chicken broth (or Bone Broth, page 345, or store-bought broth)

1 pound mushrooms, sliced

1 large onion, chopped

2 cups cubed butternut squash (omit on Wahls Paleo Plus)

1 teaspoon organic kelp powder, such as Starwest Botanicals organic kelp (optional)

½ teaspoon iodized sea salt

1 pound oysters or scallops (use 2 pounds for Wahls Paleo)

2 cups chopped cauliflower

1 cup minced fresh cilantro

❖ Place coconut milk, broth, mushrooms, onion, squash, kelp powder, and salt in a pot. Heat to simmering until squash is nearly tender, 5 to 10 minutes. Add oysters or scallops and cauliflower, bring back to a gentle simmer, and turn the heat off. Let stew sit for 10 minutes. Stir in the cilantro and serve. Add coarse ground pepper to each bowl as you like.

SALADS

I OFTEN RECOMMEND having a salad, but nutritional content can vary drastically depending on which vegetables, fruits, nuts, seeds, fat sources, and meats you choose. In general I recommend piling your plate with fresh raw leafy greens of all types, chopping other vegetables you have, and adding them (cucumber, carrots, radishes, bell peppers, mushrooms, green onions, or whatever you like, but try to include sulfur-rich vegetables to balance the greens), drizzling with a cold-pressed olive oil and a splash of fresh lemon juice or vinegar, and adding some animal protein like steak, chicken, or fish.

Salmon or Chicken Salad

SERVES 3

You can use these meat salads as a spread, side dish, or salad accent. If using salmon, find a can of wild sockeye salmon that contains the bones. By keeping the bones in the salad, you will markedly increase your calcium intake. Serve with gluten-free crackers or bread. My daughter is very fond of having this with a collard green as a wrap. You can steam the collard green for a minute to soften it before using it in place of flatbread. If you prefer, warm the salad slightly on the stove before eating. This is an easy meal that you can make from pantry foods.

1 14.7-ounce can salmon, drained, or 4 medium skinless cooked chicken breasts (about 13 ounces)
½ small onion, minced
1 clove garlic, minced
¼ cup minced celery
¼ cup chopped parsley
2 tablespoons gluten-free peanut sauce
⅓ teaspoon organic kelp powder, such as Starwest Botanicals organic kelp (optional)
¼ teaspoon iodized sea salt

❖ Put the salmon in a bowl and mash the bones. If using chicken, chop the breasts into bite-size pieces. Place salmon or chicken and onion, garlic, celery, parsley, peanut sauce, kelp powder, and salt in a food processor and pulse until the mixture reaches your desired texture. You can also chop and mix by hand.

SIDE DISHES

THESE ARE VEGETABLE DISHES to have on the side. One of the things I discovered was that by adding bacon to a dish, it cut the bitterness and made vegetables much more appealing to Zach and Zebby. When we discovered gluten-free, nitrate-free bacon, we were all much happier.

Greens and Bacon

SERVES 3

ANY TYPE OF green will work well with this recipe.

> *4 slices bacon, cut into bite-size pieces (nitrate-free)*
> *6 cups chopped greens (beet, mustard, or any other greens)*
> *3 cloves garlic, chopped*
> *1 tablespoon balsamic vinegar*
> *1 teaspoon organic kelp powder, such as Starwest Botanicals*
>   *organic kelp (optional)*
> *½ teaspoon iodized sea salt*

❖ Fry bacon. Retain all fat. Add greens, garlic, vinegar, kelp powder, and salt to the pan. Cook until greens are wilted. Serve.

Brussels Sprouts, Bacon, and Cranberries

SERVES 4

AS A CHILD, I did not care for Brussels sprouts, but now both Jackie and I are very fond of them. The trick here is not to overcook them, because they'll become bitter if you do. The cranberries are a lovely addition visually and taste-wise, and the almonds add a little more calcium to the meal. This is a quick and easy dish to prepare.

4 slices bacon (nitrate-free)
4 cups halved Brussels sprouts
1 cup whole fresh cranberries
¼ cup chopped onion
2 tablespoons balsamic vinegar
1 teaspoon organic kelp powder, such as Starwest Botanicals
  organic kelp (optional)
¼ cup raw almonds, chopped (soaked once you are doing Wahls
  Paleo or Wahls Paleo Plus)

❖ Fry bacon. Pour off half the fat (or retain all of the fat to increase your intake of healthy fats). Add Brussels sprouts, cranberries, onion, vinegar, and kelp powder to skillet. Cover and simmer for two minutes. Add the chopped almonds when you serve it.

Mashed Turnips

SERVES 4

1 pound turnips
½ cup nutritional yeast
¼ cup chopped chives
4 cloves garlic, minced
2 tablespoons coconut oil
1 teaspoon organic kelp powder, such as Starwest Botanicals
  organic kelp (optional)
¼ teaspoon iodized sea salt
¼ teaspoon ground black pepper

❖ Wash and cut up turnips into bite-size pieces. Place in a steamer basket and steam until tender, which will be 5 to 10 minutes, depending on how small you cut the pieces. When the turnips are tender, place in a bowl with the remaining ingredients and mash with a potato masher. (You can also pulse the mixture in a food processor until the desired texture is achieved.) Add more coarsely ground black pepper to individual servings if desired.

Sautéed Red Cabbage

SERVES 4

My mother was very fond of red cabbage, and introduced our family to eating it sautéed.

> *2 tablespoons coconut oil*
> *4 cups chopped red cabbage*
> *1½ tablespoons sliced fresh ginger*
> *1 tablespoon balsamic vinegar*

❖ Heat coconut oil in a skillet over medium heat. Add cabbage, ginger, and vinegar. Sauté for 2 to 4 minutes.

Quinoa and Red Peppers

SERVES 4

Zebby is fond of this recipe. We based it on a dish served at an Algerian restaurant in Elkader, Iowa.

> *1 cup quinoa*
> *1½ cups water*
> *1 cup chopped red pepper*

❖ Soak quinoa for 10 minutes and rinse carefully to remove the skin (which has a bitter coating called saponin) or sprout by soaking 6 to 24 hours and then rinse. Return to pot, add the water, cover the pan, and simmer 10 minutes. Add chopped red pepper and simmer another 5 minutes. Remove from heat and let it sit in the pot for another 5 minutes. Fluff with a fork and serve.

Cauliflower Rice

SERVES 4

1 medium cauliflower

❖ Cut cauliflower into pieces that will fit in through the food processor chute (unless you choose to grate it by hand). Place cauliflower in a steamer basket in large pot on the stove. Steam for 2 to 4 minutes. Put the grating blade in the food processor. Run the steamed cauliflower, including stems and leaves, through the food processor. This is a great substitute for rice. You could also put it through the processor to make mashed cauliflower, which can be eaten like mashed potatoes. This is a low-carbohydrate alternative to potatoes: It tastes great, goes with any dish that has a lovely sauce, and will not cause a rise in insulin levels.

Spaghetti Squash

SERVES 4

1 large spaghetti squash

❖ Poke holes in the squash to allow steam to escape. Bake in oven at 375 degrees for 1 hour or in a Crock-Pot on low for 10 hours. The squash is done when a carving fork can easily pierce the skin. Split the squash in half and scoop out and discard the seeds. Scrape out the squash, which will look like noodles, and serve.

Sweet Potato or Winter Squash

MAKE ½ TO 1 SWEET POTATO OR
SQUASH PER SERVING, DEPENDING ON SIZE

❖ Cut up and steam for 10 to 15 minutes or until a carving fork can easily pierce the skin. Place sweet potatoes or squash in serving dish and serve.

Beet and Red Cabbage Mixture

SERVES 1

You can make this two ways. Use the freshly grated ginger or the cinnamon-cocoa combination, or you can omit the spices and simply have the beet-red cabbage mixture. The beets and cabbage are excellent for mitochondria and detoxification. Ginger, cinnamon, and cocoa are all powerhouse spices that add even more mitochondrial and detoxification support, which is why I started adding them to more of my foods.

¼ *cup beets, raw*
¼ *cup chopped red cabbage*
1 tablespoon flaxseed or hemp oil
1 tablespoon olive oil
1 teaspoon ground cinnamon (optional)
¼ *teaspoon unsweetened cocoa (optional) or 1 teaspoon grated*
    fresh ginger (instead of the cocoa-cinnamon combination)

❖ Combine all ingredients. Place in a food processor and pulse to your desired consistency.

Beet and Cranberry Mixture

SERVES 1

¼ *cup beets, raw*
¼ *cup fresh whole cranberries*
1½ *tablespoons sliced or grated fresh ginger*

❖ Combine all ingredients. Place in a food processor and pulse to desired consistency.

B E V E R A G E S

Bone Broth Tea

I LIKE TO COMBINE Bone Broth and coconut milk to make a warm drink for my mornings, especially during the winter. The basis is a cup of hot Bone Broth and ⅓ of a can of full-fat coconut milk. Then I add spices (like turmeric) and some vegetables (like carrots or garlic). The Vitamix can handle anything, so I add vegetables raw or cooked and put the entire mixture on high until blended smooth. If it seems too thick, I add more broth until it reaches my desired thickness. Again, experiment with spices and your local in-season vegetables.

Turmeric Tea

SERVES 1

1 cup Bone Broth (page 345)
⅓ can (or more) full-fat coconut milk
½ tablespoon ground turmeric
1 clove garlic, peeled and crushed

❖ Bring the Bone Broth to a simmer over medium heat. Add remaining ingredients, then blend in a Vitamix or other high-speed blender.

Hot Cocoa

SERVES 1

OUR GREAT-GREAT-GRANDMOTHERS AND -grandfathers knew to use spices to make foods seem sweeter. Spices that have a little heat, such as cinnamon, cloves, mint, and ginger, will help reduce the perceived bitterness of food and improve the relative sweetness. I make hot cocoa using just organic cocoa powder, cinnamon, and coconut milk. There is no sugar in the cocoa, but the cinnamon cuts the bitterness nicely. The longer you are away from sugar, the more your taste buds and taste sensibility will change. You will likely find your foods tasting sweeter, and you may find bitter tastes more appealing. If this chocolate seems too bitter for your taste, add a very ripe banana or some of the approved sweeteners, such as a teaspoon of honey. Stevia leaves are certainly fine, but once stevia is processed, I am not certain about the impact of the processing, so I do not use it.

¼–1 teaspoon unsweetened cocoa
½–1 teaspoon ground cinnamon
½ can full-fat coconut milk
½ cup water
Optional: Make a mint cocoa by adding a few drops of oil of mint

❖ Combine all ingredients in a blender, and blend until smooth. (Stirring alone will not produce a smooth cocoa.) Heat gently in a saucepan over medium heat on the stove.

FERMENTED FOODS

FERMENTED FOODS WERE a long tradition in most of our great-grandmothers' kitchens. They are not hard to make and add a lot of nutrition to your diet. Here are some easy recipes that I enjoy. Fermented foods are an acquired taste, so start slowly. Kombucha is the easiest. Then add other fermented foods as condiments to your meals.

Kombucha Tea

MAKES 16 CUPS

You CAN PURCHASE KOMBUCHA TEA at the store, but for the freshest possible tea where you control the ingredients, make it yourself. To make a gallon of tea, you can either add tea bags to heated water or make sun tea. Either way, you must ensure that there is no chlorine in your water or you'll kill the kombucha "mother," or SCOBY, which is responsible for fermenting the tea. I always use reverse-osmosis water, but if you don't have that type of filter, you can also let the water sit uncovered for 24 hours or boil it for 5 minutes to get rid of the chlorine. The metals from your pans may also disrupt the kombucha, so you should use a nonreactive container such as a one-gallon glass jar to make the tea. Make sure to wash all of your containers with hot, soapy water before starting. You can order kombucha mothers through the Internet (find both mothers and supplies at Kombucha Kamp, www.kombuchakamp .com), or if you are lucky, you can get a mother from a friend.

I drink Kombucha tea regularly; however, there have been a couple of reported cases of people becoming ill from too much acid in their bloodstreams attributed to drinking kombucha. If you have any kidney or liver disease, or diabetes, you are at a higher risk to have problems with kombucha. Start with drinking just a ¼ cup when you first begin to confirm that you have no problems with it. Then you can increase to ½ cup and then a full cup or more each day.

1 gallon black tea, green tea, rooibos tea, or yerba maté
1 cup white granulated sugar
1 mother

❖ Add the sugar while the tea is still warm and stir until dissolved. After the tea has cooled to room temperature, remove the tea bags. Pour the tea into a gallon jar that holds the mother or SCOBY. Place a mesh bag over the jar and cover the jar with a towel to let the mixture breathe. Store the mixture at room temperature in a well-ventilated area without light for 7 to 10 days, though fermentation time can vary. You can check whether it's done by taste or by using a pH strip to see if its pH is between 2.6 and 4.0. Discard any kombucha that smells rancid or looks to be contaminated with mold or insects. A well-fermented batch will be cloudy and fizzy with stringy, brown pieces from the SCOBY. Pour the kombucha into quart jars, seal them, let them sit on the counter for another day, then place them in the refrigerator. Consume within the month. Leave 1 to 2 cups of tea with the mother and put the mother back in the refrigerator to reuse. You can make a fresh batch of kombucha every other weekend, but kombucha that has been fermented too long turns into usable vinegar. Because of its acidity, the tea should not be prepared or stored in lead-glazed ceramic or lead crystal containers, as toxic elements can leach into the tea.

Beet Kvass

SERVES 3

EASTERN EUROPE HAS a long history of fermenting foods, including root vegetables. The fermentation process increases the production of vitamins and enzymes, and it helps put the correct health-promoting bacteria back in your bowels. Beets are traditionally an excellent support for your detoxification enzymes, and fermented beets offer even more support to the detoxification process. I like to alternate between drinking kombucha and beet kvass, and I dilute the beet kvass with an equal amount of water when I drink it. It is very important to use organic beets for the kvass and water that has absolutely no chlorine. You also need a starter from some fermented beets or a single probiotic capsule, like an acidolphilus capsule you can buy at your grocery store or pharmacy, with the supplements. Open the capsule and dump it into the mix. Get one with as large a number of different species as possible. (The one I use has fifteen different strains of health-promoting bacteria in it.)

1 cup coarsely sliced or chopped beets
1 tablespoon grated ginger
1 tablespoon grated orange peel
1 tablespoon iodized sea salt
1 probiotic capsule
2½ cups water

❖ Clean a canning jar and lid carefully in hot soapy water. Rinse well. Place beet pieces in the jar, sprinkling ginger, orange zest, and salt as you go. Open the probiotic capsule and sprinkle the contents on beets to introduce the helpful bacteria. Fill with water. Place a jar with a diameter smaller than the opening of the canning jar on the beets to keep them submerged. After 2 to 3 days, the fermentation should be sufficient, and the jar can be sealed and placed in the refrigerator. Drain the liquid and drink it. (You can also eat the beets, or discard them, but they are good in smoothies or salads.)

Sauerkraut and Fermented Vegetables

THIS IS A VERY EASY fermented food recipe and was a staple for American settlers. Both my grandmothers would have made fermented root vegetables and pickles regularly. (All vegetables need to be organic.)

> *1 small organic cabbage*
> *Organic carrots, garlic, and/or onions, to taste*
> *Ginger, to taste*
> *Hot peppers, chopped or whole, to taste*
> *1 tablespoon iodized sea salt*
> *1 probiotic capsule*

❖ Clean a wide-mouth canning jar and lid carefully in hot soapy water. Rinse carefully. Wash the cabbage and vegetables. The goal is to have 80 percent or more grated cabbage in the mixture. Grate the cabbage and carrots. Grate the ginger. Place the cabbage in the jar, sprinkling ginger, hot peppers, other root vegetables (to taste), and salt as you go. Pack the vegetables into the canning jar with a spoon. Open the probiotic capsule and sprinkle on the cabbage. Place a jar with a diameter smaller than the opening of the canning jar on the cabbage to submerge it below the brine. Place the jar in another container to catch any brine that overflows during the fermemtation process, and store in a cool, dark place. Check the jar periodically to remove any unsubmerged pieces of vegetables or mold that has appeared. If the level of brine is below the top of the vegetables, add additional salted water until the vegetables are completely submerged (2 teaspoons salt to 1 cup filtered water. Remember, tap water has chlorine and will kill the friendly bacteria.) After a week, the fermentation should be sufficient and the jar can be sealed and placed in the refrigerator. Fermentation time can vary; if desired, the vegetables can be fermented longer until the desired taste and texture have been achieved.

DESSERTS

You do get to have some treats. Your taste buds will adjust and you will discover new flavors in your foods. These are some wonderful desserts using dried fruit, fresh berries, and spices to accent and sweeten the dish.

Fruit Pudding

SERVES 2

In this recipe, the spices enhance the fruit's natural sweetness. After you've gone two weeks without sugar, your cravings for sweets will fade.

- *1 cup full-fat coconut milk*
- *1 cup any berries, or combination of berries (such as blackberries, blueberries, raspberries, and strawberries)*
- *1 medium Hass avocado, peeled, pitted, and chopped*
- *1 teaspoon ground cardamom*
- *1 teaspoon ground cinnamon*

❖ Bring coconut milk to a boil. Add hot coconut milk, berries, avocado, and spices to a Vitamix and blend for 3 minutes. Pour into a bowl and refrigerate.

Raspberry-Flaxseed Pudding

SERVES 2

Once you get to Wahls Paleo, the flaxseeds should be soaked for 2 to 6 hours before use to eliminate phytates and lectins. This will make them softer and easier to blend, so you won't have to grind the seeds separately. If you're not on Wahls Paleo or Wahls Paleo Plus, grind the flaxseeds immediately before use in a coffee grinder. That way the omega-3 fatty acids won't have broken down. You may increase or decrease the flaxseed to make the pudding your desired level of firmness. Fresh berries and a tablespoon of full-fat coconut milk make a lovely garnish for serving.

> ¼ *cup flaxseeds*
> *1 cup full-fat coconut milk*
> *1 cup raspberries*
> *1 teaspoon ground cardamom*
> *1 teaspoon ground cinnamon*

❖ Grind flaxseeds just prior to use (Wahls Diet) or soak seeds for 2 to 6 hours prior to use (Wahls Paleo and Wahls Paleo Plus). Bring the coconut milk to a boil. Place ground flaxseeds or whole soaked flaxseeds, hot coconut milk, raspberries, and spices in a Vitamix or other high-speed blender, and blend for 3 minutes. Pour into a bowl and refrigerate.

Wahls Fudge

MAKES 20 SERVINGS

WE USE THIS RECIPE when people are losing too much weight. We have people eat as much fudge as they need to maintain a healthy weight. This is a marvelous sweet treat with raisins, but you can use any dried fruit, like plums, dates, or cherries. The coconut oil keeps the carbohydrates from entering your bloodstream too quickly. This is an excellent treat that will hopefully help you to adjust to a new way of eating. For those who are following Paleo Plus and reducing their carbohydrate intake, omit the raisins, though you will have to cut back considerably on cocoa to keep the fudge from being too bitter. (Start with ¼ teaspoon.) If you are still losing too much weight, you may need to increase the carbs, even if you're on Paleo Plus. If so, add raisins and don't be concerned about whether you are in ketosis.

1 cup coconut oil

1 cup raisins

1 cup walnuts (soaked once you are doing Wahls Paleo)

1 medium Hass avocado, peeled and pitted

½ cup dried unsweetened coconut

1–2 teaspoons ground cinnamon

1 teaspoon unsweetened cocoa powder

❖ Put everything in a food processor and blend on high until smooth. Press mixture into an 8 × 8 glass baking dish, and place in the refrigerator. Keep refrigerated.

Appendix A
THE WAHLS PROTOCOL
COMPLETE FOOD LISTS

THE FIRST STEP we give our study subjects is to go through their homes and eating environments and remove all of the prohibited foods. Donate them to a food bank, give them to a neighbor, or toss them—whatever seems appropriate to you. Completing that step dramatically increases the probability of success. To help you do this, I am starting with the list of prohibited foods for the Wahls Diet, and then I'll tell you what you would be removing for Wahls Paleo and Wahls Paleo Plus. After that, I'll provide a table summarizing the three plans, followed by the list of foods you can eat by category.

PROHIBITED FOODS
All gluten-containing foods

1. Wheat, rye, malt, most commercial oats (unless specifically labeled gluten-free), and all products made from these:
   - Bread; most baked goods, like muffins, cookies, cake, rolls, biscuits, and croissants; most pasta; most crackers; flour tortillas; and any breakfast cereal containing wheat or other gluten grains
   - Many packaged foods contain wheat or other gluten-containing grains, so check the label! Foods that contain gluten but aren't obviously made of wheat include soy sauce (tamari is okay), seitan, and many brands of veggie "meats," like veggie burgers, veggie hot dogs, and veggie "chicken." Words to look for include: brominated flour, durum flour, enriched flour, farina, flour, graham flour, phosphate flour, plain flour, self-rising flour, semolina, white flour, teff, einkorn, emmer, kamut, and spelt
2. Barley
   - Barley, including pearl barley, like the kind you might put in soup
   - All beer that isn't specifically labeled gluten-free

- Cider and other fermented beverages (Note: Distilled non-grain-based alcohol, such as vodka or gin, is gluten-free, and some fermented ciders are gluten-free, but check the label. Most wine is also gluten-free.)
- Malt products (malt syrup, malt extract, malt flavoring, malted beverages, and malted milk)

All dairy products

- All cow, sheep, and goat milks
- All products made from those milks, like cheese, yogurt, cream, and ice cream
- All products containing milk proteins, such as baked goods, pudding, and snacks containing cheese
- Many packaged foods contain milk or milk components, such as casein and whey, so check the label.

Other foods to avoid

- Chicken and duck eggs, omega-3 eggs, and all foods containing eggs
- Nonorganic soy products
- Processed meats—like hot dogs, bologna, and salami—that contain gluten or nitrates
- All oils other than the permitted oils listed in the following pages. Do not consume corn, soybean, canola, or grapeseed oils. Also, do not consume any trans fats, hydrogenated or partially hydrogenated oils, or any type of margarine.
- All foods sweetened with sugar, high-fructose corn syrup, or other refined sweeteners, including artificial sweetener. This includes:
  - Desserts and snacks sweetened with sugar
  - Regular or diet soda
  - Sweetened juice drinks
  - Sports drinks
  - Fruit canned or frozen with added sugar or artificial sweetener
  - Any drink or foods made with sugar, high-fructose corn syrup, or artificial sweetener
- Any foods made with monosodium glutamate (MSG)
- Do not microwave any food you intend to eat!

- With Wahls Paleo, reduce your intake of gluten-free grains, legumes, and potatoes to two servings a week, and remove soy milk completely.
- At the Wahls Paleo Plus level, remove all grains, legumes, peanuts, and soy.

WAHLS PROTOCOL FOOD RULES

That last section was about what you can't eat, but this section is what you *can* eat! Here are the general food rules for the three diet plans. After the summary, I provide a table comparing the three diets and then the list of foodstuffs contained in each of the various food categories. Make sure to vary the foods within each group that you consume each day.

Wahls Diet

- Remove all prohibited foods from your diet, as specified previously.
- Eat 9 cups of vegetables and fruit (3 cups greens, 3 cups sulfur-rich, 3 cups color).
- You may reduce your 9 cups in proportion to one another if it is making you feel uncomfortably full or giving you digestive trouble; in other words, if you reduce your intake to 6 cups, you should get 2 cups from each category. Or, eat up to 12 cups!
- Eat high-quality protein, preferably animal, as desired (6 to 12 ounces daily according to gender and size). Gluten-free, nitrate-free processed meats are acceptable.
- Vegetarians are encouraged to soak, and preferably sprout, the grains and legumes consumed. (See chapter 6, "Wahls Paleo," for more information on the difference between the two.)
- Eating organic is encouraged.
- Limit gluten-free grain products to one per day.
- Limit sweeteners to 1 teaspoon.
- Avoid all artificial sweeteners.
- Avoid vegetable oils high in omega-6 fatty acids, like corn, soybean, canola, grapeseed, and palm kernel oils.
- Avoid hydrogenated fats.
- If constipated, use flaxseed or chia seed as needed to have soft bowel movements daily.
- Eat to satiety.

The food groups added in Wahls Paleo (soaked nuts and seeds, seaweed, organ meats, and fermented foods) are also permitted if desired in the Wahls Diet.

Wahls Paleo

- Continue eating 9 cups of vegetables and fruit and being gluten-, dairy-, and egg-free, as in the Wahls Diet.
- Increase protein to 9 to 21 ounces of meat daily, with 12 ounces of organ meat and 16 ounces of high omega-3 fish each week.
- Reduce all gluten-free grain products, potatoes, and legumes to two servings per week (soaked if consumed).
- Add seaweed and algae daily.
- Add lacto-fermented food daily.
- Add soaked nuts and seeds.
- Avoid soy and rice milk.
- Switch to coconut milk and soaked nut milks.

Wahls Paleo Plus

- Continue eating vegetables and fruit, and being gluten-, dairy-, and egg-free, as in the Wahls Diet. Continue with the fermented foods, organ meats, soaked nuts and seeds, coconut milk, soaked nut milks, seaweed, and algae as in Wahls Paleo.
- You may reduce your 9 cups to 6 cups, but retain an even distribution between leafy green, color, and sulfur categories. Remove apples, pears, and bananas. Raw starchy colored vegetables may be consumed as part of the color allotment. Limit fruit to one cup per day with a preference for berries and low-carbohydrate fruits. Avoid all dried and canned fruit and fruit juices.
- Avoid all legumes, grains, and white potatoes.
- Reduce protein back down to 6 to 12 ounces according to size and gender.
- Increase fat to a can of full-fat coconut milk (about 14 ounces) or 4 to 5 tablespoons coconut oil per day. Have full-fat coconut milk or coconut oil with each meal.
- Reduce cooked starchy vegetables and starchy fruit to 2 servings per week eaten with coconut milk/fat and protein. If you are losing too much weight, you may gradually add starchy cooked vegetables back into your diet to determine which level is right for you.

- Eliminate legumes, including pea pods and green beans.
- Eliminate even gluten-free soy sauce (coconut aminos are a good substitute).
- Limit alcohol to special occasions because of the carb content.
- If not showing urine ketones, you may need to reduce your intake of starchy vegetables and fruits and/or increase your fat intake.
- Note: The transition to Wahls Paleo Plus should occur over several weeks to avoid problems with nausea, vomiting, or diarrhea with the shift to a fat-burning metabolism.

The following chart summarizes the food categories and the goal for each food group. Note the colors are broken down into high-carbohydrate and low-carbohydrate foods. Remember that Wahls Paleo Plus stresses low-carbohydrate colors and limits high-carbohydrate vegetables and fruits.

Food Category	Wahls Diet	Wahls Paleo	Wahls Paleo Plus
Fruits and Vegetables	Goal	Goal	Goal
Leafy greens (6 cups raw)	3 cups/day	3 cups/day	2–3 cups/day
Sulfur-rich (raw or cooked)	3 cups/day	3 cups/day	2–3 cups/day
Nonstarchy colorful (raw or cooked)	3 cups/day	3 cups/day	2–3 cups/day
Starchy color (raw or cooked) as part of the 3 cups color category	As part of 3 cups color	As part of 3 cups of color	Raw as part of 2–3 cups of color; cooked 2 servings/week maximum
Apple, pear, bananas	After 9 cups	After 9 cups	Avoid
Protein Sources			
Organ meats	As desired	12 ounces/week	12 ounces/week
Wild cold-water fish	As desired	16 ounces/week	16 ounces/week
Other meat, poultry, game	6–12 ounces/day	9–21 ounces/day	6–12 ounces/day
Beans, legumes, peas, lentils, peanuts	As desired	2 servings/week maximum	Avoid
Raw nuts and seeds	4 ounces/day maximum	Soaked 4 ounces/day maximum	Soaked 4 ounces/day maximum
Eggs	Avoid	Avoid	Avoid

Food Category	Wahls Diet	Wahls Paleo	Wahls Paleo Plus
Fats and Oils			
Flax, hemp, walnut	2 tablespoons/day maximum	2 tablespoons/day maximum	2 tablespoons/day maximum
Olive	As desired	As desired	As desired
Coconut (coconut oil, coconut butter)	As desired	As desired	4–6 tablespoons/day or more (or 1¾ cups full-fat coconut milk)
Animal fat (clarified butter, lard, bacon grease)	As desired	As desired	As desired
Milk and Milk Substitutes			
Full-fat coconut milk	As desired	As desired	1¾ cups/day (or 4–6 tablespoons coconut oil) or more
Rice (organic preferred)	As desired	Avoid	Avoid
Soy (organic only)	As desired	Avoid	Avoid
Nut and seed (almond, hazelnut, hemp)	As desired	Soaked, as desired	Soaked, as desired
Animal (cow, goat, sheep)	Avoid	Avoid	Avoid
Grains			
Gluten-free (rice, oat, quinoa, amaranth, buckwheat, corn)	1 serving/day maximum	2 servings/week maximum	Avoid
Gluten grains (wheat, rye, barley)	Avoid	Avoid	Avoid
Additional Items			
Seaweed	Permitted, up to 1 serving/day (serving = 2.5 ounces fresh or reconstituted, 1 teaspoon flakes, or ¼ teaspoon powder)	Up to 1 serving/day	Up to 1 serving/day
Dried algae (chlorella, spirulina, blue-green)	Up to 1 teaspoon chlorella or spirulina or ½ teaspoon blue-green	Up to 1 teaspoon/day	Up to 1 teaspoon/day
Nutritional yeast	1–2 tablespoons/day	1–2 tablespoons/day	1–2 tablespoons/day
Fermented non-dairy, non-grain foods	As desired	1 or more servings/day	1 or more servings/day

COMPLETE FOOD LISTS FOR ALL LEVELS OF THE WAHLS PROTOCOL

Dark green leafy vegetables (3 cups cooked or 6 cups raw, daily):

(* = Vegetables high in calcium)

- Arugula*
- Beet greens
- Bok choy* and other Asian greens
- Chard, all colors
- Chicory
- Cilantro
- Collard greens*
- Dandelion greens*
- Endive
- Escarole
- Kale,* all types (curly, lacinto/dinosaur, red, etc.)
- Lettuce, all types of deep-green, bright-green, and red-leaf (no iceberg)
- Mizuna
- Mustard greens*
- Parsley
- Radicchio
- Radish leaves
- Romaine lettuce
- Spinach*
- Tatsoi*
- Turnip greens*
- Watercress
- Wheatgrass

Colored vegetables and fruits (3 cups daily):

Even though they have white flesh, we allow zucchini and cucumbers because they are low in carbohydrates and their skins, which you should eat, are very high in antioxidants. Consume at least three difference colors daily. Note: While on Wahls Paleo Plus, switch colors to the low-carbohydrate vegetables and fruits. Limit starchy produce to two servings per week eaten with 1 to 2 tablespoons of fat and protein. If not in nutritional ketosis, you may need to eliminate the higher-carbohydrate vegetables and fruits and/or increase coconut milk. Note: For the following lists, any food containing 30 grams of carbohydrates or more per cup qualifies it as a higher-carb choice.

Green

LOWER/MODERATE-CARBOHYDRATE

- Artichoke
- Asparagus
- Avocado
- Beans, green (avoid on Wahls Paleo Plus)
- Cabbage, green
- Celery
- Cucumber, with skin
- Grapes, green
- Green peas (avoid on Wahls Paleo Plus)
- Honeydew melon
- Kiwi, green
- Limes
- Okra
- Olives, green
- Peppers, green
- Snow peas (avoid on Wahls Paleo Plus)
- Sugar snap peas (avoid on Wahls Paleo Plus)
- Zucchini with skin

HIGHER-CARBOHYDRATE

- Commercial juices (avoid on Wahls Paleo Plus)

Red

LOWER/MODERATE-CARBOHYDRATE

- Beets
- Blood oranges
- Cabbage, red
- Cherries
- Cranberries
- Currants, red
- Grapefruit, red
- Grapes, red
- Peppers, red
- Radicchio
- Raspberries, red
- Rhubarb
- Strawberries
- Tomatoes, red
- Watermelon

HIGHER-CARBOHYDRATE

- Commercial juices (avoid on Wahls Paleo Plus)
- Dried cranberries and other dried fruit (avoid on Wahls Paleo Plus)
- Pomegranate

Blue/Purple/Black

LOWER/MODERATE-CARBOHYDRATE

- Aronia berries
- Blackberries
- Blueberries
- Currants, black
- Eggplant
- Elderberries
- Grapes, black
- Grapes, purple
- Kale, purple
- Olives, black
- Plums
- Raspberries, black

HIGHER-CARBOHYDRATE

- Commercial juice (avoid on Wahls Paleo Plus)
- Dates (avoid on Wahls Paleo Plus)
- Dried currants (avoid on Wahls Paleo Plus)
- Figs, purple (avoid on Wahls Paleo Plus)
- Prunes (avoid on Wahls Paleo Plus)
- Raisins (avoid on Wahls Paleo Plus)

Yellow/Orange

LOWER-/MODERATE-CARBOHYDRATE

- Apricots
- Carrots
- Grapefruit
- Kiwi, golden
- Lemon
- Mango
- Muskmelon
- Nectarines
- Oranges
- Papaya
- Peaches
- Peppers, orange and yellow
- Pineapple
- Pumpkin
- Squash, summer and winter
- Sweet potatoes
- Tangerines
- Tomatoes, yellow
- Yams

HIGHER-CARBOHYDRATE

- Acorn squash
- Commercial juice (avoid on Wahls Paleo Plus)
- Dried apricots, pineapple, or other dried fruit (avoid on Wahls Paleo Plus)
- Figs
- Sweet potatoes, cooked

Sulfur-rich vegetables (3 cups daily):

(* = Vegetables high in calcium)

- Arugula*
- Asparagus
- Bok choy*
- Broccoli
- Broccoli rabe (rapini)
- Brussels sprouts
- Cabbage
- Cauliflower
- Chives
- Collard greens*
- Daikon
- Garlic, all types (two cloves = 1 serving)
- Kale*
- Kohlrabi
- Leeks
- Mizuna
- Mushrooms
- Mustard greens
- Onions, red, yellow, and white
- Radishes
- Rutabagas
- Scallions
- Shallots
- Tatsoi
- Turnip greens*
- Turnips
- Watercress

Starchy fruits not included in the 9 cups (white flesh). Consume only after 9 cups are finished:

- Apple (avoid on Wahls Paleo Plus)
- Banana (avoid on Wahls Paleo Plus)
- Pear (avoid on Wahls Paleo Plus)

Other white nonstarchy vegetables may be consumed after the 9 cups have been eaten:

- Bamboo shoots
- Cucumbers without skin
- Jicama
- Water chestnuts (canned)
- Zucchini without skin

Sea vegetables/algae (introduced with Wahls Paleo and Wahls Paleo Plus):

Algae (serving = 1 teaspoon spirulina or chlorella or ½ teaspoon blue-green)

- Blue-green algae
- Chlorella
- Spirulina

Seaweed (1 serving = 2.5 ounces fresh or reconstituted, 1 teaspoon flakes, or ¼ teaspoon powder)

Red
- Dulse
- Irish moss
- Nori

Brown
- Bladderwrack
- Kelp
- Kombu
- Wakame

Green
- Sea lettuce

Animal protein (strongly recommended in the Wahls Diet, mandatory for Wahls Paleo and Wahls Paleo Plus; prefer organic if possible, wild or grass-fed ideal):

- Beef
- Buffalo/bison
- Chicken
- Duck
- Elk
- Fish, all kinds (salmon, tuna, cod, sardines, mackerel, tilapia, sea bass, herring, etc.)
- Lamb
- Pork
- Processed meat with no gluten, nitrates, or monosodium glutamate
- Shellfish, all kinds (shrimp, crab, lobster, scallops, etc.)
- Turkey
- Veal
- Venison, rabbit, pheasant, quail, and other wild game

Organ meat (12 ounces per week; introduced with Wahls Paleo and continued in Wahls Paleo Plus):

- Brain
- Gizzard
- Heart
- Kidney
- Liver
- Sweetbreads
- Tongue
- Tripe

Omega-3 rich fish (16 ounces a week; encouraged in the Wahls Diet, mandatory with Wahls Paleo and Wahls Paleo Plus)

- Anchovies
- Clams
- Halibut
- Herring
- Mackerel
- Mussels
- Oysters
- Salmon
- Sardines
- Trout
- Tuna (fresh)

Dairy substitutes (organic preferred)

- Organic full-fat coconut milk, canned
- Organic unsweetened nut milk (like almond, hazelnut, or hemp milk; homemade soaked nut milk is strongly preferred for Wahls Paleo and Wahls Paleo Plus)
- Unsweetened coconut milk in a carton (for Wahls Diet and Wahls Paleo only, not for use on Wahls Paleo Plus. This is different from canned coconut milk, with much less fat and added fillers.)
- Organic soy milk (avoid on Wahls Paleo and Wahls Paleo Plus)
- Yogurts and other products made from coconut milk, nut milks, or organic soy (Wahls Diet only), but watch the sugar content.

Non-gluten grains and potatoes (eaten only after meeting your 9 cups goal: 1 serving per day on the Wahls Diet, 2 servings per week on Wahls Paleo, *avoid on Wahls Paleo Plus*):

- Almond and other nut flours
- Amaranth
- Arrowroot
- Brown rice
- Buckwheat
- Chickpea flour
- Coconut flour
- Coconut meat, fresh or unsweetened dried (shredded or flaked)
- Corn
- Flaxseeds and flax meal
- Millet
- Oatmeal (certified gluten-free brands only)
- Quinoa
- Sago
- Sorghum
- Soy flour
- Tapioca

- White potatoes (Yukon gold or heirloom red or black potatoes)
- Wild rice

Legumes (2 servings per week maximum on Wahls Paleo, avoid on Wahls Paleo Plus):

- Any dried beans (black, white, pinto, lima, peanuts, peanut butter, etc.)
- Lentils
- Pea pods and green beans

Nuts and seeds (sprouting of nuts and seeds introduced with Wahls Paleo and continued with Wahls Paleo Plus)

† = good source of fiber

* = high in calcium

- Tree nuts (unless you are allergic to them, including almonds,* walnuts, hazelnuts, cashews, Brazil nuts, and pistachios), maximum 4 ounces of nuts and seeds per day
- Seeds (sunflower, pumpkin, sesame, flax,† and chia†)
- Peanuts (unless you are allergic to them; peanuts are technically a legume, so avoid on Wahls Paleo and Wahls Paleo Plus)
- Peas (green, split peas, black-eyed peas; avoid on Wahls Paleo Plus)
- Tahini (sesame butter)
- Sunflower butter
- Almond butter

Cold-pressed oils (do not fry with or heat these oils):

- Avocado oil
- Flax oil
- Hemp oil
- Olive oil, extra virgin
- Walnut oil

Cooking oils:

- Clarified butter/ghee
- Coconut oil, extra virgin
- Rendered animal fats (e.g., lard, chicken fat, duck fat)
- Other oil/seed butters: Very occasional use of organic sesame oil. Coconut fat sources (use as desired on the Wahls Diet and Wahls Paleo, but required on Wahls Paleo Plus; these are used to increase the intake of medium-chain triglycerides to assist in achieving nutritional ketosis)

Condiments/flavorings:

- Brewer's yeast—though I prefer nutritional yeast because it has B_{12} added
- Coconut aminos (a soy-sauce-like condiment; one popular brand is Coconut Secret Raw Vegan Aminos)
- Herbs/spices without added sugar or salt
- Horseradish
- Miso (brown rice and soy versions only, not barley or other miso containing gluten); avoid on Wahls Paleo and Wahls Paleo Plus
- Mustard
- Nutritional yeast (Make sure it is gluten-free; if it causes headaches or fatigue, add it to your "prohibited" list.)
- Pickles
- Sauerkraut
- Sea salt (iodized or regular)
- Tamari (Make sure it's gluten-free, preferably fermented instead of hydrolyzed.)
- Wasabi (The powder is gluten-free, but the paste may have gluten, so be sure to read the label.)

Sweeteners (limit to 1 teaspoon per day and avoid on Wahls Paleo Plus):

- Honey
- Real maple syrup, organic (Do not use "pancake syrup" or anything containing high-fructose corn syrup. Organic maple syrup is important—formaldehyde may have been added to nonorganic brands.)
- Molasses* (high in calcium)
- Sorghum

- Stevia leaves or extract
- Raw sugar, evaporated cane juice, or other relatively unrefined forms of cane sugar (I prefer that you choose one of the other sweeteners, if possible, and avoid sugar entirely. *Do not* consume white sugar.)

Fermented foods (introduced with Wahls Paleo and Wahls Paleo Plus; start with one serving per day for Paleo and two servings per day for Paleo Plus, though additional servings are fine. You can find these in the refrigerator section of grocery and natural food stores, or, of course, you can make them yourself using the recipes in this book.)

- ½ cup lacto-fermented almond, soy, and coconut milk cultures
- ½ cup kombucha tea
- ½ cup beet kvass
- ¼ cup kimchi
- ¼ cup lacto-fermented cabbage, sauerkraut, pickles, or other vegetables

Beverages

- Water
- Club soda
- Coffee
- Tea (black or green, white, red rooibos, oolong, matcha, herbal)
- Yerba maté
- Kombucha tea
- Unsweetened 100% fruit juice (Avoid on Wahls Paleo Plus; have smoothies blended with water and/or coconut milk instead.)
- 100% vegetable juice
- 100% vegetable/fruit juice unsweetened (Avoid fruit juice on Wahls Paleo Plus; have smoothies blended with water instead.)
- Alcohol (daily limit to no more than one drink for women and two for men—special occasions only on Wahls Paleo Plus):
  - Gluten-free beer
  - Non-grain-based alcohol (like potato vodka)
  - Wine

Appendix B
NUTRIENT COMPARISON TABLES

Wahls versus the average US intake mean for females aged 50–59

The following table summarizes the nutrient comparison of the average US dietary intake for a woman my age and the intake for the one-week menus of the Wahls Diet, Wahls Paleo, and Wahls Paleo Plus. The nutrients with ** are the key thirty-one nutrients per the Bourre and Bowman articles. The additional micro- and macronutrients are provided to demonstrate how healthful the Wahls Diets are in comparison to the average US diet.

I have also provided information about the macronutrient content, glycemic index, and glycemic load from the three weeks of menus we provided to show that all three Wahls diets are more nutrient-dense than the average American diet.

Key Brain Nutrient Comparison of the US, Wahls Diet, Wahls Paleo Diet, Wahls Paleo Plus Diets					
Nutrients	*US**	*Wahls Diet*	*Wahls Paleo*	*Wahls Paleo Plus*	*Dietary Reference Intakes†*
Macronutrients and Dietary Fiber					
Energy, kcal	1,759	2,009	1,991	2,012	
Protein, g	70	107	158	84	46
Fat, g	66	80	80	152	
Carbohydrate, g	219	244	178	103	130
Dietary fiber, g	17	52	40	31	*21*
Protein, % energy	16	20	32	16	
Fat, % energy	33	34	35	65	
Carbohydrate, % energy	50	46	33	19	
Glycemic Index (≤55 is low; ≥70 is high)	n/a	52	53	38	
Glycemic Load (<80 is low; 100 is moderate)	n/a	100	74	28	

Nutrients	US*	Wahls Diet	Wahls Paleo	Wahls Paleo Plus	Dietary Reference Intakes†
Cholesterol and Fatty Acids					
Cholesterol, mg**	228	165	567	351	
Trans-fatty acids, g**	2.06‡	0.46	0.62	0.38	
Palmitic acid 16:0, g**	11.36	9.41	10.82	16.47	
Linoleic acid 18:2, g**	13.51	15.94	10.99	11.08	*11*
Linolenic acid 18:3, g**	1.47	3.16	3.09	2.32	
Arachidonic acid 20:4, g**	0.12	0.10	0.50	0.33	
Eicosapentaenoic acid 20:5 (EPA), g**	0.03	0.27	0.37	0.40	
Docosahexaenoic acid 22:6 (DHA), g**	0.07	0.44	0.59	0.46	
Vitamins					
Retinol, mcg**	420	341	1,406	1,388	
Vitamin B_1 (thiamin), mg **	1.4	9.3	8.7	2.7	1.1
Vitamin B_2 (riboflavin), mg**	1.9	10.4	9.7	3.8	1.1
Vitamin B_3 (niacin), mg**	21.5	72.2	84.2	38.3	14††
Vitamin B_6 (pyridoxine), mg**	1.8	10.7	10.8	3.9	1.5
Vitamin B_9 (folic acid), mcg DFE**	487	947	1137	872	400
Vitamin B_{12} (cobalamin), mcg**	4.8	19.3	23.1	14.4	2.4
Vitamin C (ascorbic acid), mg**	99	440	561	337	75
Vitamin D, mcg**	4.6	12.8	8.8	10.1	*15*
Vitamin E (total alpha-tocopherol), mg**	8.2	24.5	18.4	16.7	15
Vitamin K, mcg**	152	1,346	1,384	1,120	*90*
Minerals					
Calcium, mg**	890	1,731	957	736	1,200
Phosphorus, mg**	1,202	1,771	1,986	1,438	700
Magnesium, mg**	283	635	501	448	320
Iron, mg**	13.1	21.5	27.4	21.8	8
Zinc, mg**	9.8	16.3	31.8	18.3	8
Copper, mg**	1.2	3.0	3.6	3.2	0.9
Selenium, mcg**	95.8	118.4	209.9	129.9	55

Nutrient Comparison Tables

Nutrients	US*	Wahls Diet	Wahls Paleo	Wahls Paleo Plus	Dietary Reference Intakes†
Minerals					
Sodium, mg	2,992	2,380	3,042	2,539	*1,300*
Potassium, mg	2,592	6,140	6,234	4,807	*4,700*
Carotenoids					
Beta-carotene, mcg**	3,097	27,190	31,223	21,494	
Alpha-carotene, mcg**	490	1,510	2,745	1,717	
Beta-cryptoxanthin, mcg**	98	1,195	493	1,033	
Lutein + Zeaxanthin, mcg**	2,428	37,460	23,273	31,327	
Lycopene, mcg**	4,238	10,832	2,917	1,362	

*Mean intake for females 50–59 years in the United States, 2009–2010. Premenopausal women and men will have slightly different average intakes. http://www.ars.usda.gov/SP2UserFiles/Place/12355000/pdf/0910/Table_1_NIN_ GEN_09.pdf and http://www.ars.usda.gov/SP2UserFiles/Place/12355000/pdf/0910/Table_5_EIN_GEN_09.pdf accessed June 7, 2013.

** Key Brain Nutrients

‡ Based on median intake (third quintile) of 6,183 women ≥45 years who participated in the Women's Health Study; Annals of Neurology 72 (2012): 124–34.

† Recommended Dietary Allowances and Adequate Intakes for females 51–70 years; usual intake at or above these levels have a low probability of inadequacy. Adequate Intake values are in italics. http://www.iom.edu/Activities/ Nutrition/SummaryDRIs/DRI-Tables.aspx

†† mg niacin equivalents

Appendix C
RESOURCES

WAHLS RESOURCES

On the following pages find information for all the products and services mentioned in this book. Because resources are ever-changing, check my website, www.thewahlsprotocol.com, for the most up-to-date product and supplement recommendations.

Electrical therapy devices for NMES

https://www.djoglobal.com/products/empi/empi-continuum

I used the 300 PV manufactured by Empi initially and then transitioned to a newer device called the Continuum that also delivers NEMS to stimulate your muscles and TENS for pain control. You can go to their website to learn how to obtain an electrical therapy device, and guidance for how to obtain a prescription for the device. You can also contact Empi and purchase without a prescription. You will still need a physical therapist to design the exercise program and the electrical training program.

Functional electrical therapy cycles

http://www.restorative-therapies.com

Cycles that are powered by hand (ergonomic) or legs (bicycle) are augmented with electrical stimulation of muscles. This is another excellent training device with case examples of patients with multiple sclerosis and spinal cord injury who have benefited from using functional electrical stimulation to support the use of cycling exercise machines.

FES devices

EMPI DEVICES

http://www.djoglobal.com/products/empi/empi-continuum

This company distributes a variety of e-stim and orthopedic devices.

WALK AID
http://www.walkaide.com/en-US/Pages/default.aspx

BIONESS
http://www.bioness.com/Home.php

These devices use functional electrical stimulation, or FES. A sequential firing of the device helps the person contract muscles in the leg, pick up their toes, and flex their ankle upward as they swing their leg forward. Bioness also has devices to improve the function of the thigh muscles and improve hand function.

Whole-body vibration machines

http://www.slimvibes.com/compare.html

This site allows the consumer to compare several manufacturer and models. You will need to assemble the device once it is delivered to your home.

http://www.powerplate.com

Power Plate is a company that will deliver the device and set it up in your home.

Endless Pools

http://www.endlesspools.com

Community-supported agriculture

LOCAL HARVEST INC.
http://www.localharvest.org/csa/

This website is focused on organic and local foods. It will help you find a farmer who offers shares in a community-sponsored agriculture near you.

Omega-3 fatty acid supplements

GREEN PASTURE
http://www.greenpasture.org/public/Home/index.cfm

This company uses traditional fermentation to create fermented cod-liver oil and skate-liver oil. It also has casein-free butter oil that is particularly high in vitamin K_2 as well as coconut oil.

Organ meat capsules

DR. RUN'S ULTRA-PURE

http://www.drrons.com

If you can't get used to eating organ meat, you could consider capsules of dried organ meat. He also has a number of vitamin and other supplements.

Nutrition products based on nutrigenomics

METAGENICS

http://www.metagenics.com

Metagenics is a nutrition company that was founded by Dr. Jeffrey Bland, a nutritional biochemist who based it on the principle of using nutrition to overcome the less effective enzymes a person has because of their particular DNA.

Seaweed

MAINE COAST SEA VEGETABLES

http://www.seaveg.com/shop

High-performance blending machines

VITAMIX

http://www.Vitamix.com

Enter the code 06-004969 to get free standard shipping when ordering online.

These will cost $200 to $600 depending on the features you choose. I waited until my blender died and got a Vitamix. After that, I wondered why I had waited so long. You can look for the refurbished models and save some money that way.

HEALTH MASTER

http://www.myhealthmaster.com

Montel Williams has the Health Master, another high-performance blending machine. I have not used it, however.

Food-processing machines

Cuisinart has several food processors that you can consider. We have used the Custom 14.

http://www.cuisinart.com/products/food_processors.html

Dehydrators

Many virtual and brick-and-mortar sporting goods and camping supply stores will carry dehydrators. Prices will likely range from approximately $100 to $300 or more, depending on the features you choose.

- Open Country and Nesco are round dehydrators. You can get additional trays to make the dehydrator taller.
- Excalibur is a rectangular dehydrator that has nine trays.

Melatonin enhancing

https://www.lowbluelights.com/index.asp?

Low Blue Lights sells products to boost melatonin production naturally. This is done by limiting your exposure to light in the blue frequency range. Products will include amber-tinted glasses and amber lightbulbs.

Books

ELECTRICAL THERAPY TEXTBOOKS

- Verbová G, Hudlicka D, *Application of Muscle/Nerve Stimulation in Health and Disease (Advances in Muscle Research)* Centofanti K. New York: Springer, 2008.
  This is a reference book for the research on the use of electrical therapy to recover from injury and restore function, including the setting-in of progressive brain and spinal cord disorders. It also includes a chapter that is written as a how-to for performing electrical stimulation for the lay individual.

GROWING YOUR OWN FOOD

- Bartholomew M. *All New Square Foot Gardening.* Brentwood, TN: Cool Springs Press, 2006.
  This book is an excellent resource for growing more of your own food with less work.

IMPACT OF CHRONIC MOLD AND OTHER BIOTOXIN-RELATED PROBLEMS

- Shoemaker R. *Surviving Mold: Life in the Era of Dangerous Buildings.* Baltimore, MD: Otter Bay Books, 2010.
  The presence of mold in the internal environment of a building's ventila-

tion, heating, and cooling systems can, in the genetically susceptible person, lead to chronic fatigue and numerous medical, neurological, and psychological symptoms.

ATHEROSCLEROSIS (BLOOD VESSEL HEALTH)

- Houston M. *What Your Doctor May Not Tell You About Heart Disease.* New York: Grand Central Life and Style, 2012.

  Atherosclerosis (clogging of the arteries and veins) is very common in those with autoimmune problems.

Labs for nutritional and other functional laboratory testing

ENTEROLAB

https://www.enterolab.com/default.aspx

This lab offers testing for sensitivities to a variety of foods, including gluten, dairy, and other foods such as soy and nightshades. It also offers genetic testing for the genes that put that person at a high risk for developing a severe type of food sensitivity reaction. A physician's prescription is not required for these tests. This is how I convinced my family to go gluten- and dairy-free.

Such labs offer a wide variety of nutritional and functional medicine assessments. They have information for patients and clinicians on their web pages and can assist the layperson with finding a health care practitioner who can oversee a functional medicine evaluation.

GENOVA DIAGNOSTICS AND METAMETRIX

http://www.gdx.net/ and http://www.metametrix.com

These two companies have merged into one company. At present they still have two websites, but that will likely evolve into one website over the next two years. The tests must be ordered by a health care practitioner. They can assist the consumer with finding a health care practitioner with whom to work.

Organizations

THE VITAMIN D COUNCIL

http://www.vitamindcouncil.org

This website provides information about vitamin D deficiency, toxicity, health conditions related to vitamin D, and vitamin D supplementation for public and health professionals. You can also request a home test kit to obtain your vitamin D level without a doctor's order.

INSTITUTE FOR FUNCTIONAL MEDICINE
http://www.functionalmedicine.org

You can search the site for more information about functional medicine and use the "Find a Functional Medicine Practitioner" page to search for a provider.

ANCESTRAL HEALTH SOCIETY
http://www.ancestryfoundation.org

The Ancestral Health Society fosters interdisciplinary collaboration among scientists, health care professionals, and laypersons to promote an evolutionary perspective on current health challenges. They have many fascinating materials for anyone interested in the concepts of ancestral health and how they can apply them today.

WAHLS FOUNDATION
http://www.thewahlsfoundation.org

The Wahls Foundation, Inc. is a nonprofit entity created on May 11, 2011, whose mission is to educate the public and health care practitioners about the benefits of the Wahls diet plans, exercise, neuromuscular electrical stimulation, and other health-promoting behaviors, and to support research via the Wahls Research Fund (www.thewahlsprotocol.com).

It costs $3,000,000 to test the effectiveness of the Wahls Protocol using a randomized control. It is randomized clinical trials that are used to establish the standard of care. If you wish to become part of the team and make a tax-deductible donation to the Wahls Research Fund to help me continue my research and education program, you may do so by going to www.the wahlsprotocol.com and using the donate button there. The University of Iowa Foundation has created a special account to support the innovative work that I am doing:

https://www.givetoIowa.org/GiveToIowa/WebObjects/GiveToIowa.woa/wa/go To?area=wahls

If you wish to donate by writing a check you may do so by making it out to the University of Iowa Foundation and putting "Dr. Terry Wahls Research Account" on the memo line. Checks should be mailed to:

University of Iowa Foundation
P.O. Box 4550
Iowa City, IA 52244 U.S.A.

ACKNOWLEDGMENTS

I GOT MY LIFE BACK. I write this book so that you can get yours back, too.

This book would not be possible without the love and support of my wife, Jackie, and our children, Zach and Zebby. They are my sustenance.

There are many others who have given me critical support and encouragement in this journey. It was a global village of named and unnamed who made this work possible. There are multiple parallel journeys: the memoir, my recovery, the research, the teaching, the public outreach. All have been necessary to give birth to this book. The work on the memoir began when I thought that all I could do was create a legacy for my children, for that time when I'd no longer be there, physically or cognitively. How lucky and glad I am to be with them still, in both capacities! Critical support came from the Patient Voices Project with the University of Iowa and the editors Paul Cassel and Kate Gleeson, who worked closely with me for over a year to shape my early storytelling. Kate Gleeson connected me with my literary agent, Lynn Franklin, who saw the possibilities in my work years ahead of everyone else. Without their early guidance and support, this work would never have blossomed.

My discovery and creation of the Wahls Protocol is of course critical to this book and could not have happened without my discovery of Dr. Ashton Embry. It was his organization, the Direct-MS charity of Canada, that encouraged the very first steps in my journey back to health. This could not have happened without Dr. Lael Stone, the physician who first directed me to look at Dr. Ashton Embry's work. Through Dr. Embry, I found Loren Cordain and then eventually the Ancestral Health movement. Next I discovered the role of neuromuscular electrical stimulation through Dr. Richard Shields's work and the Institute for Functional Medicine and their community of health professionals. I especially need to thank Drs. Jeff Bland, David Jones, Catherine Willner, Jay Lombardi, David Perlmutter, Mark Hyman, Michael

Stone, Kristi Hughes, and Laurie Hoffman, their president. I have to thank my personal physicians, Drs. Lael Stone, E. Torage Shivapour, and Gwen Beck, for their willingness to work with me through the years.

In the development of the research program I have many to thank, and they include Drs. Paul Rothman, Warren Darling, Kathryn Chaloner, Linda Snetselaar, Susan Lutgendorf, Ergun Uc, E. Torage Shivapour, Garry Buettner, Jeff Murray, Zuhair Ballas, John Cowdery, Peter Cram, Nicole Nisly, and Cathy Swanson. I must specifically thank Babita Bisht, who was my first research assistant and was critical to our lab's success. I also have to thank the many undergraduate students who volunteered their time in the lab.

Big thanks to Cathy Chenard, the registered dietitian who works in my research lab and has provided critical support to the development of our study diets and this manuscript, and to Tom Nelson, our graphic designer, who created the wonderful illustrations for this book. My editor, Marisa Vigilante, has been invaluable from the beginning, nursing the early concepts for this book all the way to its current form. I must also thank Jonathan Sabin and Leanne Ely, who were key mentors as I developed my business so that I could create a website and begin spreading my message to a wider audience. Teaching the public began with an e-mail to Theresa Carbrey, the person in charge of education at the local organic food co-op, pitching the idea of giving a lecture about how changing my diet led to improvement in my MS. Theresa agreed, and over the next several years I taught many courses for the co-op. In 2011, Cliff Missen gave me the opportunity to give a presentation at the TEDx talk in November. That same summer Eve Adamson approached me as I stood in line to pick up that week's vegetables from my local CSA, suggested that we write a book together and helped me rework my book proposal. My TEDx talk went viral, and I soon had a book contract for *The Wahls Protocol*. That meant, of course, that I now had to write while also working full-time in clinic and doing my research. Fortunately for me, Eve is a tremendous writer with a vast amount of experience in crafting a how-to book for the public. It is the beginning of a partnership that I hope will produce many books.

This brings me back to all of you, the public. Every day we receive countless messages through social media, e-mails, and phone calls from people whose lives have been helped by the Wahls Protocol. It is the global village that made this work possible, and it is the global village that will reclaim its health by teaching one another that we are in charge of the food we eat and how we choose to live. With hearts filled with gratitude for having our lives back again, we teach, and the teaching spreads around the world.

NOTES

Introduction

1 Cordain L. *The Paleo Diet: Lose Weight and Get Healthy by Eating the Foods You Were Designed to Eat.* New York: John Wiley & Sons, 2002.

2 Lin Y, Desbois A, Jiang S, Hou ST. Group B vitamins protect murine cerebellar granule cells from glutamate/NMDA toxicity. *Neuroreport* 15 (2004): 2241–44.

3 Beal MF. Bioenergetic approaches for neuroprotection in Parkinson's disease. *Ann Neurol* 53, Suppl 3 (2003): S39–S47; Zhang W, Narayanan M, Friedlander RM. Additive neuroprotective effects of minocycline with creatine in a mouse model of ALS. *Ann Neurol* 53 (2003): 267–70.

4 Bisht B; Darling WG; Grossmann RE; Shivapour ET; Lutgendorf SK; Snetselaar LG; Hall MJ; Zimmerman MB; Wahls TL. A multimodal intervention for patients with secondary progressive multiple sclerosis: feasibility and effect on fatigue. *J Altern Complement Med* 20 (2014).

Chapter 1

1 Willett WC. Balancing life-style and genomics research for disease prevention. *Science* 296 (2002): 695–98.

2 Alberts B, Johnson A, Lewis J, Raff M, Roberts K, Walter P. *Molecular Biology of the Cell.* 4th ed. New York: Garland Publishing, 2002.

3 Ibid.

4 Drug Influences on Nutrient Levels and Depletion. *Natural Medicines Comprehensive Database* (serial online) 2012; available from Therapeutic Research Faculty (accessed November 16, 2012).

5 Montagna P, Sacquegna T, Martinelli P et al. Mitochondrial abnormalities in migraine. Preliminary findings. *Headache* 28 (1988): 477–80; Stuart S, Griffiths LR. A possible role for mitochondrial dysfunction in migraine. *Mol Genet Genomics* 287 (2012): 837–44; Welch KM, Ramadan NM. Mitochondria, magnesium and migraine. *J Neurol Sci* 134 (1995): 9–14.

6   Pieczenik SR, Neustadt J. Mitochondrial dysfunction and molecular pathways of disease. *Exp Mol Pathol* 83 (2007): 84–92.

7   Alberts, et al. *Molecular Biology of the Cell.*

8   Ibid.

9   Ames BN, Liu J. Delaying the mitochondrial decay of aging with acetylcarnitine. *Ann NY Acad Sci* 1033 (2004): 108–16; Ames BN. Prevention of mutation, cancer, and other age-associated diseases by optimizing micronutrient intake. *J Nucleic Acids* (2010): pii: 725071. doi: 10.4061/2010/725071.

10 Ames BN. Prevention of mutation.

11 Bowman GL, Silbert LC, Howieson D, et al. Nutrient biomarker patterns, cognitive function, and MRI measures of brain aging. *Neurology* 78 (2012): 241–49.

12 Ibid.

13 Bourre JM. Effects of nutrients (in food) on the structure and function of the nervous system: update on dietary requirements for brain. Part 2: macronutrients. *J Nutr Health Aging* 10 (2006): 386–99; Bourre JM. Effects of nutrients (in food) on the structure and function of the nervous system: update on dietary requirements for brain. Part 1: micronutrients. *J Nutr Health Aging* 10 (2006): 377–85.

14 Ames, Liu. Delaying the mitochondrial decay, 108–16.

15 Bourre. Effects of nutrients (in food), part 2: macronutrients, 386–99; Bourre. Effects of nutrients (in food): part 1: micronutrients, 377–85.

16 Mateljan G. *The World's Healthiest Foods.* Seattle, Washington: World's Healthiest Foods, 2006; Higden J, Drake V. *An Evidence-Based Approach to Dietary Phytochemicals* [serial online], 2012.

17 Ibid.; The World's Healthiest Foods, www.whfoods.com, updated March 24, 2013; The George Mateljan Foundation (accessed May 22, 2013); Ground Beef Calculator, http://ndb.nal.usda.gov/ndb/beef/show, updated January 13, 2012; Nutrient Data Laboratory United States Department of Agriculture (accessed March 5, 2013; online interactive database); Linus Pauling Institute Micronutrient Research for Optimum Health, Oregon State University, http://lpi.ore gonstate.edu/infocenter (accessed May 22, 2013).

18 Frankl V. *Man's Search for Meaning.* Rev., updated ed., Boston: Beacon Press, 2006.

Chapter 2

1   Wucherpfennig KW. Structural basis of molecular mimicry. *J Autoimmun* 16 (2001): 293–302.

2   Ramagopalan SV, Sadovnick AD. Epidemiology of multiple sclerosis. *Neurol Clin* 29 (2011): 207–17.

3   Zamboni P, Menegatti E, Bartolomei I, et al. Intracranial venous haemodynamics in multiple sclerosis. *Curr Neurovasc Res* 4 (2007): 252–58; Zamboni P, Galeotti R, Menegatti E, et al. Chronic cerebrospinal venous insufficiency in patients with multiple sclerosis. *J Neurol Neurosurg Psychiatry* 80 (2009): 392–99.

4   Malagoni AM, Galeotti R, Menegatti E, et al. Is chronic fatigue the symptom of venous insufficiency associated with multiple sclerosis? A longitudinal pilot study. *Int Angiol* 29 (2010): 176–82.

5   Mandato KD, Hegener PF, Siskin GP, et al. Safety of endovascular treatment of chronic cerebrospinal venous insufficiency: a report of 240 patients with multiple sclerosis. *J Vasc Interv Radiol* 23 (2012): 55–59; Zamboni P, Galeotti R, Weinstock-Guttman B, Kennedy C, Salvi F, Zivadinov R. Venous angioplasty in patients with multiple sclerosis: results of a pilot study. *Eur J Vasc Endovasc Surg* 43 (2012): 116–22.

6   Marder E, Gupta P, Greenberg BM, et al. No cerebral or cervical venous insufficiency in US veterans with multiple sclerosis. *Arch Neurol* 68 (2011): 1521–25.

7   Blasi C. The autoimmune origin of atherosclerosis. *Atherosclerosis* 201 (2008): 17–32.

8   Virtanen JK, Rissanen TH, Voutilainen S, Tuomainen TP. Mercury as a risk factor for cardiovascular diseases. *J Nutr Biochem* 18 (2007): 75–85.

9   Blasi F, Tarsia P, Arosio C, Fagetti L, Allegra L. Epidemiology of *Chlamydia pneumoniae*. *Clin Microbiol Infect* 4 Suppl 4 (1998): S1–S6.

10 Dyslipidemia: Nutritional and Nutraceutical Functional Medicine Approach. Cardiometabolic Module, 2012 Annual International Symposium, Institute for Functional Medicine, Gig Harbor, Washington, June 1, 2012.

11 The New Era of Managing Cardiovascular Disease, Metabolic Dysfunctions and Obesity. Cardiometabolic Module, 2012 Annual International Symposium, Institute for Functional Medicine, Scottsdale, Arizona, May 31, 2012.

12 Fire in the Hole: The Metabolic Connecting Points Between Major Chronic Diseases. Cardiometabolic Module, 2012 Annual International Symposium, Institute for Functional Medicine, Scottsdale, Arizona, May 30, 2012.

13 Bland JS, Levin B, Costarella L, et al. *Clinical Nutrition: A Functional Approach.* 2nd ed. Gig Harbor, Washington: Institute for Functional Medicine, 2004.

14 Fire in the Hole: The Metabolic Connecting Points Between Major Chronic Diseases. Cardiometabolic Module, 2012 Annual International Symposium, Institute for Functional Medicine, Scottsdale, Arizona, May 30, 2012.

15 Dean B. Understanding the role of inflammatory-related pathways in the pathophysiology and treatment of psychiatric disorders: evidence from human peripheral studies and CNS studies. *Int J Neuropsychopharmacol* 14 (2011): 997–1012; Suvisaari J, Loo BM, Saarni SE, et al. Inflammation in psychotic disorders: a population-based study. *Psychiatry Res* 189 (2011): 305–11.

16 Kaptoge S, Di Angelantonio E, Lowe G, et al. C-reactive protein concentration and risk of coronary heart disease, stroke, and mortality: an individual participant meta-analysis. *Lancet* 375 (2010): 132–40.

17 Lord RS, Bralley A. *Laboratory Evaluations for Integrative and Functional Medicine*, 2nd ed. Atlanta, GA: Metametrix Institute, 2008.

18 Ames, BN. Prevention of mutation; Ames. Delaying the mitochondrial decay, 108–61; Ames. Prevention of mutation; Ames. Optimal micronutrients delay mitochondrial decay and age-associated diseases. *Mech Ageing Dev* 131 (2010): 473–79.

19 Dyslipidemia: Nutritional and Nutraceutical Functional Medicine Approach. Cardiometabolic Module, 2012 Annual International symposium, Institute for Functional Medicine, Gig Harbor, Washington, June 1, 2012; The New Era of Managing Cardiovascular Disease, Metabolic Dysunctions and Obesity. Cardiometabolic Module, 2012 Annual International Symposium, Institute for Functional Medicine, Scottsdale, Arizona, May 31, 2012; Fire in the Hole: The Metabolic Connecting Points Between Major Chronic Diseases. Cardiometabolic Module, 2012 Annual International Symposium, Institute for Functional Medicine, Scottsdale, Arizona, May 30, 2012.

20 Ibid.

Chapter 3

1 Koizumi M, Ito H, Kaneko Y, Motohashi Y. Effect of having a sense of purpose in life on the risk of death from cardiovascular diseases. *J Epidemiol* 18 (2008): 191–96.

2 Ventegodt S, Andersen NJ, Merrick J. The life mission theory II. The structure of the life purpose and the ego. *Scientific World Journal* 3 (2003): 1277–85.

3 Emmons R, McCullough E. *The Psychology of Gratitude*. New York: Oxford University Press, 2004.

Chapter 4

1 Adams KM, Lindell KC, Kohlmeier M, Zeisel SH. Status of nutrition education in medical schools. *Am J Clin Nutr* 83 (2006): 941S–944S.

2 Cordain L, Eaton SB, Sebastian A, Mann N, Lindeberg S, Watkins BA, O'Keefe JH et al., eds. Origins and evolution of the Western diet: health implications for the 21st century, *Am J Clin Nutr* 81:2 (2005): 341–45; Cordain L, Eaton SB, Miller JB, Mann N, Hill K. The paradoxical nature of hunter-gatherer diets: meat-based, yet non-atherogenic. *Eur J Clin Nutr* 56, Suppl 1 (2002): S42–S52; Cordain L, Eades MR, Eades MD. Hyperinsulinemic diseases of civilization: more than just Syndrome X. *Comp Biochem Physiol A Mol Integr Physiol* 36 (2003): 95–112; Eaton SB, Konner M, Shostak M. Stone agers in the fast lane: chronic degenerative diseases in evolutionary perspective. *Am J Med* 84 (1988): 739–49.

3 Gurven M, Kaplan H. Longevity Among Hunter-Gatherers: A Cross-Cultural Examination. *Population and Development Review* 33 (2007): 321–65.

4 Mummert A, Esche E, Robinson J, Armelagos GJ. Stature and robusticity during the agricultural transition: evidence from the bioarchaeological record. *Econ Hum Biol* 9 (2011): 284-301; Sajantila A. Major historical dietary changes are reflected in the dental microbiome of ancient skeletons. *Investig Genet* 4 (2013): 10.

5 Gurven M, Kaplan H. Longevity Among Hunter-Gatherers, 321–65; Mummert A, Esche E, Robinson J, Armelagos GJ. Stature and robusticity during the agricultural transition: evidence from the bioarchaeological record. *Econ Hum Biol* 9 (2011): 284-301.

6 Sajantila A. Major historical dietary changes are reflected in the dental microbiome of ancient skeletons. *Investig Genet* 4 (2013): 10; Egger G. Health, "illth," and economic growth: medicine, environment, and economics at the crossroads. *Am J Prev Med* 37 (2009): 78–83.

7 Obesity and Overweight (updated May 13, 2012), Centers for Disease Control and Prevention, http://www.cdc.gov/nchs/fastats/overwt.htm (accessed August 18, 2013).

8 Frassetto LA, Schloetter M, Mietus-Synder M, Morris RC, Jr., Sebastian A. Metabolic and physiologic improvements from consuming a paleolithic, hunter-gatherer type diet. *Eur J Clin Nutr* 63 (2009): 947–55; Osterdahl M, Kocturk T, Koochek A, Wandell PE. Effects of a short-term intervention with a paleolithic diet in healthy volunteers. *Eur J Clin Nutr* 62 (2008): 682–85.

9 Jonsson T, Granfeldt Y, Ahren B, et al. Beneficial effects of a Paleolithic diet on cardiovascular risk factors in type 2 diabetes: a randomized cross-over pilot study. *Cardiovasc Diabetol* 8 (2009): 35.

10 Fasano A. Leaky gut and autoimmune diseases. *Clin Rev Allergy Immunol* 42

(2012): 71–78; Guandalini S, Newland C. Differentiating food allergies from food intolerances. *Curr Gastroenterol Rep* 13 (2011): 426–34.

11 Sanfilippo, D. *Practical Paleo: A Customized Approach to Health and a Whole-Foods Lifestyle.* Auberry, CA: Victory Belt Publishing, 2012.

12 Calton, M, Calton J. *Naked Calories: The Caltons' Simple 3 Step Plan to Micronutrient Sufficiency.* Cleveland, Ohio: Changing Lives Press, 2013.

13 Treem WR. Emerging concepts in celiac disease. *Curr Opin Pediatr* 16 (2004): 552–59.

14 Fallon S, Enig MG. *Nourishing Traditions.*

Chapter 5

1 Moriya M, Nakatsuji Y, Okuno T, Hamasaki T, Sawada M, Sakoda S. Vitamin K2 ameliorates experimental autoimmune encephalomyelitis in Lewis rats. *J Neuroimmunol* 170 (2005): 11–20.

2 Ferland G. Vitamin K and the nervous system: an overview of its actions. *Adv Nutr* 3 (2012): 204–12; Ferland G. Vitamin K, an emerging nutrient in brain function. *Biofactors* 38 (2012): 151–57.

3 Watzl B. Anti-inflammatory effects of plant-based foods and of their constituents. *Int J Vitam Nutr Res* 78 (2008): 293–98; Shukitt-Hale B, Lau FC, Joseph JA. Berry fruit supplementation and the aging brain. *J Agric Food Chem* 56 (2008): 636–41; Joseph J, Cole G, Head E, Ingram D. Nutrition, brain aging, and neurodegeneration. *J Neurosci* 29 (2009): 12:795–801; Holt EM, Steffen LM, Moran A, et al. Fruit and vegetable consumption and its relation to markers of inflammation and oxidative stress in adolescents. *J Am Diet Assoc* 109 (2009): 414–21.

4 Webb AJ, Patel N, Loukogeorgakis S, et al. Acute blood pressure lowering, vasoprotective, and antiplatelet properties of dietary nitrate via bioconversion to nitrite. *Hypertension* 51 (2008): 784–90.

5 Frostegard J. *Arteriosler Thromb Vasc Biol.* 9 (2005): 1776–85.

6 Guerrero-Beltran CE, Calderon-Oliver M, Pedraza-Chaverri J, Chirino YI. Protective effect of sulforaphane against oxidative stress: recent advances. *Exp Toxicol Pathol* 64 (2012): 503–508; Morihara N, Sumioka I, Moriguchi T, Uda N, Kyo E. Aged garlic extract enhances production of nitric oxide. *Life Sci* 71 (2002): 509–17; Noyan-Ashraf MH, Sadeghinejad Z, Juurlink BH. Dietary approach to decrease aging-related CNS inflammation. *Nutr Neurosci* 8 (2005): 101–10; Ping Z, Liu W, Kang Z et al. Sulforaphane protects brains against hypoxic-ischemic injury through induction of Nrf2-dependent phase 2 enzyme.

Brain Res 1343 (2010): 178–85; Thakur AK, Chatterjee SS, Kumar V. Beneficial effects of Brassica juncea on cognitive functions in rats. *Pharm Biol* 51 (2013): 1304–10; Holt EM, Steffen LM, Moran A, et al. Fruit and vegetable consumption and its relation to markers of inflammation and oxidative stress in adolescents. *J Am Diet Assoc* 109 (2009): 414–21; Vasanthi HR, Mukherjee S, Das DK. Potential health benefits of broccoli: a chemico-biological overview. *Mini Rev Med Chem* 9 (2009): 749–59; Wierinckx A, Breve J, Mercier D, Schultzberg M, Drukarch B, Van Dam AM. Detoxication enzyme inducers modify cytokine production in rat mixed glial cells. *J Neuroimmunol* 166 (2005): 132–43.

7   Guerrero-Beltran CE, Calderon-Oliver M, Pedraza-Chaverri J, Chirino YI. Protective effect of sulforaphane against oxidative stress: recent advances. *Exp Toxicol Pathol* 64 (2012): 503–508; Latte KP, Appel KE, Lampen A. Health benefits and possible risks of broccoli: an overview. *Food Chem Toxicol* 49 (2011): 3287–3309; Vasanthi HR, Mukherjee S, Das DK. Potential health benefits of broccoli, 749–59; Williams MJ, Sutherland WH, McCormick MP, Yeoman DJ, de Jong SA. Aged garlic extract improves endothelial function in men with coronary artery disease. *Phytother Res* 19 (2005): 314–19.

8   Borek C. Garlic reduces dementia and heart-disease risk. *J Nutr* 136 (2006): 810S–812S; Chauhan NB. Multiplicity of garlic health effects and Alzheimer's disease. *J Nutr Health Aging* 9 (2005): 421–32.

9   Borek C. Antioxidant health effects of aged garlic extract. *J Nutr* 131 (2001): 1010S–1015S; Borek C. Garlic reduces dementia, 810S–812S; Williams MJ, Sutherland WH, McCormick MP, Yeoman DJ, de Jong SA. Aged garlic extract improves endothelial function, 314–19.

10 Akramiene D, Kondrotas A, Didziapetriene J, Kevelaitis E. Effects of beta-glucans on the immune system. *Medicina* (Kaunas, Lithuania) 43 (2007): 597–606.

11 Lull C, Wichers HJ, Savelkoul HF. Antiinflammatory and immunomodulating properties of fungal metabolites. *Mediators Inflamm* June 9, 2005(2): 63-80; Borek C. Antioxidant health effects; 1010S–1015S; Akramiene D, Kondrotas A, Didziapetriene J, Kevelaitis E. Effects of beta-glucans on the immune system. *Medicina* (Kaunas, Lithuania) 43 (2007): 597–606.

12 Chatrou ML, Winckers K, Hackeng TM, Reutelingsperger CP, Schurgers LJ. Vascular calcification: the price to pay for anticoagulation therapy with vitamin K-antagonists. *Blood Rev* 26 (2012): 155–66; Shea MK, Holden RM. Vitamin K status and vascular calcification: evidence from observational and clinical studies. *Adv Nutr* 3 (2012): 158–65.

13 Huebner FR, Lieberman KW, Rubino RP, Wall JS. Demonstration of high opioid-like activity in isolated peptides from wheat gluten hydrolysates. *Peptides* 5 (1984): 1139–47; Teschemacher H, Koch G. Opioids in the milk. *Endocr Regul* 25 (1991): 147–50.

14 Gearhardt AN, Davis C, Kuschner R, Brownell KD. The addiction potential of hyperpalatable foods. *Curr Drug Abuse Rev* 4 (2011): 140–45.

15 *Textbook of Functional Medicine.* Gig Harbor, Washington: Institute for Functional Medicine, 2010; Brown AC. Gluten sensitivity: problems of an emerging condition separate from celiac disease. *Expert Rev Gastroenterol Hepatol* 6 (2012): 43–55; Cascella NG, Kryszak D, Bhatti B et al. Prevalence of celiac disease and gluten sensitivity in the United States clinical antipsychotic trials of intervention effectiveness study population. *Schizophr Bull* 37 (2011): 94–100; da Silva Neves MM, Gonzalez-Garcia MB, Nouws HP, Delerue-Matos C, Santos-Silva A, Costa-Garcia A. Celiac disease diagnosis and gluten-free food analytical control. *Anal Bioanal Chem* 397 (2010): 1743–53; Hadjivassiliou M, Grunewald RA, Lawden M, Davies-Jones GA, Powell T, Smith CM. Headache and CNS white matter abnormalities associated with gluten sensitivity. *Neurology* 56 (2001): 385–88; Hadjivassiliou M, Sanders DS, Grunewald RA, Woodroofe N, Boscolo S, Aeschlimann D. Gluten sensitivity: from gut to brain. *Lancet Neurol* 9 (2010: 318–30; Humbert P, Pelletier F, Dreno B, Puzenat E, Aubin F. Gluten intolerance and skin diseases. *Eur J Dermatol* 16 (2006): 4–11; Jackson JR, Eaton WW, Cascella NG, Fasano A, Kelly DL. Neurologic and psychiatric manifestations of celiac disease and gluten sensitivity. *Psychiatr Q* 83 (2012): 91–102; Valentino R, Savastano S, Maglio M, et al. Markers of potential coeliac disease in patients with Hashimoto's thyroiditis. *Eur J Endocrinol* 146 (2002): 479–83; Vereckei E, Szodoray P, Poor G, Kiss E. Genetic and immunological processes in the pathomechanism of gluten-sensitive enteropathy and associated metabolic bone disorders. *Autoimmun Rev* 10 (2011): 336–40.

16 *Textbook of Functional Medicine.* Gig Harbor, Washington: Institute for Functional Medicine, 2010.

Chapter 6

1 Miller GJ, Field RA, Riley ML. Lipids in wild ruminant animals and steers. *J Food Qual* 9 (1986): 331–41.

2 The New Era of Managing Cardiovascular Disease, Metabolic Dysfunctions and Obesity. Cardiometabolic Module, 2012 Annual International Symposium, Institute for Functional Medicine, Scottsdale, Arizona, May 31, 2012.

3 Simopoulos AP. Human requirement for N-3 polyunsaturated fatty acids. *Poult Sci* 79 (2000): 961–70.

4 Simopoulos AP. The importance of the omega-6/omega-3 fatty acid ratio in cardiovascular disease and other chronic diseases. *Exp Biol Med (Maywood)* 233 (2008): 674–88; Simopoulos AP. Importance of the omega-6/omega-3 balance in health and disease: evolutionary aspects of diet. *World Rev Nutr Diet* 102 (2011): 10–21.

5 Simopoulos AP. The importance of the omega-6/omega-3 fatty acid ratio, 674–88.

6 Deal CL, Moskowitz RW. Nutraceuticals as therapeutic agents in osteoarthritis. The role of glucosamine, chondroitin sulfate, and collagen hydrolysate. *Rheum Dis Clin North Am* 25 (1999): 379–95.

7 Replace and Replenish: Treatment of Digestive Dysfunction. Advance Practice Module: Restoring Gastrointestinal Equilibrium: Practical Applications for Understanding, Assessing and Treating GI Dysfunction. Conference, Institute for Functional Medicine, Scottsdale, Arizona, December 9, 2011.

8 Young GS, Conquer JA, Thomas R. Effect of randomized supplementation with high dose olive, flax or fish oil on serum phospholipid fatty acid levels in adults with attention deficit hyperactivity disorder. *Reprod Nutr Dev* 45 (2005): 549–58.

9 Tripoli E, Giammanco M, Tabacchi G, Di Majo D, Giammanco S, La Guardia M. The phenolic compounds of olive oil: structure, biological activity and beneficial effects on human health. *Nutr Res Rev* 18 (2005): 98–112.

10 Muskiet FAJ. Fat Detection, Taste, Texture, and Post Ingestive Effects, Chapter 2, 19–79, in Pathophysiology and Evolutionary Aspects of Dietary Fats and Long-Chain Polyunsaturated Fatty Acids Across the Life Cycle. Boca Raton, FL: CRC Press, 2009; Kavanagh K, Jones KL, Sawyer J, et al. Trans fat diet induces abdominal obesity and changes in insulin sensitivity in monkeys. *Obesity (Silver Spring)* 15 (2007): 1675–84.

11 Bowman GL, Silbert LC, Howieson D, et al. Nutrient biomarker patterns, 241–49.

12 Ibid.

13 Urbano G, Lopez-Jurado M, Aranda P, Vidal-Valverde C, Tenorio E, Porres J. The role of phytic acid in legumes: antinutrient or beneficial function? *J Physiol Biochem* 56 (2000): 283–94.

14 Cordain L, Toohey L, Smith MJ, Hickey MS. Modulation of immune function by dietary lectins in rheumatoid arthritis. *Br J Nutr* 83 (2000): 207–17.

15 Flavin DF. The effects of soybean trypsin inhibitors on the pancreas of animals and man: a review. *Vet Hum Toxicol* 24 (1982): 25–28.

16 Mensah P, Tomkins A. Household-level technologies to improve the availability and preparation of adequate and safe complementary foods. *Food Nutr Bull* 24 (2003): 104–25.

17 Gasnier C, Dumont C, Benachour N, Clair E, Chagnon MC, Seralini GE. Glyphosate-based herbicides are toxic and endocrine disruptors in human cell lines. *Toxicology* 262 (2009): 184–91; Richard S, Moslemi S, Sipahutar H, Benachour N, Seralini GE. Differential effects of glyphosate and roundup on human placental cells and aromatase. *Environ Health Perspect* 113 (2005): 716–20.

18 Samsel A, Seneff S. Glyphosate's Suppression of Cytochrome P450 Enzymes and Amino Acid Biosynthesis by the Gut Microbiome: Pathways to Modern Diseases. *Entropy* (2013) 15: 1416–63.

19 McEvoy M. Organic 101: Can GMOs Be Used in Organic Products? (updated May 13, 2013), United States Department of Agriculture, http://blogs.usda.gov /2013/05/17/organic-101-can-gmos-be-used-in-organic-products (accessed July 21, 2013).

20 Cordain L, Toohey L, Smith MJ, Hickey MS. Modulation of immune function by dietary lectins, 207–17.

21 Berk Z. Technology of production of edible flours and protein products from soybeans, 1992. Rome, Food and Agriculture Organization of the United Nations (updated July 8, 2012); http://www.fao.org/docrep/t0532e/t0532e00.htm (accessed June 15, 2013).

22 Tang G. Bioconversion of dietary provitamin A carotenoids to vitamin A in humans. *Am J Clin Nutr* 91 (2010): 1468S–1473S.

23 Carmel R. Nutritional vitamin-B12 deficiency. Possible contributory role of subtle vitamin-B12 malabsorption. *Ann Intern Med* 88 (1978): 647–49; Dastur DK, Santhadevi N, Quadros EV, et al. Interrelationships between the B-vitamins in B12-deficiency neuromyelopathy. A possible malabsorption-malnutrition syndrome. *Am J Clin Nutr* 28 (1975): 1255–70.

24 Blumenschine RJ, Cavallo JA. Scavenging and human evolution. *Sci Am* 267 (1992): 90–96.

25 Cooksley VG. *Seaweed: Nature's Secret to Balancing Your Metabolism, Fighting Disease, and Revitalizing Body & Soul.* New York: Stewart, Tabori & Chang, 2007.

26 Brownstein D. *Iodine: Why You Need It, Why You Can't Live Without It.* 3rd ed. West Bloomfield, IN: Medical Alternative Press, 2004.

27 Ibid.

28 Becker G, Osterloh K, Schafer S, et al. Influence of fucoidan on the intestinal absorption of iron, cobalt, manganese and zinc in rats. *Digestion* 21 (1981): 6–12; Tanaka Y, Waldron-Edward D, Skoryna SC. Studies on inhibition of intestinal absorption of radioactive strontium. VII. Relationship of biological activity to chemical composition of alginates obtained from North American seaweeds. *Can Med Assoc J* 99 (1968): 169–75.

29 Damonte EB, Matulewicz MC, Cerezo AS. Sulfated seaweed polysaccharides as antiviral agents. *Curr Med Chem* 11 (2004): 2399–2419.

30 Price WA. *Nutrition and Physical Degeneration.* 8th ed. Lemon Grove, CA, Price Pottinger Nutrition, 2008; Fallon S, Enig MG. *Nourishing Traditions: The Cookbook that Challenges Politically Correct Nutrition and the Diet Dictocrats.* Rev. second ed. Washington, DC: New Trends, 2007.

31 Fallon S, Enig MG. *Nourishing Traditions.*

32 Ibid.

33 Ibid.

34 Howell E. *Enzyme Nutrition.* Garden City Park, New York: Avery Publishing Group, 1995.

35 Holmes E, Li JV, Marchesi JR, Nicholson JK. Gut microbiota composition and activity in relation to host metabolic phenotype and disease risk. *Cell Metab* 16 (2012): 559–64; Moschen AR, Wieser V, Tilg H. Dietary Factors: Major Regulators of the Gut's Microbiota. *Gut Liver* 6 (2012): 411–16.

36 Cordain L, Eaton SB, Sebastian A, Mann N, Lindeberg S, Watkins BA, O'Keefe JH, et al., eds. Origins and evolution of the Western diet: health implications for the 21st century. *Am J Clin Nutr* 81 (2005): 341–45.

37 Benito-Leon J, Pisa D, Alonso R, Calleja P, Diaz-Sanchez M, Carrasco L. Association between multiple sclerosis and Candida species: evidence from a case-control study. *Eur J Clin Microbiol Infect Dis* 29 (2010): 1139–45.

38 *Neuroprotection: A Functional Medicine Approach for Common and Uncommon Neurologic Syndromes.* Institute for Functional Medicine, San Diego, California, February 11–13, 2005 (conference and continuing education module, including DVDs).

39 *Textbook of Functional Medicine.* Gig Harbor, Washington: Institute for Functional Medicine, 2010; *Clinical Nutrition: A Functional Approach.* 2 ed. Levin JS, Levin B, Costarella L, et al. Gig Harbor, Washington: Institute for Functional Medicine, 2004.

Chapter 7

1 Guelpa G. La lutte contre l'épilepsie par la désintoxication et par la rééduca-
tion alimentaire. *Rev Ther Medico-Chirurgicale* 78 (1911): 8–13.

2 Wilder RM. High fat diets in epilepsy. *Mayo Clin Bull* 2 (1921):308. see Wilder
RM. High fat diets in epilepsy. *Mayo Clin Bull* 2 (1921):308.

3 Peterman MG. The ketogenic diet in epilepsy. JAMA 84 (1925): 1979–83.

4 Huttenlocher PR, Wilbourn AJ, Signore JM. Medium-chain triglycerides as a
therapy for intractable childhood epilepsy. *Neurology* 21 (1971): 1097–1103.

5 Balietti M, Casoli T, Di Stefano G, Giorgetti B, Aicardi G, Fattoretti P. Ketogenic diets: an historical antiepileptic therapy with promising potentialities for
the aging brain. *Ageing Res Rev* 9 (2010): 273–79; Maalouf M, Rho JM, Mattson
MP. The neuroprotective properties of calorie restriction, the ketogenic diet,
and ketone bodies. *Brain Res Rev* 59 (2009): 293–315; Milder J, Patel M. Modulation of oxidative stress and mitochondrial function by the ketogenic diet.
Epilepsy Res 100 (2012): 295–303; Rho JM, Stafstrom CE. The ketogenic diet:
what has science taught us? *Epilepsy Res* 100 (2012): 210–17; Stafstrom CE, Rho
JM. The ketogenic diet as a treatment paradigm for diverse neurological disorders. *Front Pharmacol* 3 (2012): 59; Zhao Z, Lange DJ, Voustianiouk A, et al. A
ketogenic diet as a potential novel therapeutic intervention in amyotrophic
lateral sclerosis. BMC *Neurosci* 7 (2006): 29.

6 Seyfried T. *Cancer as a Metabolic Disease: On the Origin, Management, and
Prevention of Cancer.* New York: John Wiley & Sons, 2012.

7 *Neuroprotection: A Functional Medicine Approach for Common and Uncommon
Neurologic Syndromes.* Institute for Functional Medicine, San Diego, California, February 11–13, 2005 (conference and continuing education module, including DVDs).

8 Fontan-Lozano A, Lopez-Lluch G, Delgado-Garcia JM, Navas P, Carrion AM.
Molecular bases of caloric restriction regulation of neuronal synaptic plasticity.
Mol Neurobiol 38 (2008): 167–77.

Chapter 8

1 Carson R. *Silent Spring.* Orlando, FL: Houghton Mifflin Harcourt, 1962.

2 Toxicity: Mechanisms of Toxic Insult and Recognizable Patterns. Detoxifica-
tion Advanced Practice Module Detox: Understanding Biotransformation and
Recognizing Toxicity, Evaluation and Treatment in the Functional Medicine
Model, Institute for Functional Medicine, 2011 conference, Phoenix, Arizona,
December 9, 2011.

3 Ibid.

4 Choi AL, Sun G, Zhang Y, Grandjean P. Developmental fluoride neurotoxicity: a systematic review and meta-analysis. *Environ Health Perspect* 120 (2012): 1362–8.

Chapter 9

1 Velikonja O, Curic K, Ozura A, Jazbec SS. Influence of sports climbing and yoga on spasticity, cognitive function, mood and fatigue in patients with multiple sclerosis. *Clin Neurol Neurosurg* 112 (2010): 597–601.

2 Dalgas U, Stenager E, Jakobsen J, et al. Resistance training improves muscle strength and functional capacity in multiple sclerosis. *Neurology* 73 (2009): 1478–84; Dalgas U, Stenager E, Jakobsen J, et al. Fatigue, mood and quality of life improve in MS patients after progressive resistance training. *Mult Scler* 16 (2010): 480–90.

3 Kileff J, Ashburn A. A pilot study of the effect of aerobic exercise on people with moderate disability multiple sclerosis. *Clin Rehabil* 19 (2005): 165–69.

4 Carro E, Trejo JL, Busiguina S, Torres-Aleman I. Circulating insulin-like growth factor I mediates the protective effects of physical exercise against brain insults of different etiology and anatomy. *J Neurosci* 21 (2001): 5678–84; Carro E, Trejo JL, Nunez A, Torres-Aleman I. Brain repair and neuroprotection by serum insulin-like growth factor I. *Mol Neurobiol* 27 (2003): 153–62; Cotman CW, Berchtold NC, Christie LA. Exercise builds brain health: key roles of growth factor cascades and inflammation. *Trends Neurosci* 30 (2007): 464–72; White LJ, Castellano V. Exercise and brain health: implications for multiple sclerosis. Part II: immune factors and stress hormones. *Sports Med* 38 (2008): 179–86.

5 de la Cerda P, Cervello E, Cocca A, Viciana J. Effect of an aerobic training program as complementary therapy in patients with moderate depression. *Percept Mot Skills* 112 (2011): 761–69.

6 White LJ, Castellano V. Exercise and brain health, 179–86; Cotman CW, Berchtold NC, Christie LA. Exercise builds brain health, 464–72.

7 Rojas Vega S, Knicker A, Hollmann W, Bloch W, Struder HK. Effect of resistance exercise on serum levels of growth factors in humans. *Horm Metab Res* 42 (2010): 982–86.

8 Velikonja O, Curic K, Ozura A, Jazbec SS. Influence of sports climbing and yoga, 597–601.

9 Gorgey AS, Mather KJ, Cupp HR, Gater DR. Effects of resistance training on

adiposity and metabolism after spinal cord injury. *Med Sci Sports Exerc* 44 (2012): 165–74.

10 Sitja-Rabert M, Rigau D, Fort Vanmeerghaeghe A, Romero-Rodriguez D, Bonastre Subirana M, Bonfill X. Efficacy of whole body vibration exercise in older people: a systematic review. *Disabil Rehabil* 34 (2012): 883–93.

11 Arena R, Pinkstaff S, Wheeler E, Peberdy MA, Guazzi M, Myers J. Neuromuscular electrical stimulation and inspiratory muscle training as potential adjunctive rehabilitation options for patients with heart failure. *J Cardiopulm Rehabil Prev* 30 (2010): 209–23; Quittan M, Wiesinger GF, Sturm B, et al. Improvement of thigh muscles by neuromuscular electrical stimulation in patients with refractory heart failure: a single-blind, randomized, controlled trial. *Am J Phys Med Rehabil* 80 (2001): 206–14.

12 Sillen MJ, Speksnijder CM, Eterman RM, Janssen PP, Wagers SS, Wouters EF, Uszko-Lencer NH, Spruit MA. Effects of neuromuscular electrical stimulation of muscles of ambulation in patients with chronic heart failure or COPD: a systematic review of the English-language literature. *Chest.*, 136 (2009):44–61. doi: 10.1378/chest.08-2481.

13 Talbot LA, Gaines JM, Ling SM, Metter EJ. A home-based protocol of electrical muscle stimulation for quadriceps muscle strength in older adults with osteoarthritis of the knee. *J Rheumatol* 30 (2003): 1571–78; Palmieri-Smith RM, Thomas AC, Karvonen-Gutierrez C, Sowers M. A clinical trial of neuromuscular electrical stimulation in improving quadriceps muscle strength and activation among women with mild and moderate osteoarthritis. *Phys Ther* 90 (2010): 1441–52; Gaines JM, Metter EJ, Talbot LA. The effect of neuromuscular electrical stimulation on arthritis knee pain in older adults with osteoarthritis of the knee. *Appl Nurs Res* 17 (2004): 201–6.

14 Piva SR, Goodnite EA, Azuma K, et al. Neuromuscular electrical stimulation and volitional exercise for individuals with rheumatoid arthritis: a multiple-patient case report. *Phys Ther* 87 (2007): 1064–77.

15 Santos M, Zahner LH, McKiernan BJ, Mahnken JD, Quaney B. Neuromuscular electrical stimulation improves severe hand dysfunction for individuals with chronic stroke: a pilot study. *J Neurol Phys Ther* 30 (2006): 175–83; Sullivan JE, Hedman LD. A home program of sensory and neuromuscular electrical stimulation with upper-limb task practice in a patient 5 years after a stroke. *Phys Ther* 84 (2004): 1045–54.

16 Stackhouse SK, Binder-Macleod SA, Stackhouse CA, McCarthy JJ, Prosser LA, Lee SC. Neuromuscular electrical stimulation versus volitional isometric

strength training in children with spastic diplegic cerebral palsy: a preliminary study. *Neurorehabil Neural Repair* 21 (2007): 475–85; Carmick J. Clinical use of neuromuscular electrical stimulation for children with cerebral palsy, Part 1, 505–13; Carmick J. Clinical use of neuromuscular electrical stimulation for children with cerebral palsy, Part 2: Upper extremity. *Phys Ther* 73 (1993): 514–22; Scheker LR, Chesher SP, Ramirez S. Neuromuscular electrical stimulation, 226–32.

17 Wahls, TL, Reese D, Kaplan D, Darling WG. Rehabilitation with neuromuscular electrical stimulation leads to functional gains in patients with secondary progressive and primary progressive multiple sclerosis: a case series report. *J Altern Complement Med* 16 (2010): 1343–49.

18 Burridge J, Taylor P, Hagan S, Swain I. Experience of clinical use of the Odstock dropped foot stimulator. *Artif Organs* 21 (1997): 254–60; Taylor PN, Burridge JH, Dunkerley AL, et al. Clinical use of the Odstock dropped foot stimulator: its effect on the speed and effort of walking. *Arch Phys Med Rehabil* 80 (1999): 1577–83.

19 Courtney AM, Castro-Borrero W, Davis SL, Frohman TC, Frohman EM. Functional treatments in multiple sclerosis. *Curr Opin Neurol* 24 (2011): 250–54; McClurg D, Ashe RG, Marshall K, Lowe-Strong AS. Comparison of pelvic floor muscle training, electromyography biofeedback, and neuromuscular electrical stimulation for bladder dysfunction in people with multiple sclerosis: a randomized pilot study. *Neurourol Urodyn* 25 (2006): 337–48.

20 Szecsi J, Schlick C, Schiller M, Pollmann W, Koenig N, Straube A. Functional electrical stimulation-assisted cycling of patients with multiple sclerosis: biomechanical and functional outcome: a pilot study. *J Rehabil Med* 41 (2009): 674–80; Ratchford JN, Shore W, Hammond ER, et al. A pilot study of functional electrical stimulation cycling in progressive multiple sclerosis. *NeuroRehabilitation* 27 (2010): 121–28.

Chapter 10

1 Smolders J. Vitamin D and multiple sclerosis: correlation, causality, and controversy. *Autoimmune Dis* 2011 (2011): 629538; Mowry EM. Vitamin D: evidence for its role as a prognostic factor in multiple sclerosis. *J Neurol Sci* 311 (2011): 19–22.

2 Yang CY, Leung PS, Adamopoulos IE, Gershwin ME. The implication of vitamin D and autoimmunity: a comprehensive review. *Clin Rev Allergy Immunol* 45 (2013):217–26; Pludowski P, Holick MF, Pilz S, et al. Vitamin D effects on mus-

culoskeletal health, immunity, autoimmunity, cardiovascular disease, cancer, fertility, pregnancy, dementia and mortality: a review of recent evidence. *Auto-immun Rev* 12 (2013): 976–89.

3   Milliken SV, Wassall H, Lewis BJ, et al. Effects of ultraviolet light on human serum 25-hydroxyvitamin D and systemic immune function. *J Allergy Clin Im-munol* 129 (2012): 1554–61.

4   Faridar A, Eskandari G, Sahraian MA, Minagar A, Azimi A. Vitamin D and multiple sclerosis: a critical review and recommendations on treatment. *Acta Neurol Belg* 112 (2012): 327–33.

5   Kumar A, Singh RB, Saxena M, et al. Effect of carni Q-gel (ubiquinol and carnitine) on cytokines in patients with heart failure in the Tishcon study. *Acta Cardiol* 62 (2007): 349–54; Sacher HL, Sacher ML, Landau SW, et al. The clinical and hemodynamic effects of coenzyme Q10 in congestive cardiomyop-athy. *Am J Ther* 4 (1997): 66–72; Singh RB, Niaz MA, Rastogi V, Rastogi SS. Coenzyme Q in cardiovascular disease. *J Assoc Physicians India* 46 (1998): 299–306; Kumar A, Singh RB, Saxena M, et al. Effect of carni Q-gel (ubiquinol and carnitine) on cytokines in patients with heart failure in the Tishcon study. *Acta Cardiol* 62 (2007): 349–54.

6   Muller T, Buttner T, Gholipour AF, Kuhn W. Coenzyme Q10 supplementation provides mild symptomatic benefit in patients with Parkinson's disease. *Neuro-sci Lett* 341 (2003): 201–4.

7   Brewer GJ. Copper excess, zinc deficiency, and cognition loss in Alzheimer's disease. *Biofactors* 38 (2012): 107–13; Loef M, von Stillfried, N, Walach H. Zinc diet and Alzheimer's disease: a systematic review. *Nutr Neurosci* 15 (2012): 2–12.

8   Ziegler D, Low PA, Litchy WJ, et al. Efficacy and safety of antioxidant treat-ment with alpha-lipoic acid over 4 years in diabetic polyneuropathy: the NA-THAN 1 trial. *Diabetes Care* 34 (2011): 2054–60.

9   Muller T, Buttner T, Gholipour AF, Kuhn W. Coenzyme Q10 supplementation provides mild symptomatic benefit in patients with Parkinson's disease. *Neuro-sci Lett* 341 (2003): 201–4.

10 Liu J. The effects and mechanisms of mitochondrial nutrient alpha-lipoic acid on improving age-associated mitochondrial and cognitive dysfunction: an overview. *Neurochem Res* 33 (2008): 194–203; Milgram NW, Araujo JA, Hagen TM, Treadwell BV, Ames BN. Acetyl-L-carnitine and alpha-lipoic acid supple-mentation of aged beagle dogs improves learning in two landmark discrimina-tion tests. *FASEB J* 21 (2007): 3756–62.

11 Kumar A, Singh RB, Saxena M, et al. Effect of carni Q-gel (ubiquinol and

carnitine) on cytokines in patients with heart failure in the Tishcon study. *Acta Cardiol* 62 (2007): 349–54; Sacher HL, Sacher ML, Landau SW, et al. The clinical and hemodynamic effects of coenzyme Q10, 66–72; Singh RB, Niaz MA, Rastogi V, Rastogi SS. Coenzyme Q in cardiovascular disease, 299–306.

12 Pallas M, Verdaguer E, Tajes M, Gutierrez-Cuesta J, Camins A. Modulation of sirtuins: new targets for antiageing. *Recent Pat CNS Drug Discov* 3 (2008): 61–69.

13 James D, Devaraj S, Bellur P, Lakkanna S, Vicini J, Boddupalli S. Novel concepts of broccoli sulforaphanes and disease: induction of phase II antioxidant and detoxification enzymes by enhanced-glucoraphanin broccoli. *Nutr Rev* 70 (2012): 654–65; Applying Oral Chelation. Advanced Practice Module Detox: Understanding Biotransformation and Recognizing Toxicity, Evaluation and Treatment in the Functional Medicine Model, Institute for Functional Medicine, 2011 conference, Phoenix, Arizona, December 10, 2011.

14 Larijani VN, Ahmadi N, Zeb I, Khan F, Flores F, Budoff M. Beneficial effects of aged garlic extract and coenzyme Q10 on vascular elasticity and endothelial function: The FAITH randomized clinical trial. *Nutrition* 29 (2012): 71–5. Weiss N, Papatheodorou L, Morihara N, Hilge R, Ide N. Aged garlic extract restores nitric oxide bioavailability in cultured human endothelial cells even under conditions of homocysteine elevation. *J Ethnopharmacol* 145 (2012): 162–7.

15 Anderson JG, Taylor AG. Effects of healing touch in clinical practice: a systematic review of randomized clinical trials. *J Holist Nurs* 29 (2011): 221–28; Anderson JG, Taylor AG. Biofield therapies and cancer pain. *Clin J Oncol Nurs* 16 (2012): 43–48.

16 Rapaport MH, Schettler P, Bresee C. A preliminary study of the effects of repeated massage on hypothalamic-pituitary-adrenal and immune function in healthy individuals: a study of mechanisms of action and dosage. *J Altern Complement Med* 18 (2012): 789–97.

17 Hughes CM, Smyth S, Lowe-Strong AS. Reflexology for the treatment of pain in people with multiple sclerosis: a double-blind randomised sham-controlled clinical trial. *Mult Scler* 15 (2009): 1329–38.

18 Elster E. Eighty-one patients with multiple sclerosis and Parkinson's disease undergo upper cervical chiropractic care to correct vertebral subluxation: a retrospective analysis. *Journal Vetebral Subluxation Research* 23 (2004): 1–9.

19 Foroughipour M, Bahrami Taghanaki HR, Saeidi M, Khazaei M, Sasannezhad P, Shoeibi A. Amantadine and the place of acupuncture in the treatment of

fatigue in patients with multiple sclerosis: an observational study. *Acupunct Med* 31 (2013): 27–30.

20 Quispe-Cabanillas JG, Damasceno A, von Glehn F, et al. Impact of electroacupuncture on quality of life for patients with Relapsing-Remitting Multiple Sclerosis under treatment with immunomodulators: a randomized study. *BMC Complement Altern Med* 12 (2012): 209.

21 Lappin MS, Lawrie FW, Richards TL, Kramer ED. Effects of a pulsed electromagnetic therapy on multiple sclerosis fatigue and quality of life: a double-blind, placebo controlled trial. *Altern Ther Health Med* 9 (2003): 38–48.

22 Piatkowski J, Kern S, Ziemssen T. Effect of BEMER magnetic field therapy on the level of fatigue in patients with multiple sclerosis: a randomized, double-blind controlled trial. *J Altern Complement Med* 15 (2009): 507–11; Ziemssen T, Piatkowski J, Haase R. Long-term effects of Bio-Electromagnetic-Energy Regulation therapy on fatigue in patients with multiple sclerosis. *Altern Ther Health Med* 17 (2011): 22–28.

23 Mirshafiey A. Venom therapy in multiple sclerosis. *Neuropharmacology* 53 (2007): 353–61.

24 Zamboni P, Galeotti R, Weinstock-Guttman B, Kennedy C, Salvi F, Zivadinov R. Venous angioplasty in patients with multiple sclerosis, 116–22.

Chapter 11

1 Sabayan B, Foroughinia F, Mowla A, Borhanihaghighi A. Role of insulin metabolism disturbances in the development of Alzheimer's disease: mini review. *Am J Alzheimer's Dis Other Demen* 23 (2008): 192–99.

2 The New Era of Managing Cardiovascular Disease, Metabolic Dysunctions and Obesity. Cardiometabolic Module, 2012 Annual International Symposium, Institute for Functional Medicine, Scottsdale, Arizona, May 31, 2012; Fire in the Hole: The Metabolic Connecting Points Between Major Chronic Diseases. Cardiometabolic Module, 2012 Annual International Symposium, Institute for Functional Medicine, Scottsdale, Arizona, May 30, 2012.

3 Hyman M. *The Blood Sugar Solution.* New York: Little Brown and Company, 2012.

4 Rapaport MH, Schettler P, Bresee C. A preliminary study of the effects of repeated massage on hypothalamic-pituitary-adrenal and immune function in healthy individuals: a study of mechanisms of action and dosage. *J Altern Complement Med* 18 (2012): 789–97.

5   Bixler E. Sleep and society: an epidemiological perspective. *Sleep Med* 10, Suppl 1 (2009): S3–S6.

6   Bamer AM, Johnson KL, Amtmann D, Kraft GH. Prevalence of sleep problems in individuals with multiple sclerosis. *Mult Scler* 14 (2008): 1127–30; Manconi M, Ferini-Strambi L, Filippi M, et al. Multicenter case-control study on restless legs syndrome in multiple sclerosis: the REMS study. *Sleep* 31 (2008): 944–52; Moreira NC, Damasceno RS, Medeiros CA et al. Restless leg syndrome, sleep quality and fatigue in multiple sclerosis patients. *Braz J Med Biol Res* 41 (2008): 932–37.

7   Khong TP, de Vries F, Goldenberg JS, et al. Potential impact of benzodiazepine use on the rate of hip fractures in five large European countries and the United States. *Calcif TVOL. Int* 91 (2012): 24–31; Sylvestre MP, Abrahamowicz M, Capek R, Tamblyn R. Assessing the cumulative effects of exposure to selected benzodiazepines on the risk of fall-related injuries in the elderly. *Int Psychogeriatr* 24 (2012): 577–88.

Chapter 12

1   Alberts B, Johnson A, Lewis J, Raff M, Roberts K, Walter P. *Molecular Biology of the Cell.* 4th ed. New York: Garland Publishing, 2002.

2   *Textbook of Functional Medicine.* Gig Harbor, Washington: Institute for Functional Medicine, 2010.

3   Coca AF. *The Pulse Test.* 5th ed. New York: St. Martin's Press, 1996.

4   Morrison HI, Ellison LF, Taylor GW. Periodontal disease and risk of fatal coronary heart and cerebrovascular diseases. *J Cardiovasc Risk* 6 (1999): 7–11; Seymour GJ, Ford PJ, Cullinan MP, Leishman S, Yamazaki K. Relationship between periodontal infections and systemic disease. *Clin Microbiol Infect* 13, Suppl 4 (2007): 3–10.

5   Chronic Infections and Neurological Disease: The Challenge of Emerging Infections in the 21st Century—Tolerance, Terrain, Susceptibility, 2011 International Annual Symposium Institute for Functional Medicine, Bellevue, Washington, April 30, 2011.

6   Ibid.; The Role of Chlamydophila in Autoimmune Disease. The Challenge of Emerging Infections in the 21st Century—Tolerance, Terrain, Susceptibility, 2011 International Annual Symposium Institute for Functional Medicine, Bellevue, Washington, April 30, 2011.

INDEX

Page numbers in **bold** indicate tables; those in *italics* indicate figures.

Abrahams, Charlie and Jim, 193
acupuncture, 291
adenosine triphosphate (ATP), 29–30, 31, 279
adrenals, 295, 297, 301, 302, 327
aerobic training, 224, 232, 233, 234, 235, 249–51, 306
African-Americans, 270, 277, 300
aging, 24, 30, 31, 32, 34, 35, 36, **39**, 65, 256
alcohol, 143, 210, 212, 305
algae, 226, 266, 280–81, **283**, 337, *371*
Algerian Chicken/Algerian Vegetarian (recipe), 340–41
alpha-carotene, **39**, 111–12, **383**
alpha-linolenic acid (ALA), **40**, 156, 160, 205
alternative medicine, 261, 287–94
Alzheimer's disease, 233, 284, 300
American standard diet, 93, 100, 107, **108**, 150–51, **151**, 189–90, **190**, 201, 381–84
Ames, Bruce, 35–36
amino acids, 10, 35, 37, 154–56, 158, *222*, 223
annual tests, 266, **267–68**
antibiotics, 33, 137, 155, 181, 183
Antigen Leukocyte Cellular Antibody Test (ALCAT), 324
antinutrients, 36, 38, **40**, 95, 99, 134, 150, 163, 165, 178
antioxidants, 10, 30, 31, 35, 36, 38, **39**, 54, 62, 65, 93, 94, 110, 112, 113–14, 118, 159, 161, 179, 285–86
apoptosis (cell death), 28–29, *29*, 30, 300
"Applying Functional Medicine in Clinical Practice" (Institute for Functional Medicine), 328
arachidonic acid (AA), **40**, 205–6, 277, **382**
arthritis, 52, 117, 254, 272, 346
artificial sweeteners, 141, 143
Asian culture, 96, 112, 118, 120, 165, 172, 212
atherosclerosis, 113, 118, 119, 157, 162, 296, 300

attention deficit hyperactivity disorder (ADHD), 19, 160, 308
autism, 46, 131, 193, 283
autoimmunity, 46–66
autonomic nervous system, 296–98, 301
Avocado–Bone Broth Soup (recipe), 346

baclofen, 236, 260, 309
Bacon, Brussels Sprouts, and Cranberries (recipe), 353–54
Bacon and Greens (recipe), 353
bacteria (bad), 32, 54, 90, 91
balance training, 234, 235, 239–41, *240*, 243, 251
Basic Meat and Greens Skillet (recipe), 338–40
Basic Smoothie (recipe), 335–36
Beans, Red Chili with (recipe), 350
Beet and Cranberry Mixture (recipe), 357
Beet Kvass (recipe), 361–62
Beet and Red Cabbage Mixture (recipe), 357
beetroot juice study, 114
benzodiazepines, 33, 305, 309
beta-carotene, **39**, 111–12, 166, **383**
beverages (recipes), 358–59
biochemistry of cells and disease, 23, 25, 26, 34, 46–47, 49–50, 64–66
Bio-Electromagnetic-Energy-Regulation (BEMER) therapy, 292
biofield therapies, 289–90
blood-brain barrier, 91, 191
blood vessel health, 36, **40**, 60, 61, 63–64, 65, 91, 111, 112, 113, 114, 116, 117–18, 119, 121, 128, 157, 162, 204, 224, 297, 298, 300, 311, 313
bodywork therapy, 197, 290, 302–3
bone broth, 127, 158, 159, 230, 272, 287
Bone Broth (recipes), 345–48
Bone Broth Tea (recipe), 358
bone health, 157–59, 166, 252, 311
Bowman, G. L., 162
Brain Aging Study, Oregon, 36, 162
brain-derived neurotrophic factor (BDNF), 233, 252

brain fog, 5, 22, 30, 46, 62, 69, 167, 168, 183,
    199, 275, 326
brain grade scale, 79
brain health, 37–38, 38, **39–40,** 63, 93, 102,
    110, 122, 130
Brussels Sprouts, Bacon, and Cranberries
    (recipe), 353–54
B vitamins, 10, 25, 31, 33, 35, 107, 111, 120,
    174, 182, 266, 273, 278–79, **283,** 284,
    309, 313, **382**
    See also specific B vitamins

cabbage, 118, 142, 170, 182, 285, 337
Cabbage (Red), Sautéed (recipe), 355
Cabbage (Red) and Beet Mixture (recipe), 357
calcium, **108,** 112, 135, **151,** 163, 165, 170, **190,**
    197, **267,** 274–75, **283,** 309, **382**
Calton, Jayson and Mira, 8, 10, 23, 26–35, 29,
    38, **39, 40,** 47, 61, 62, 63, 64, 65–66, 86,
    93
cancers, 24, 36, 54, 65, 85, 112, 113, 114, 116,
    118, 119, 120, 121, 164, 193, 200, 220,
    269, 271, 272, 285, 296, 320
Candida, 90, 91, 182, 183
carbohydrates, 6, 54, 68, 87, 91, 99–100, 102,
    103, 122, 141, 151–53, 169, 181, 190,
    191, 192, 193–95, 196, 197, 202, 207,
    208, 209, 211, 229, **267, 268,** 277, 281,
    299, 300, **383, 384**
cardiovascular training, 224, 232, 233, 234,
    235, 249–51, 306
carnitine, 8, **39,** 174, 284
Carrot–Bone Broth Soup (recipe), 347
Carson, Rachel, 220
casein, 91, 98, 130, 131, 134
Cauliflower Rice (recipe), 356
Cauliflower–Turmeric Bone Broth Soup
    (recipe), 347
cell function
    biochemistry of cells and disease, 23, 25, 26,
        34, 46–47, 49–50, 64–66
    building blocks, 21–22, 23, 24, 25, 26–30,
        29, 35, 45
    free radicals, 30, 31, 61, 64, 114, 179
    nutrition importance, 5–6, 11, 13, 21, 22, 23,
        24, 25, 26–30, 29, 35–37, 38, **39–40,** 41,
        53, 56, 63, 86, 105
    See also mitochondria; Wahls Protocol
cerebrospinal venous insufficiency (CCSVI)
    theory, 60, 61, 63–64, 118, 293–94
Charcot, Jean-Martin, 58
Chicken, Algerian (recipe), 340–41

Chicken Rosemary (recipe), 341
Chicken Salad (recipe), 352
Chili (Red) with Beans (recipe), 350
chiropractic care, 291
cholecalciferol (vitamin D), 25, 36, 38, **39,** 62,
    108, 151, 166, 168, 174, **190,** 197, 266,
    267, **267,** 268–74, 276, **283, 382**
cholesterol, 12, 32–33, **40,** 90, 174, 196, 263,
    267, 268, 277, **382**
clay toxin binders, 286–87
clinical trials, Wahls Protocol, 197–99,
    200–201, 332–33
cobalamin (vitamin B$_{12}$), 36, 37, **39, 108, 151,**
    166–67, 174, 182, **190,** 222, **267,** 279,
    382
Coca, Arthur F., 324
Cocoa, Hot (recipe), 358–59
Coconut Milk–Fish Soup (recipe), 348
coconut oil/milk, 103, 120, 127, 135, 136, 161,
    164, 184, 188, 193, 196, 197, 202–3, 207,
    208, 210, 211–12, 231, 265, 285, **371**
cod liver oil, 166, 273, 274, 276, **283**
coenzyme Q10 (ubiquinone), 8, 30, 31, 32–33,
    38, **40,** 101, 174, 223, 279–80, **283,** 284,
    313
colonics/cleanses/chelation, 222, 292–93
community-supported agriculture (CSA),
    123–24, 155
Compendium of Cookery, 173, 342
complementary medicine, 261, 287–94
complete blood count (CBC), 266, **267**
Complete Food Lists, 366–80, **370–71, 372,**
    373–80
conventional medicine, 2, 5, 7, 14, 19–20, 47,
    49, 50, 52–53, 54, 55–56, 57, 60–61
Copaxone, 4, 20, 22, 34, 57, 60
copper, **39,** 170, 284, **382**
Cordain, Loren, 6, 92, 93
cortisol, 47, 295, 299, 302, 315
Coumadin, 128–29, 276
Cranberries, Brussels Sprouts, and Bacon
    (recipe), 353–54
Cranberry and Beet Mixture (recipe), 357
creatine, 8, 30, **40,** 174, **267,** 280, 284
Curl-Ups (exercise), 248, *248*
cytokines, 201, 233, 278, 300

dairy-free (Wahls Diet part two), 86, 88, 90,
    91, 95, 96–99, 107, 126–27, 129, 130,
    131, 133–36, 140–41, 149, 184, 367
dementia, 36, 114, 119, 193, 227, 233, 234, 284,
    300

depression, 19, 20, 37, 46, 53, 117, 233, 291, 298, 315
desserts (recipes), 363–65
detoxification, 118, 121, 221–26, *222*, 285, 292–93
diabetes, 12, 19, 33, 46, 56, 89, 90, 99, 158, 220, 227, 234, 283, 284, 296, 299–300, 308, 313, 315, 326
diagnoses and treatments, 47–49, 59
diagnosis of MS, 1, 2–4, 44, 58, 59
diet. *See* Wahls Diet; Wahls Paleo; Wahls Paleo Plus
digestive enzymes, 127, 129, 175, 176, 281–82, **283**
Direct-MS, 5, 6, 333
disease. *See* science of life, disease, and you
docosahexaenoic acid (DHA), 37, **40**, 137, 156, 160, 169, 205, 275, 276, **283**, 346, 382
Downward-Facing Bridge (exercise), 246, *246*
drugs, supplements, and alternative medicine, 41, 42–43, 261–94
drug therapy, 4, 19–20, 22, 34, 47–48, 49, 52–53, 54, 55–56, 56–57, 57, 60, 61, 62

Edison, Thomas, 2
eggs, 95, 137, 141, 143, 184, 205, **370**
eicosapentaenoic acid (EPA), **40**, 160, 205, 275, 276, 277, **283**, 382
elimination diets, 323–24
Embry, Ashton, 5, 6
endocrine disruptors, 220, 227, 229
endotoxins, 220–21, *222*
environmental aspect of disease, 20, 23–25, 53, 55–56, 57, 58, *58*, 59, 63
epilepsy, 34, 193, 298
Epsom salt baths, 303–4, 306
Erector Spinae #1 and #2 (exercises), 239, *239*
essential fatty acids, 10, 35, 36, 37, 38, **40**, 54, 62, 63, 87, 93, 156–57, **157**, 159, 160, 161, 174, 204, 205–6, 266, 275–77, **283**, 309
e-stim (neuromuscular electrical stimulation), 9, 12, 34, 42, 197, 252, 253–60, *254*, 312
exercise and electricity, 41, 42, 232–60
expectations, recovery, 311–15
exposure to toxins, minimizing, 221, 227–31
Extension (exercise), 244, *244*
eye health, 27, 58, 61, 62, 92, 111, 113, 116

fatigue, 20, 32, 50, 53, 56, 60, 63, 120, 200, 225, 291, 292, 297, 304, 312, 324, 326

fats and oils. *See* Wahls Diet; Wahls Paleo; Wahls Paleo Plus
fermentable oligosaccharides, disaccharides, monosaccharides, and polyols (FODMAPs), 122
fermentation, 191–92
fermented foods addition (Wahls Paleo part four), 101–2, 120, 142, 150, *150*, 175, 180–84, 202, 282, **371**
fermented recipes, 359–63
fillings (dental), 175, 220, 229–31
fish. *See* Wahls Diet; Wahls Paleo; Wahls Paleo Plus
Fish–Coconut Milk Soup (recipe), 348
fish oils, 160, 276, **283**
Flaxseed-Raspberry Pudding (recipe), 363–64
Flexion (exercise), 244, *244*
fluoride, 170, 231
focused, getting, 67–81
folic acid (vitamin B$_9$), 36, 37, **39**, 107, **108**, 111, **151**, 171, **190**, 222, **267**, 279, **382**
food allergies, 10, 19, 54, 63, 130, 135, 179, 315, 323–25, 328, 329
Food Lists, 366–80, **370–71**, **372**, **373–80**
foods (real), 35–37, 38, **39–40**
See also nutrition importance; Wahls Diet; Wahls Paleo; Wahls Paleo Plus
Frankl, Viktor, 44
free radicals, 30, 31, 61, 64, 114, 179
Fruit Pudding (recipe), 363
fruits. *See* Wahls Diet; Wahls Paleo; Wahls Paleo Plus
Fudge, Wahls (recipe), 209, 364–65
fueling your cells, 27–29, *29*
functional electric stimulation (FES), 258, 259
functional medicine, 9–11, 13, 25, 43, 49–50, 53–57, 61–64, 264, 318–29

gamma-aminobutyric acid (GABA), 236, 306, 309
gamma-linolenic acid (GLA), **40**, 156, 206, 266, 275–77
genetically modified organisms (GMOs), 142, 161, 165
genetic aspect of disease, 10, 20, 22–24, 25, 26, 58, *58*, 59, 60, 138
genetic tests, 320–21
glucosamine/glycan, 157, 158, 287, 346
glucose, 29, **39**, 54, 201, 299
Gluteal Stretch (exercise), 237, *237*

gluten-free (Wahls Diet part two), 88, 91, 95, 96–99, 107, 126–27, 129–34, 140–41, 149, 184, 366–67
glycemic index, 124, 189, 194, 195, 208, 272, 336, **381**
grains, legumes, potatoes. *See* Wahls Diet; Wahls Paleo; Wahls Paleo Plus
"Green-BACK," 111, 112
Greens and Bacon (recipe), 353
Greens and Meat Basic Skillet (recipe), 338–40
growth hormones, 137, 139, 155
Gurven, M., 88

Hamstring Stretch (exercise), 237, *237*
Healing Touch, 289–90, 312
healing yourself, 20, 44–45, 311, 329, 333–34
health, 21–25, 35
heart health, 19, 25, 28, 33, 36, 46, 52, 63, 64–65, 68, 89, 99, 112, 114, 118, 119, 121, 157, 167, 170, 220, 234, 269, 279, 280, 283, 304, 311, 313–14, 326
heavy metals, 54, 170, 171, 220, 221, 222, 224, 227, 280
hemoglobin A₁C, 201, **268**, 277
herbs, 223–24, 338
high blood pressure, 12, 19, 36, 52, 63, 65, 90, 112, 313
high-density lipoprotein (HDL), 196, **267**, 277, 300
higher purpose for your life, 68, 70–71, 302
high-fructose corn syrup, 87, 141, 143, 219
highly sensitive C-reactive protein (CRP), 201, **267, 277**
high-sugar, high-starch diets, 6, 32, 54, 56, 87, 89, 90, 91, 100, 192, 219, 281
homocysteine, 201, **267, 279,** 285, 287
Homo/Homo sapiens, 86, 156
hormonal balance, 10, 25, 50, 54, 57, 62, 63, 113, 121, 300, 326–27
Hot Cocoa (recipe), 358–59
Huntington's disease, 199, 320, 334
Hyman, Mark, 302

"idiopathic" symptoms, 4, 47, 158
immune cells reactivity, 51–52, 54, 61, 62, 91
immune system, 3, 6, 10, 37, 116, 120, 166, 326
    See also autoimmunity
immune system hyperreactivity, 54, 55, 97, 111, 126
infections, 25, **39,** 53, 54, 55, 56, 58, 62, 63, 325–26

inflammation, 6, 10, **40,** 47, 54, 62, 64–65, 68, 91, 113, 126, 156, 157, 158, 162, 163, 165, 195, 201, 233, 275, 277, 285, 296, 298, 299, 300, 304, 313, 315
inflammatory bowel disease (IBD), 47, 122, 127, 131, 314
Institute for Functional Medicine, 10, 113, 121, 220, 236, 328, 329
insulin resistance, 90, 152, 298–300, 313
iodine, 37, 38, **39,** 169–70, 171, 223
iron, 30, **39,** 107, **108, 151,** 171, 190, 284, 309, **382**
irradiated food, 141, 143
irritable bowel syndrome (IBS), 131, 314

joint health, 52, 53, 157–59, 272, 287, 346
journaling, 302, 306
    See also Wahls Diary

Kale-Sausage Soup (recipe), 349–50
Kaplan, H., 88
ketogenic diets, 29, 102, 103, 190–95, 202
ketosis, 191, 195–98, 202, 207–8, 209, 210, 211
kidney health, 222, 222–23, 224, 272, 285, 292, 311
Kombucha Tea (recipe), 182, 359–61

lacto-fermentation, 101, 125–26, 180, 181, 182, 184
Lateral Flexion (exercise), 245, *245*
lead, 30, 54, 61, 170, 278
leaky brain, 91, 297
leaky gut syndrome, 6, 10, 91, 96–97, 158, 167, 297, 324
lectins, 6, 99, 126, 134, 163, 165
legumes. *See* Wahls Diet; Wahls Paleo; Wahls Paleo Plus
lesions, 36–37, 57, 59, 62, 117, 263, 291
lifestyle aspect of disease, 20, 23–25, 53, 55–56, 57
linoleic acid (LA), **40,** 156, 205–6, **382**
lipids, 201, 277, 313
lipoic acid, **40,** 280, 284, 309
liver, eating, 166, 167, 168, 173, 174
Liver, Onion, and Mushrooms (recipe), 342
liver health, 28, 65, 113, 121, 191, 196, 210, 222, 222, 224, 292, 311
Liver Pâté (recipe), 342–43
L-methylfolate (levomefolic acid), **283**
Lou Gehrig's disease (ALS), 193, 199, 334
low-density lipoprotein (LDL), 196, 277

lupus, 19, 46, 47, 52, 118
Lyme disease, 62, 170, 326

magnesium, 30, 38, **39**, 108, **151**, 163, 165,
 171, 174, **190**, 275, **283**, 304, 309, **382**
magnetic resonance imaging (MRI) scans, 36,
 37, 55, 57, 59, 62, 263, 289
Man's Search for Meaning (Frankl), 44
Mashed Turnips (recipe), 354
massage, 12, 197, 290, 302–3, 306
meat. *See* Wahls Diet; Wahls Paleo; Wahls
 Paleo Plus
Meat and Greens Basic Skillet (recipe),
 338–40
Medical Symptoms Questionnaire (MSQ),
 74–78, 311, 315, 316–17, 318
medications. *See* drugs, supplements, and
 alternative medicine
meditation/prayer, 12, 197, 301–2, 306
medium-chain triglycerides (MCTs), 193–94,
 196
melatonin, 307–8
memory loss, 34, 50, 102, 283, 298, 304
menaquinone-7 (vitamin K$_2$), 128–29
mental health problems, 24, 54, 64, 130, 157,
 193, 200, 268, 269, 296
mercury, 30, 54, 61, 170, 175, 220, 229–31
methyl B$_{12}$, 167, 266, **283**
methylsulfonylmethane (MSM), 117, 287, 346
microbiome health, 90, 152, 328, 329
micronutrients, 37–38, 38, **39–40**, 63, 93, 102,
 110, 122, 130
 See also specific micronutrients
microwaved food, 141, 142, 143, 184, 200
*Minding My Mitochondria: How I Overcame
 Secondary Progressive Multiple Sclerosis
 (MS) and Got out of My Wheelchair*
 (Wahls), 286
"Minding Your Mitochondria" (Wahls), 13,
 92
minerals and nutrition, 29–30, 31, 33, 35, 36,
 37, 38, **39**, 62, 63, 65, 87, 93, 94, 107,
 108, **151**, 159, 170–71, 223
 See also specific minerals
mitochondria, 26–35
 mitochondrial strain, 31–35, 43–44, 61, 62,
  63, 64, 65–66
 See also cell function; Wahls Protocol
mobility improvement, 312–13
modified elimination diet, 323–24
molecular mimicry, 6, 55
monosodium glutamate, 141, 143

monounsaturated fats (MUFA), 203, 204, 205
mood disorders, 12, 25, 33–34, 37, 46, 52, 56,
 63, 91, 220, 233, 234, 283
motivation, 67–68, 69, 70–71
movement importance, 25, 41, 42, 53, 54, 56,
 63, 232, 233–34, 260, 290
muds/clays for detoxification, 224–26, 230
multiple sclerosis (MS), 1–15, 57–64
 See also Wahls Protocol
mushrooms, 120–21, 124, 142, 181, 183
Mushrooms, Liver, and Onions (recipe), 342
myelin, 37, 38, **39, 40**, 51, 58, 59, 94, 111, 112,
 179, 275, 311
My Healthy Plate (USDA), 201

N-acetylcysteine (NAC), 222, 285, 309
*Naked Calories: The Calton's Simple 3-Step Plan
 for Micronutrient Sufficiency* (Calton
 and Calton), 93
nature, spending time in, 301, 302, 303
nerve growth factor (NGF), 233, 234, 252, 295
neurodegenerative diseases, 32–33, 193, 199,
 200, 220, 227, 284
*Neuromuscular electrical stimulation and dietary
 interventions...a case report,* 257
neuromuscular electrical stimulation (e-stim),
 9, 12, 34, 42, 197, 252, 253–60, 254, 312
neuromuscular reeducation, 243–49, 244, 245,
 246, 247, 248, 249
neuropathy, 34, 158, 283, 308
*Neuroprotection: A Functional Medicine
 Approach for Common and Uncommon
 Neurologic Syndromes* (Institute for
 Functional Medicine), 10
niacin (vitamin B$_3$), 29, 36, **39**, 107, **108**, **151**,
 171, **190**, 222, 266, **382**
Nutrient Comparison Tables, **108**, **151**, **190**,
 381, **381–84**
nutritional ketosis, 191–92, 194, 195, 196–97,
 198, 207–8, 209, 210, 211
nutritional testing, 321–22
nutritional yeast, 182, 183, **371**
nutrition importance, 5–6, 11, 13, 21, 22, 23,
 24, 25, 26–30, 29, 35–37, 38, **39–40**, 41,
 53, 56, 63, 86, 105
 See also Wahls Diet; Wahls Paleo; Wahls
  Paleo Plus; Wahls Protocol
nuts/seeds. *See* Wahls Diet; Wahls Paleo;
 Wahls Paleo Plus

obesity, 19, 56, 63, 65, 89, 99, 200–201, 227,
 234, 296, 304, 315

omega-3 fatty acids, 37, 38, **40**, 54, 137, 143, 156, **157**, 160, 161, 174, 204, 205, 275–77, **283**, 309

omega-6 fatty acids, 40, 54, 143, 156, 160, 161, 204, 205–6, 277

Onions, Liver, and Mushrooms (recipe), 342

onions, 118–19, 120, 142, 181

osteoporosis, 167, 272

oxidation, 31, 54, *222*, 223

Paleo Diet, The (Cordain), 6, 92, 93

Paleolithic nutrition, 6, 7, 10–11, 12, 13, 86–95, 111, 137–38, 140, 152, 168–69, 329

Paleo Solution; The Original Human Diet (Wolf), 92, 93

Pan American Games in Washington, DC (1978), 1

pancreas, 281–82, 299

pantothenic acid (vitamin B$_5$), 29, **40**, 171, 266

parasympathetic system, 296, 301

Parkinson's disease (PD), 102, 193, 199, 227, 280, 283, 284, 291, 308, 322

Pepper–Bone Broth Soup (recipe), 347–48

Peppers (Red) and Quinoa (recipe), 355

periodontal (gum) disease, 62, 112

pesticides, 61, 137, 219

Peterman, M. G., 193

physical therapists, 234, 235, 236, 240, 242, 243, 251, 253–54, 255, 256, 257, 258

phytates, 99, 134, 163, 178

phytochemicals, 110, 113, 116

phytonutrients, 110, 111, 116, 121, 130

Pilates, 240, 242, 290

pizza (recipe), 343–44

plastics, 220, 224, 227, 228, 280

pollution, 25, 88, 219, 220

polycystic ovary syndrome (PCOS), 65, 227, 229, 300

polyunsaturated fats (PUFA), 162, 203, 204–5

post-traumatic stress disorder, 12, 56, 315

potatoes. *See* Wahls Diet; Wahls Paleo; Wahls Paleo Plus

Price, Weston A., 173

Primal Blueprint, The (Sisson), 92, 93

primary-progressive MS (PPMS), 59, 198

probiotic supplements, 181

processed foods, 36, 87, 91, 129–30, 219

progressive-relapsing MS (PRMS), 59–60

protein. *See* Wahls Diet; Wahls Paleo; Wahls Paleo Plus

Psoas Stretch (exercise), 238, *238*

pudding recipes, 363–64

pulsed electromagnetic therapy (PEMF), 292

pyridoxine (vitamin B$_6$), 36, 37, **39**, **108**, **151**, 171, **190**, *222*, 266, **382**

Quadriceps Stretch (exercise), 238, *238*

Quinoa and Red Peppers (recipe), 355

Raspberry-Flaxseed Pudding (recipe), 363–64

raw foods addition (Wahls Paleo part four), 101–2, 150, *150*, 175–86

Rawmesan (recipe), 344

recipes, 335–65

recommended daily allowances (RDAs), 93, 107, 108, **108**, 151, **151**, 190, **190**

recovery, 310–29

Red Cabbage, Sautéed (recipe), 355

Red Cabbage and Beet Mixture (recipe), 357

Red Chili with Beans (recipe), 350

Red Peppers and Quinoa (recipe), 355

reflexology, 290–91

Rehabilitation with neuromuscular electrical stimulation...a case series report, 257

Reiki/Healing Touch/Therapeutic Touch, 289–90, 312

relapsing-remitting multiple sclerosis (RRMS), 57, 58, 59, 92, 173, 252, 291, 312

resources, 385–91

restless legs syndrome (RLS), 308–9

retinol (vitamin A), 36, **39**, **108**, 111–12, **151**, 166, 171, 174, **190**, 273, 276, **382**

rheumatoid arthritis, 19, 46, 47, 118, 254, 287, 314

riboflavin (vitamin B$_2$), 29, 36, **39**, 107, **108**, **151**, 171, **190**, *222*, 266, **382**

Rice, Cauliflower (recipe), 356

Rosemary Chicken (recipe), 341

salads (recipes), 351–52

Salmon or Chicken Salad (recipe), 352

saturated fats, *203*, 204

Sauerkraut and Fermented Vegetables (recipe), 362–63

Sausage–Kale Soup/Vegetarian Kale Soup (recipe), 349–50

Sautéed Red Cabbage (recipe), 355

science of life, disease, and you, 19–45

   See also cell function; mitochondria; nutrition importance

Seafood Stew (recipe), 351

Seafood-Tomato Soup (recipe), 348–49

Seated Leg Lift (exercise), 245, *245*

seaweed addition (Wahls Paleo part three), 101, 133, 150, *150*, 168–72, 184, 202, 223, 337–38, **371**

secondary progressive MS (SPMS), 58, 59, 252, 257, 286, 312

selenium, **39**, 171, 223, **382**

self-massage, 12, 302–3, 306

"self" molecules, 51, 52, 55, 61

Shields, Richard, 251, 252

side dishes (recipes), 353–58

Silent Spring (Carson), 220

single nucleotide polymorphisms (SNPs, snips), 25, 273

Sisson, Mark, 92, 93

skillet meals (recipes), 336–43

skin health, 51, 91, 112, 113, 116, 117, 131, 220, 224–26, 227, 324

sleep importance, 62, 63, 65, 304–7, 309

Smoothie, Basic (recipe), 335–36

smoothies, 120, 124, **144, 145, 146, 147, 185, 186, 187,** 213

soaking and sprouting (nuts and seeds) addition (Wahls Paleo part four), 101–2, 133, 134, 150, *150*, 163–64, 175, 178–80, 184, **370**

Soleus/Achilles Stretch (exercise), 237, *237*

soups, 120, 125, 157, 158

soups (recipes), 345–51

soy, 135, 136, 141, 142, 143, 156, 161, 164–67, 170, 184, 205, 207

Spaghetti Squash (recipe), 356

spices, 223–24, 338

spinal cord health, 3, 4, 36, 46, 58, 59, 61, 158, 233, 259, 291, 311

sprouting (germination) process, 178–80

"standard of care," 48, 49

statin drugs, 32–33, 174, 280

Stew, Seafood (recipe), 351

stool test, 324–25

strength training, 232, 233, 234, 235, 241–43, 251

stress management, 41, 42, 295–309

stretching, 234, 235, 236–39, *237*, *238, 239*

strokes, 34, 65, 68, 193, 254, 326

sugars, 6, 32, 54, 56, 87, 89, 90, 91, 100, 129–30, 141

sulfur, 30, 37, 38, 171

sulfur-rich vegetables, three cups (Wahls Diet), 96, 107, 109, 116–21, 142, 223, 241, 272, 285, 337, **370**

sun and vitamin D, 269, 270, 273

Superman (exercise), 249, *249*

supplements, 8–9, 10, 11, 41, 42–43, 107, 110, 112, 181, 221–22, 224, 261, 264–66, 272–87, **283**

sweat glands and detoxification, 222, *222*, 223, 224, 292

Sweet Potato (recipe), 356

swimming, 168, 177, 224, 242, 250

symbiotic colony of bacteria and yeast (SCOBY), 338, 360

sympathetic nervous system, 296–97, 301, 302

symptoms
    diagnoses and, 47–48, 49, 59
    Medical Symptoms Questionnaire (MSQ), 74–78, 311, 315, 316–17, 318
    multiple sclerosis (MS), 1–2, 3–4, 5, 6, 7, 19, 22, 27, 34, 36–37, 46, 50, 55, 58, 59, 61, 62, 68, 154, 167

taurine, *222*, 306, 309

tea recipes, 358, 359–61

Technology, Entertainment, Design (TED) and TEDx, 13, 22, 50, 164, 173

thiamine (vitamin B₁), 29, 36, 37, **39**, 107, 108, **151**, 171, 190, 266, **382**

thyroid health, 51–52, 130, 169–70, 172, **268**, 297, 308, 327

Tomato-Seafood Soup (recipe), 348–49

toothbrushes and toothpaste, 231

toxic load reduction, 41, 42, 219–31

trans fats, 36, **40**, 141, 143, 161–63, 203, 204, **382**

traumatic brain injury, 12, 45, 199, 279, 298, 310

travel tips, Wahls Protocol, 281

triglycerides, 193, 196, 197, **267**, 277, 300

troubleshooting Wahls Protocol, 315–18

trypsin inhibitors, 134, 163, 165

turmeric, 285

Turmeric-Cauliflower–Bone Broth Soup (recipe), 347

Turmeric Tea (recipe), 358

Turnips, Mashed (recipe), 354

ubiquinone (coenzyme Q10), 8, 30, 31, 32–33, 38, **40**, 101, 174, 223, 279–80, **283, 284,** 313

University of Iowa, 4, 13, 201, 259

Upward-Facing Bridge (exercise), 247, *247*

vascular disease theory, MS, 60

vegetable oils, 160–63, 184, 205

vegetables. *See* Wahls Diet; Wahls Paleo; Wahls Paleo Plus

Vegetables (Fermented) and Sauerkraut
(recipe), 362–63
vegetarians
advice for, 99, 133–34, 142, 144, 155–56, 157,
159–67, 205
Algerian Vegetarian (recipe), 340–41
Vegetarian Kale Soup (recipe), 349–50
vibration exercise, 251–53
vision health, 27, 58, 61, 62, 92, 111, 166
vitamin A (retinol), 36, **39**, **108**, 111–12, **151**,
166, 171, 174, **190**, 273, 276, **382**
vitamin B₁ (thiamine), 29, 36, 37, **39**, 107,
108, **151**, 171, **190**, 266, **382**
vitamin B₂ (riboflavin), 29, 36, **39**, 107, **108**,
151, 171, **190**, *222*, 266, **382**
vitamin B₃ (niacin), 29, 36, **39**, 107, **108**, **151**,
171, **190**, *222*, 266, **382**
vitamin B₅ (pantothenic acid), 29, **40**, 171, 266
vitamin B₆ (pyridoxine), 36, 37, **39**, **108**, **151**,
171, **190**, *222*, 266, **382**
vitamin B₉ (folic acid), 36, 37, **39**, 107, **108**,
111, **151**, 171, **190**, *222*, **267**, 279, **382**
vitamin B₁₂ (cobalamin), 36, 37, **39**, **108**, **151**,
166–67, 174, 182, **190**, *222*, **267**, 279,
382
vitamin C, 36, **39**, **108**, 111, 112, **151**, 171, 273
vitamin D (cholecalciferol), 25, 36, 38, **39**, 62,
108, **151**, 166, 168, 174, **190**, 197, 266,
267, **267**, 268–74, 276, **283**, **382**
vitamin E, 36, **39**, **108**, **151**, 171, 174, 179,
190, 266, 273, 276–77, **283**, **382**
vitamin K, 36, **40**, 111, 112, 128–29, 171, 174,
273, 274, 276, **382**
vitamins and nutrition, 10, 25, 29, 31, 33, 35,
36, 37, 38, **39**, **40**, 62, 63, 65, 87, 93, 94,
108, 110, **151**, 159, 171, 272–73
See also specific vitamins

Wahls, Terry, 1–15, 70–71, 92, 286, 310–11,
331–34
See also Wahls Protocol
Wahls Diary, 69–73, 78–81, 89, 109, 152, 211,
221, 234, 235, 265, 288, 302, 311, 316,
329
Wahls Diet, 41, 85–148, 366–80, 381–83
buying produce, 94, 122–25, 141
colored vegetables and fruits, three cups, 96,
107, 109, 113–16, 142, 223, 370
compliance with, 316–18
dairy-free (part two), 86, 88, 90, 91, 95,
96–99, 107, 126–27, 129, 130, 131,
133–36, 140–41, 149, 184, 367

eggs, 95, 137, 141, 143, 184, 205, 370
fats and oils, 94, *107*, 143, **371**, **383**
fruits and vegetables, nine cups (part one),
96, 103, *107*, 108–29, 140–41, 142, 149,
181, 184, **370**
gluten-free (part two), 88, 91, 95, 96–99,
107, 126–27, 129–34, 140–41, 149, 184,
366–67
grains, legumes, potatoes, 86, 88, 90, 91, 95,
132–33, **370**, **371**
greens, three cups, 96, *107*, 109, 111–13, 142,
273, **370**
local foods emphasis, 94, 122–25, 141
mastery of, 106–48
meal plans, 143, **144–47**
milk and milk substitutes, 135–36, **371**
nutrient density, 94, **108**
nuts/seeds, *107*, 143, *370*
Paleolithic nutrition, 6, 7, 10–11, 12, 13,
86–95, 111, 137–38, 140, 152, 168–69,
329
produce preparation, 125–26, 141–42, 143
protein (organic, grass-fed, wild-caught
meat and fish) (part three), 99, 100,
101, *107*, 136–41, 142, 149, 265, 274,
275, 337, **370**, **383**
snack ideas, 148
stomach issues, 96, 126–27, 129
sulfur-rich vegetables, three cups, 96, *107*,
109, 116–21, 142, 223, 241, 272, 285,
337, **370**
summary, 41, 142–43, 368, **370**, **371**
transition into, 103–4
vegetarian advice, 99, 133–34, 142, 144,
155–56, 157, 159–67, 205
waste, stopping the, 120, 125
See also Wahls Paleo; Wahls Paleo Plus;
Wahls Protocol
Wahls Fudge (recipe), 209, 364–65
Wahls Paleo, 41, 85, 99–102, 122, 149–87,
366–80, **381–83**
fats and oils, *150*, 161, 184, **371**, **383**
fermented foods addition (part four), 101–2,
120, 142, *150*, *150*, 175, 180–84, 202,
282, **371**
grains, legumes, potatoes reduction (part
one), 99–100, 132, *150*, *150*, 151–53,
184, **370**, **371**
meal plans, **185–87**
nuts/seeds (soaking and sprouting) addition
(part four), 101–2, 133, 134, *150*, *150*,
163–64, 175, 178–80, 184, **370**

organ meat addition (part three), 101, 150, *150*, 168–69, 173–75, 177, 184, 223, 265, 274, 284, **370**

protein (organic, grass-fed, wild-caught meat and fish) daily (part two), 101, 150, *150*, 153–59, 176–78, 184, 337, **370**, **383**

raw foods addition (part four), 101–2, 150, *150*, 175, 176–78

seaweed addition (part three), 101, 133, 150, *150*, 168–72, 184, 202, 223, 337–38, **371**

See also Wahls Diet; Wahls Paleo Plus; Wahls Protocol

Wahls Paleo Plus, 41, 85, 102–3, 122, 188–216, 366–80, **381–84**

eating twice daily (part seven), 103, 202, 209–11, 212

fasting nightly (part seven), 103, 209–11, 212, 285

fats and oils addition (part one), 188, 189, *189*, 195, 197, 202–6, *203*, *204*, 207, 208, 211, 212, **371**, **384**

fruits, one serving daily (part six), 103, 188, 189, 195, 196, 197, 208, 212, **370**

grains, legumes, potatoes, elimination (part three), 102, 151, 189, *189*, 206–7, **370**, **371**

ketogenic diets, 29, 102, 103, 190–95, 202

ketosis, 191, 195–98, 202, 207–8, 209, 210, 211

meal plans, **213–16**

protein (organic, grass-fed, wild-caught meat and fish) reduction (part five), 189, *189*, 197, 202, 205, 208, 212, 337, **370**, **384**

side effects warning, 196

starchy vegetables, two servings weekly (part four), 102–3, 189, *189*, 195, 207–8, 212, **370**

vegetables reduction to six cups (part two), 102–3, 188, *189*, 195, 197, 201–2, 212, **370**

See also Wahls Diet; Wahls Paleo; Wahls Protocol

Wahls Pizza (recipe), 343–44

Wahls Protocol, 41

autoimmunity, 46–66

clinical trials, 197–99, 200–201, 332–33

Complete Food Lists, 366–80, **370–71**, **372**, **373–80**

drugs, supplements, and alternative medicine, 41, 42–43, 261–94

exercise and electricity, 41, 42, 232–60

focused, getting, 67–81

functional medicine, 9–11, 13, 25, 43, 49–50, 53–57, 61–64, 264, 318–29

healing yourself, 20, 44–45, 311, 329, 333–34

multiple sclerosis (MS) and, 1–15, 57–64

Nutrient Comparison Tables, **108**, **151**, **190**, **381**, **381–84**

nutrition importance, 5–6, 11, 13, 21, 22, 23, 24, 25, 26–30, *29*, 35–37, *38*, 39–40, 41, 53, 56, 63, 86, 105

Paleolithic nutrition, 6, 7, 10–11, 12, 13, 86–95, 111, 137–38, 140, 152, 168–69, 329

recipes, 335–65

recovery, 310–29

resources, 385–91

science of life, disease, and you, 19–45

stress management, 41, 42, 295–309

success stories, 22, 27, 34, 45, 50, 55, 57, 62, 68, 69, 92, 97, 101, 104, 117, 154, 164, 167–68, 173, 175, 177, 198, 200, 252, 278, 298, 303, 312, 322

Terry Wahls, 1–15, 70–71, 92, 286, 310–11, 331–34

thewahlsprotocol.com, 257, 333, 335, 385

toxic load reduction, 41, 42, 219–31

travel tips, 281

troubleshooting, 315–18

See also cell function; mitochondria; Wahls Diet; Wahls Paleo; Wahls Paleo Plus

walking, dragging foot, 3, 242, 243, 255

weight loss, 209, 314

Western diets, 88–89, 90, 91

Wilder, R. M., 192–93

Winter Squash (recipe), 356

Wolf, Robb, 92, 93

World War II, 156, 162, 219

xenobiotics, 219–20, 221

yeasts (bad), 32, 90, 91

yoga, 232, 240, 241, 242, 290, 302

"youthen," 15, 112

Zamboni, Paulo, 60, 63, 118, 293

zeolite, 286, 287

zinc, 30, **39**, **108**, **151**, 163, 165, 171, 174, **190**, 223, 284, **382**